A Textbook of
Bio-Nutrition
Curing Diseases Through Diet

A Textbook of
Bio-Nutrition
Curing Diseases Through Diet

S. Paul

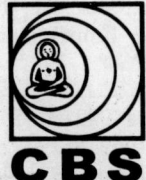

CBS

CBS Publishers & Distributors Pvt. Ltd.

New Delhi • Bengaluru • Chennai • Kochi • Kolkata • Mumbai
Hyderabad • Nagpur • Patna • Pune • Vijayawada

ISBN: 81-239-1180-7 (PB)
ISBN: 81-239-1193-9 (HB)

First Edition: 2005
Reprint: 2007, 2014, 2018

Published by **Satish Kumar Jain** and produced by **Varun Jain** for

CBS Publishers & Distributors Pvt. Ltd.,
4819/XI Prahlad Street, 24 Ansari Road, Daryaganj, New Delhi - 110002
delhi@cbspd.com, cbspubs@airtelmail.in • www.cbspd.com
Ph.: 23289259, 23266861, 23266867 • Fax: 011-23243014

Corporate Office: 204 FIE, Industrial Area, Patparganj, Delhi - 110 092
Ph: 49344934 • Fax: 011-49344935
E-mail: publishing@cbspd.com • publicity@cbspd.com

Branches:
• *Bengaluru:* 2975, 17th Cross, K.R. Road, Bansankari 2nd Stage,
  Bengaluru - 70 • Ph: +91-80-26771678/79 • Fax: +91-80-26771680
  E-mail: cbsbng@gmail.com, bangalore@cbspd.com
• *Chennai:* No. 7, Subbaraya Street, Shenoy Nagar, Chennai - 600030
  Ph: +91-44-26681266, 26680620 • Fax: +91-44-42032115
  E-mail: chennai@cbspd.com
• *Kochi:* Ashana House, 39/1904, A.M. Thomas Road, Valanjambalam,
  Ernakulum, Kochi • Ph: +91-484-4059061-65
  Fax: +91-484-4059065 • E-mail: cochin@cbspd.com
• *Kolkata:* 6-B, Ground Floor, Rameshwar Shaw Road, Kolkata - 700014
  Ph: +91-33-22891126/7/8 • E-mail: kolkata@cbspd.com
• *Mumbai:* 83-C, Dr. E. Moses Road, Worli, Mumbai - 400018
  Ph: +91-9833017933, 022-24902340/41 • E-mail: mumbai@cbspd.com

Representatives:

• Hyderabad: 0-9885175004	• Nagpur: 0-9021734563
• Patna: 0-9334159340	• Pune: 0-9623451994
• Jharkhand: 0-9811541605	• Uttarakhand: 0-9716462459

Printed at:
J.S. Offset Printers, Delhi (India)

ACKNOWLEDGEMENT

Over the years, the quasi-medical and pharmaceutical background of the author had been consistently yielding ground to Diet Therapy and Naturopathy. However, it was an attack of Arthritis at the age of 63 that set him full-blast into Clinical Nutrition, nay Bio-Nutrition. Later on, it was a three month stint at the National Institute of Nutrition, Hyderabad in 2001-02 that transformed him into a 'Zealous Evangelist' of this New Science of Bionutrition that is bound to prove as the 'Saviour' of the modern man.

All these ceaseless explorations and research had the instinctive support of my erstwhile Doctor-turned-Collaborator, Dr.(Mrs) Usha Jain, the leading Practising Naturopath and Diet Therapist of Delhi, whose greater insight and fund of practical knowledge and versatile skills became a source of continuing inspiration.

I also owe deeper gratitude to the NIN, Hyderabad Faculty, specially Ex-Director Dr. B. S. Narasinga Rao and Chief Librarian Dr. K. Sampatha Chary and who were instrumental in making me dive deep into the ocean of Bio-Nutrition and harvest undreamt of wealth from many a lesser-known source.

And vicarious gratitude to the distant cousins in America - Dr. Cherie Calbom and Dr. Bernard Jensen, whose encyclopaedic coverage of this new theme of Fruit and Vegetable Juice Therapy ever, so ever serves as a beaconlight to many a late-comer like him.

Thanks are also due to the staff of National Medical Library, Delhi and the Department of Food, as also the ICAR Libraries (both of Agriculture Ministry, Government of India), plus the CSIR Library, Delhi for helping me out with many unconventional reports and documents.

Dr. S. Paul

PREFACE

The hectic pace and tension of modern life is taking a heavy toll!

The incidence of ill-health is mounting, both in terms of morbidity and mortality. The medical sciences have no doubt made commendable progress, but the side-effects and grave complications that follow chemotherapy and other regimes play havoc with a man's psyche and his purse too. At this critical juncture, the Alternate Medicine Systems need to be explored more concertedly and promoted far more vigorously.

Grievously weighed down by the liabilities of modern medicine, many a 'Best Healer of the West' have consciously switched on to 'Nature Cure', more to the Fruit and Vegetable Juice Therapy, which also offers many additional dividends. So much so that this New Diet Therapy has come to play a very dominant role even in an advanced country like the USA. Rather, it has become a fashionable fad in the West.

Some of the pioneers in this field, viz. Drs. Bernard Jensen, Cherie Calbom, and Victor Rico have carved out very successful reputation in Diet Therapy. Rightly has Cherie Calbom been nicknamed as the 'Juice Woman'. The Wheatgrass juice has cured cases of chronic cancers. In India, the Nature Cure Centres at Uruli Kanchan (Pune), Lajpat Bhawan (Delhi) and the one at Bangalore, besides many others, have spearheaded new trends in 'Curing Disease through Diet'.

Many of the fruits and vegetables are exceptionally rich source of β-carotenes—the Nature's most potent antioxidant that can inhibit artherosclerosis and thus help prevent cardiovascular (heart) disease. Green leafy vegetables are indeed an inexpensive source of iron, besides vitamins B and C and the mineral calcium. They are all very rich in carotenoids.

These fruits and vegetables contain Bio-active agents, 'Phytochemicals'. Apart from β-carotenes found specially in oats, the other important agents include isoflavones in soyabeans, methyl allins in garlic and sulforaphane in broccoli, all of which have cancer-preventive properties. Onion and garlic juice is reputed to lower blood sugar levels, thus proving immensely beneficial to the diabetic patients. Dr. Usha Jain (Delhi) uses 'Petha' (ashgourd) and Amla (gooseberry) juice as the most effective cure for many chronic diseases. Wheatgrass juice has proved to be an outstanding success in treating cancers. Beet juice and Alfalfa sprouts are the best restorative in the armoury of the Naturopaths. By boosting man's 'immune-building' functions, this Diet Therapy can effect many miracles, beyond the ken of the conventional medical wisdom.

Nutrition, in its new incarnation, Bio-Nutrition, offers the dual benefit of providing sustenance and also helping prevent many intractable diseases. Easy availability apart, Bio-Nutrition also offers the additional plus points—lower costs and no side-effects. By now, Bio-Nutrition has emerged as the *tool nulli secundus,* to relieve man of all the diverse ailments, viz., physical, mental and psychological.

In a way, it is harking back 2400 years to the Father of Medicine: Hippocrates, who had then advised:

'*Let living foods be thy medicine*'!

The quintessence of Bio-Nutrition comes out in the historic words of another pioneering medical authority, Dr. Victor G. Rico:

'*If we eat wrongly,*

No doctor can cure us,

If we eat properly,

No doctor is needed!'

Let us shed all the mental cobwebs and come out of the stranglehold of the ever-costly, and bothersome modern treatment that may often lead the man nowhere.

This first-ever tome on Bio-Nutrition provides a ray of '*New Hope*' and '*New Life*' to the long-suffering man. Let this '*Natural Saviour*' save the Mankind!

Dr. S. Paul

CONTENTS

LIST OF DIET CHARTS

PART 1

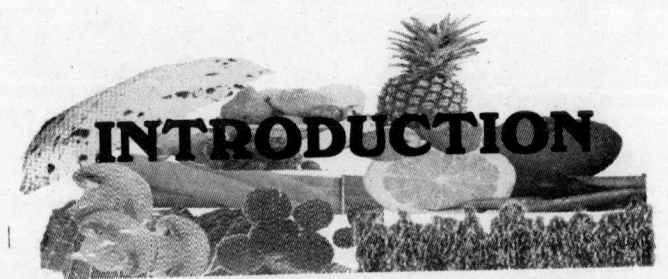

INTRODUCTION

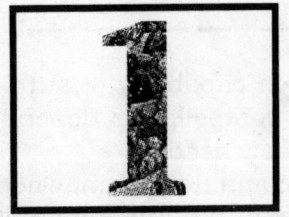

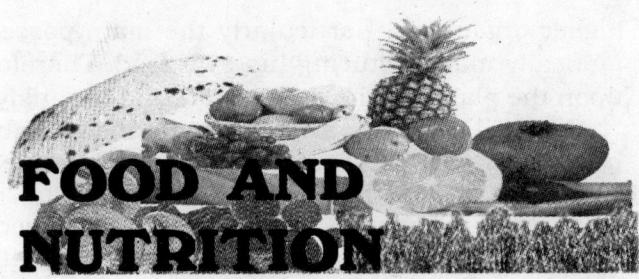

FOOD AND NUTRITION

INTRODUCTION

Food is the basic necessity of life!

Be it a high-brow business tycoon in the West or an indigent, poor landless labourer in the developing world, everyone needs food to sustain his life. Be, whatever one's economic status or calling, one does need an adequate amount of food to supply energy to the body for the most essential tasks like:

(A) Proper body growth,
(B) Maintaining and regulating the even tempo of life,
(C) For specified needs and contingencies like:

    (1) Sports and athletics
    (2) Strenuous hard labour
    (3) High altitude conditions
    (4) Convalescence
    (5) Pregnancy and lactation
    (6) For rapidly growing childhood
    (7) For the aged and the geriatrics
    (8) For those critically/terminally ill.

Apart from these physiological functions, food is also valued for its palatability and satiety effect. And then there are diverse ethnic foods that reflect the cultural differences or food habits of different groups or races in different geographic milieu. All these factors merit special consideration.

In the plant kingdom, it is the natural 'Process of Photosynthesis' that helps plants manufacture the food they need from the simple chemicals that abound in their surrounding soil and water or carbon dioxide in the air around. But higher organisms, particularly the man, possess no such capability of auto-matically manufacturing his own food. Therefore, he is compelled to depend upon the plants or the animals around to satisfy all his basic needs.

Although the wide variety of foodstuffs available to the common man may not have the same or the desired quality of nutrients, yet man has the inherent advantage, unlike the animals, to 'pick and choose' from the wide array of food resources to satisfy his general or selective needs.

Technically speaking, food may be divided into three sub-groups, viz.

(1) Energy-giving foods
(2) Body-building foods
(3) Protective/curative foods

Group one includes carbohydrates and fats which yield energy. Foods that are rich in proteins are called body-building foods. Protective or curative foods are those which have abundance of vitamins and minerals. Table 1 gives the illustrations of different foodstuffs and their important constituents:

TABLE 1.1. FOOD CLASSIFICATION

No.	Food Group	Major Nutrients
A:	**Energy-rich Foods**	
1.	Cereals, Millets and Products	Carbohydrates, Fibre, Proteins, Invisible Fat, Vitamins B_1, B_2, Folic acid and Iron
2.	Nuts and Oilseeds	Carbohydrates, Invisible Fat, Proteins, Vitamins and Minerals
3.	Vegetable Oils, Butter and Ghee	Fats, Essential Fatty acids and Fat-soluble Vitamins
4.	Sugars	Carbohydrates, viz., Glucose, Fructose, etc.
B:	**Body-building Foods**	
1.	Milk and Milk Products	Proteins, Calcium and Vitamin A, Vitamin B_2, Vitamin B_{12}
2.	Meat, Poultry and Fish	Proteins, Fats, Vitamin B complex, Iron and Iodine.
3.	Legumes and Pulses, Nuts and Oilseeds	Proteins, Invisible Fat, Vitamin B complex, Fibre, Calcium and Iron
C:	**Protective Foods**	
1.	Green Leafy Vegetables	Calcium, Iron, Folic acid, Fibre, Invisible Fat, Carotenoids and Antioxidants
2.	Other Vegetables	Fibre, Carotenoids, Folic acid, Calcium and Antioxidants
3.	Milk and Milk Products Meat, Poultry and Fish	Proteins, Calcium and Vitamin A, Vitamin B_2, Vitamin B_{12}, Iron and Iodine

And in the words of the eminent Indian nutritionist, Dr. C. Gopalan:

'Satisfaction of hunger is usually the primary criteria of adequate food intake. But the satisfaction of hunger itself is not a sage guide for the selection of proper foods. For sustaining healthy life, diet should be planned on sound 'Nutritional Principles'.

While every body eats food, the scientists and more so the nutritionists are concerned about the type or variety of food consumed, its passage through the body, its digestion, absorption and storage and the ultimate effect it has on his or her overall well-being. That is where the quintessential role of the 'Science and Art of Nutrition' comes in. Today, the emphasis is on its nutritive value and its role in the maintenance of optimal health and resistance to disease.

Technically speaking, Nutrition may be defined as the scientific study of food and its relation to the health of a man. Others have defined Nutrition as a science which deals with the processes, both physiological and biochemical, by which human/animal body utilizes food for energy and other essential requirements. The Biological Equation, enunciated by Dr. Francis Moore in 1963 (cf. The Special Supplement at the end of this Chapter) summarises all these reactions and processes in the body.

DIET THERAPY

It was the French chemist, Antoine-Laurent Lavoisier, who first initiated systematic studies in Nutrition in the eighteenth century. Rightly has Lavoisier been called 'The Father of Science of Nutrition'. However, it was the development of the science of Chemistry and later on, Bio-chemistry that helped unravel many an unanswered question pertaining to the nitty-gritty of foods that we take. Of the many illustrious scientists who made notable contribution to the modern food science are Lusk, Atwater, McCollum, Benedict, Rose and Rubner.

FOOD IN INDIAN MYTHOLOGY

In the ancient Indian literature, food has been given an unduly high spiritual significance. In fact, *Ayurveda*, the oldest scripture in the world, deals with the 'Science of Life'. It prescribes diet, medicine and a regimen of life, all of which if properly followed, will lead to maintaining the equilibrium of '*Dhatus*' (Tissue elements) that would eventually contribute to perfect sound health.

In Chapter 1, para 28.41, *Ayurveda* categorically states:

'The body is constituted of food. Hence, one must take wholesome food.'

It further lists eight factors of 'Dietetics', which must be taken into account for the proper nourishment of '*Dhatus*' in Chapter 3 (No. 1.21). These are

1. Prakrti   - Nature of food articles
2. Karana   - Method of their processing
3. Samyoga   - Combination of different foods
4. Rasi   - Quantity of food to be taken
5. Desa   - Habitat or the environment in which it is cultivated
6. Kala   - The time of cultivation of those foods
7. Upayogasamstha - Rules governing the intake of food
8. Upayokta   - The individual (consumer) himself.

Then there is the 'Ayurvedic Rasayana', which may be called the progenitor of the modern science of Gerontology, since it deals with the problem of 'Aging'. In Sanskrit language, the word used is 'Vayahsthapana'. Not only that it categorically names 'Amalaki'* fruits for rejuvenation, it also specifically mentions the season when its consumption (Kevalamalarasayana) will produce the most efficacious results—'Pausa, Magha and Phalgun' (corresponding to the months December, January and February). Efficacy of Diet therapy comes out in the inspiring eulogy: 'One can live for as many thousands of years with youth regained, depending upon as many Amalaki fruits as he has taken.'

The Miracle Plant

'Soma' is the plant extolled as the 'Lord of the Medicinal Herbs'! In Sasrut Samhita, this miracle plant is described as the 'Greatest Rejuvenator'—by implication, the aphrodisiac. There are 24 species listed of this plant and the juice expressed out of these plants rejuvenates the system. To quote from this ancient treatise:

'It enables him to witness ten thousand summers on earth in the full enjoyment of a new youthful body. And he is invested with a beauty of frame which belongs to Kandarpa (God of Love) and his complexion vies with the beams of Full Moon.'

Another great treatise on ancient medicine: 'Charakasamhita', in para 7 of Chapter 6.14, lauds the plus points of 'Soma'—the 'Excellent Rejuvenator' is an aesthetic imagery reminiscent of Kalidasa, nay a modern Keats or a Shakespeare:

'Within six months, he regains youthfulness, luminosity, lustre, voice, physical form, strength and aura like gods. And he gains mastery over his speech.'

It is indeed very gratifying to note that in the Ayurveda, one finds specific instructions regarding the appropriate choice of foods for quick recovery from diseases, as well as preventing any further complications thereof.

All these eulogies to foods and fruits in particular in the ancient literature bring out in sharp focus the greatness and glory this Science of Dietetics enjoyed in the Indian Culture in the hoary past.

Gita, another Indian classic, beautifully sums up the Indian philosophy in Chapter 4 in the following words:

'As the Food, so the Mind;
As the Mind, so the Man!'

In the common man's parlance of the Twenty-first century, it means

'Jaisa khaye ann,
Vaisa hoye mann!'
(You are what you eat!)

---

*The ancient Sanskrit name Amalaki means Amla or Gooseberry.

In India, some of the 'Ancient Nutritional Wisdom' has been handed over from one generation to another in the form of traditional recipes and culinary practices. And most of these 'Eating norms' had perfect scientific rationale for their being well-balanced and seasonally well-adapted. Dr. Pushpangadan, Director, National Botanical Research Institute, Lucknow (India) is very articulate in supporting the South Indian custom of greater use of 'Tamarind', unlike the North Indian dependence on tomatoes or ketchup etc. Similarly, greater use of onions in the hot summer weather counters the risk of heat strokes. And such like culinary practices can be multiplied manifold in each and every sub-region of the continent.

EVOLUTION OF DIETETICS

In the early part of the Twentieth Century, the scientists' interest in nutrition, *prima facie*, was concerned with the energy needs of the human body, as to how much energy is made available by different staple constituent of food, say proteins, fats and carbohydrates. Later on, vitamins and minerals were studied and explored in depth for their respective '*Enhancing Effect*' or supplementation to the nutritive values of different staple diets. And then came the amino acids, fats and fatty acids, trace elements and the hormones. It is the cumulative effect of all these ethnic practices and scientific explorations that have eventually grown into the modern science of Nutrition, nay the newly evolving Bio-Nutrition.

That way, the Food Science and its corollary, Dietetics have come to play a very important role in the life of the modern man. Man has now come to realize the full implications of nutrition and further the fact that in the ultimate analysis, the quality of his health (as also cultural or spiritual well-being) depends solely upon the food that he eats. But the dietary habits of an individual are prone to many a wide fluctuation, depending upon a host of environmental factors that guide and shape the destiny of man.

Overall, there are ten major factors that influence human nutrition. These factors, in the descending order of their values, as shown in Fig. 1.1, are:

1. Economic status
2. Regional agri-horticultural development
3. Local traditions and culture
4. Climate and weather
5. Religion and Family history
6. Age factor
7. Educational background
8. Science and technology status
9. Health status
10. Medical requirements.

Economic Status

Regional Agriculture

Local Traditions and Culture

Climate and Weather

Religion and Ethnic History

Age Factor

Educational Background

S & T Status

Health Status

Medical Requirements

NUTRITION

Nutrition is the ultimate balance-sheet of all the processes by which the animal or human system utilizes food for providing energy for growth and maintenance, as also other specified needs. The word nutrition comes from the Latin root 'nutr', which means to nurture or nourish. The Art and Science of Nutrition, prima *facie*, focuses on nourishing and sustaining life. Right from the moment of conception until death, the body needs to carry out an array of vital functions, breathing being the most subtle of them all.

Man needs energy to support all the diverse physical activity, even when he is sleeping. As such, he is required to constantly replenish these energy needs with proper food to carry on and sustain life. And in a very subtle manner, the food that he consumes also nourishes his spirit-hence the expression, '*Sattavik*' food in the Indian lore.

According to the American Medical Association:

'Nutrition is the science of food, the nutrients and other substances therein, their action, and interaction and balance in relation to health and disease, and the processes by which the organism ingests, digests, absorbs, transports and utilizes and finally excretes food substances. In addition, nutrition may be concerned with social, economic, cultural and psychological implications of food and eating.'

Optimal Nutrition

Optimal Nutrition means that an individual is getting/utilizing all the 'Essential' nutrients for maintaining his well-being at the highest possible level and in a manner that is most efficient and satisfying too.

Holistic Health

Holistic health signifies a system of preventive medicine that takes into account all the needs, requirements and physical aspirations of an individual.

Diet Therapy

Medical Nutrition Therapy (Diet Therapy) is the system of treating all the diverse maladies through the progressively greater use of Nutrition Therapy, preferably by a Registered Dietician (RD). In its latest incarnation, Diet Therapy, resting solely on Fruit (+Vegetable) Juices, as cogently proved in this treatise, is called Bio-Nutrition.

Nutrients

A nutrient is the basic chemical component or substance that is present in the food and is needed by the body. The two main functions of nutrients are:

(a) To provide material for growth as also repair of tissues that eventually maintain the basic structure of our body.

(*b*) To support the body with the energy required to perform all the mundane tasks, besides carrying on many a not-so-visible internal activity.

Nutrients are of two types:

1. Macro-nutrients like carbohydrates, fats and proteins, which supply the much-needed energy and also build tissues.
2. Micro-nutrients like vitamins, minerals and trace elements, are needed in small quantity, but they play a crucial role to regulate and control body processes.

Water is the overall vital nutrient that sustains all our life processes. In all, there are over two scores of nutrients needed by the body. These may be broadly classified into four sub-groups, viz. major nutrients, vitamins, minerals and trace elements:

1. Major Nutrients, viz., carbohydrates, fats and proteins
2. Micronutrients

   (*a*) Vitamins:
   - Fat-soluble vitamins, viz., A, D, E and K.
   - Water-soluble vitamins, viz., C and B group.

   (*b*) Minerals and Trace Elements:
   - Macro-minerals (8): These include metallic elements whose daily requirements is more than 100 mg, e.g. Ca, P, Na, K, Cl, Mg and S.
   - Micro-minerals (13): These include nutrients whose daily requirements range from 1 mg to 100 mg, e.g. Fe, Cu, Zn, Mn, I, Mb, Se, F, Br, Cr, Co, and Si.
   - Trace Elements: Whose requirement is just a few micrograms, e.g. B, Sn, Ni, Ge, V (Vanadium), W (Tungsten) and Pb.

Levels of Nutrition

Depending upon an individual's living situation as also the available food supply and health conditions, the nutritional status varies. The three levels of nutrition could be Ideal nutrition, Border-line nutrition and Malnutrition:

Ideal Nutrition

When it is ideal nutrition, it shows up in the form of

(1) A buoyant, well-developed body,
(2) An ideal weight and height,
(3) A good muscular development and tone.

Ideal nutrition reflects all-round robustness. In a perfect situation of Ideal Nutrition, the points that strike one are

(1) The skin is smooth and clear,

(2) The hair is glossy,

(3) The eyes are clear and bright,

(4) The general posture is good,

(5) The facial expression is alert.

A man has good appetite and normal digestion and so are his bowel movements. Overall, well-nourished persons are likely to be more alert, both mentally and physically. They are not only able to meet their day-to-day needs, but are also able to maintain their essential nutrient reserve for resisting infection and disease. That way, they are able to prolong their years of normal, say optimum functioning.

Borderline Nutrition

Persons with borderline nutritional status just manage to scrape through from day-to-day with barest minimum needs met. They lack the much-needed nutritional reserves to meet any extra physiological contingencies or illness. This normally happens in persons who have developed poor eating habits, or else are being made to do with poor economic conditions. Such persons need not necessarily be under-nourished, but they are prone to the risk of greater ill-health. In the normal course, human body possesses great adaptability to such lowered nutritional status. But then it can sustain only a given amount of physiological stress and that too for a limited period before the signs of malnutrition surface up.

Even in a country like USA, nearly one-third of its population is living below the optimum level of nutrition!

Malnutrition

When the energy intake is grossly inadequate and the limited nutritional reserves are depleted, else unable to meet the day-to-day needs or the added metabolic stress, it indicates the state of Malnutrition and/or Under-nutrition. This is a ubiquitous phenomenon in the resource-poor countries of Asia and Africa. It normally occurs in a large number of high-risk poverty conditions. This malnutrition status influences the health of all the persons involved, but it severely impinges upon the lives of more vulnerable sections like the infants, the pregnant women and also the aged. Herein, infant mortality rate rises very high. They suffer from stunted growth and anaemia, and are prone to greater risk of disease. In fact, this incidence of malnutrition manifests at its worst in the low-income Sub-Saharan Africa (cf. Appendices at the end of the Chapter).

Technically speaking, the terms Malnutrition and Under-nutrition are not co-terminous. Malnutrition refers to the physical ill-effects of the prolonged inadequacy of diet - an inadequacy that could be either quantitative or qualitative or both. On the other hand, Under-nutrition specifically points to the quantitative shortcoming. In plain language, it means 'Low Food intake'—something which, in the long run, has serious repercussions on the well-being of a person and could lead to many deficiency diseases.

The critical unit of food energy intake may be expressed as under:

$$1.2 \times BMR$$

where BMR represents the basic minimum energy expenditure necessary for body maintenance at rest, with no physical activity.

The statistical configurations of malnutrition are too galling a phenomenon to be just wished away. World-wide, *about 40,000-50,000 people die each day of malnutrition.* Cumulatively, more than 1000 million continue to suffer from severe malnutrition in the Third World. The 1985 Physician Task Force on Hunger in America reported that at least 20 million Americans suffer hunger some days each month.

Such is this universal blight of Malnutrition!

Over-nutrition

This condition of over-nutrition, now brazenly manifesting even in the affluent West, is another form of malnutrition, when excess calories produce obesity and overweight conditions. And this predisposes such persons to the risk of many chronic diseases. Over-nutrition is also occasioned in men using 'Megadoses' of nutrition supplements, which eventually damage the tissue. Table 1.2 gives a very comprehensive over-view of the nutritional status of different regions of the world.

TABLE 1.2: GLOBAL MICRONUTRIENT MALNUTRITION (PERCENTAGE)

Region	Vitamin A (%)	Iodine (%)	Iron (%)	Zinc (%)
South East Asia	69	41	99	71.2
West Pacific	27	31	72	18.6
Africa	49	48	73	68.0
East Mediterranean	22	74	72	73.5
VERSUS				
Americas	20	25	34	45.8
Europe	–	32	17	18.0

Source: Usha Ramakrishnan in *Nutrition Review,* May, 2002.

BIO-NUTRITION PYRAMID

The US Department of Agriculture, as also of Health and Human Service have drawn up a 'Nutrition Food Pyramid'. This pyramid is an outline of what to eat each day. Although it is not a rigid prescription, yet it is a general guide to help you choose a good, healthy diet that suits your tastes pre-eminently. This pyramid calls for eating a variety of foods so that you get all the needed nutrients and at the same time, you are provided with the requisite calories to maintain a good

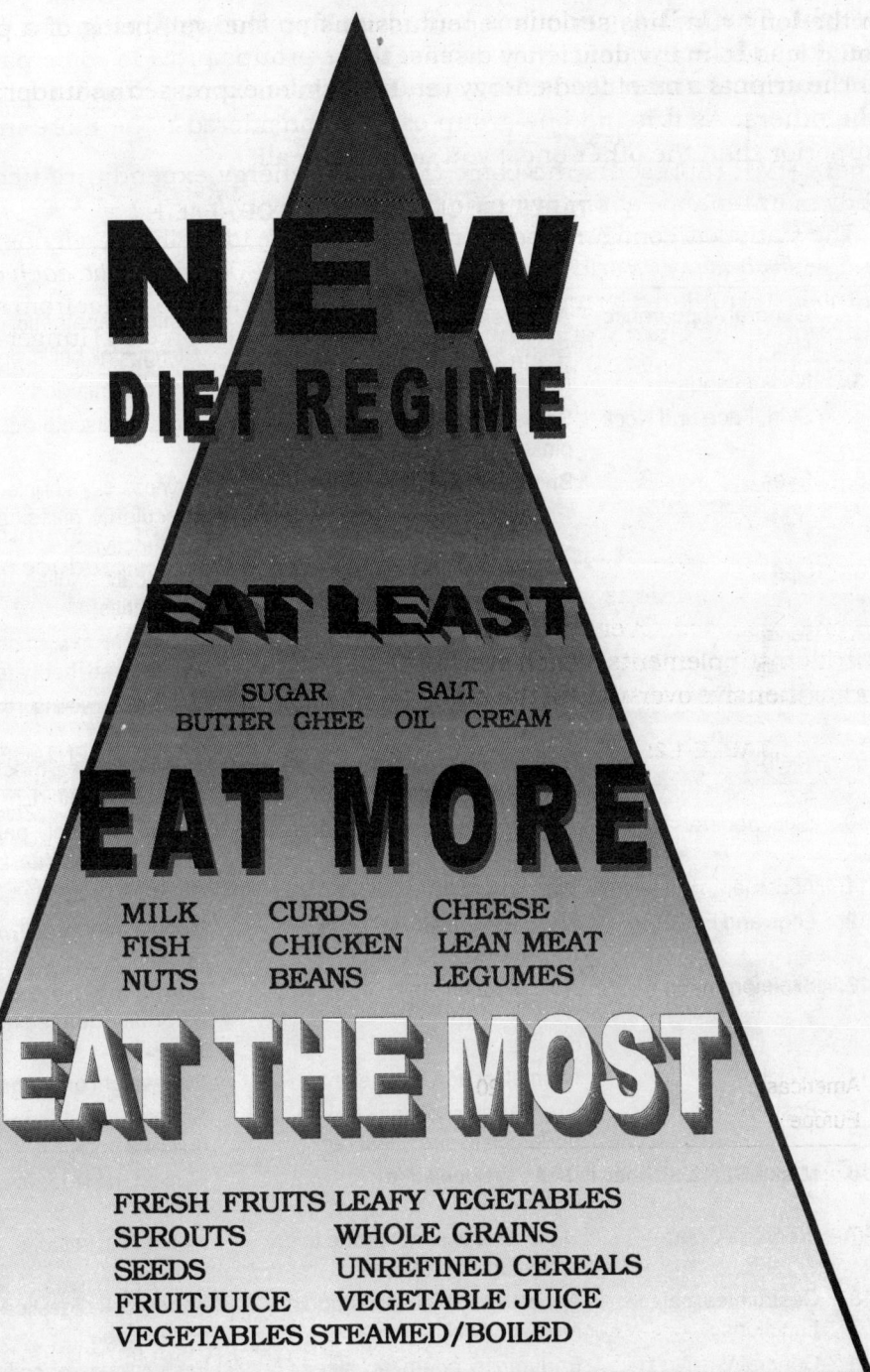

Fig. 1.2: The Bio-Nutrition Pyramid

weight. The USDA guidelines had given five food groups in the lower three sections of the Pyramid. Now each of these groups provide some part, if not all the nutrients a man needs. However, foods in one group cannot replace those in the others. As it is, no one group can be considered to be more important or superior than the other ones; you need them all.

TABLE 1.3: CLINICAL SIGNS OF HEALTH

	Features	Good	Poor
1.	General Appearance	Alert, responsive	Listless, apathetic, cachexia
2.	Hair	Shiny, lustrous; healthy scalp	Stringy, dull, brittle, dry, depigmented
3.	Neck Glands	No enlargement	Thyroid enlarged
4.	Skin, Face and Neck	Smooth, slightly moist; good color, pink-red mucous membranes	Greasy, discolored, scaly
5.	Eyes	Bright, clear; no fatigue circles	Dryness, signs of infection; increased vascularity, glassiness, thickened conjunctivae
6.	Lips	Good color, moist	Dry, scaly, swollen; angular lesions (stomatitis)
7.	Tongue	Good pink color, no lesions, surface papillae present	Papillary atrophy, smooth appearance, swollen red, beefy (glossitis)
8.	Gums	Good pink color, no swelling no bleeding, firm	Slight red, swelling, receding, spongy
9.	Teeth	Straight, no crowding, well-shaped jaws, no discoloration	Unfilled cavities, missing teeth, worn surfaces, mottled, malpositioned
10.	Skin, general	Smooth, slightly moist, good color	Rough, dry, scaly, pale, pigmented, irritated, petechiae, bruises
11.	Abdomen	Flat	Swollen
12.	Legs and Feet	No tenderness/weakness, no swelling; good color	Edema, tender calf, tingling; weakness
13.	Skeleton	No malformation	Bowed legs, knock knees, chest deformity, beaded ribs, prominent scapulae
14.	Weight	Normal for age and height	Overweight or underweight
15.	Posture	Erect arms and legs straight, abdomen in and chest out	Sagging shoulders, sunken chest, humped back
16.	Muscles	Well developed, firm	Flaccid, poor tone, undeveloped, tender
17.	Nervous Control	Quite attentive, not prone to cry, not irritable or restless	Inattentive, irritable
18.	Gastrointestinal Functions	Appetite and digestion good, regular bowel movements	Anorexia, indigestion, constipation or diarrhoea
19.	General Vitality	Endurance, energetic, sleeps well at night; vigorous	Easily fatigues, no energy, falls asleep in office, looks tired, apathetic

Source: Adapted from *Essentials of Nutrition and Diet Therapy,* Pub. Mosby.

However, the '*New mantra*' of Bio-Nutrition provides a definitive set of priorities that the 'New Millennium Man' must accord if he has to counter all the stress and strain of the hectic modern life. Herein, fruits and vegetables, unrefined cereals, seeds and sprouts emerge as the top-spinners in the modern diet charts. As mentioned in the 'Preface', and also in the summation in Chapter 24, at the end of this book, it is this New Bio-Nutrition (Diet) Regime that would soon become the 'Real Saviour' on the health front. The pyramid figure alongside categorically illustrates this new Bio-Nutrition philosophy that focuses on the relative merit of different foodstuffs.

But the Third World contingencies demand that you have to adopt a 'Cafetraia *Approach*—of offering an adaptable mix of diverse foods. In this 'Exchange System' of dietary management, since foods in each group are equal to one another in the portions indicated, they could be meaningfully exchanged within their respective groups (as practiced in India). This way, it would help maintain fairly uniform food values and calorie level too. This exchange also permits greater freedom in planning meals and snacks for different people in different situations. This approach could indeed prove a big boon in 'Enteral Nutrition', particularly for those critically ill.

In Table 1.4, we give a very comprehensive list of mircronutrient-rich foods commonly used in India. This illustrative grouping brings out the contrast, nay the human neglect, as shown earlier in Table 1.2. It only goes to show that there are available, in every region, some or the other food resources, often not-so-well-known, that could provide the basic needs of a common man.

TABLE 1.4: MICRONUTRIENT-RICH FOODS IN INDIA

Cereals and Millets	Pulses and Legumes	Nuts and Oil seeds	Vegetables Green Leafy	Other	Fruits	Spices
Ragi	Blackgram	Gingelly	Amaranth	Cluster beans	Amla	Raisins
Bajra	Bengalgram	Mustard/ Rape seed	Agathi	Dondakeri	Lime	Turmeric
Jowar	Cow pea	Niger leaves	Coriander	Ladyfinger	Tomato	Fenugreeek seeds
	Greengram	Niger	Curry leaves	Colocasia	Papaya	Coriander
	Redgram	Coconut dry	Mint	Carrots	Guava	Poppy seeds
	Horsegram	Groundnut	Mustard	Green Chillies	Lemon	
	Rajma		Ponna-ganni	Yam wild	Coconut Fresh	
	Soyabeans		Fenugreek Leaves Drumstick Leaves			

BIO-NUTRITION AND NUTRIFICATION

Bio-Nutrition is the new Food Science that amalgamates and harmoniously blends the basics of the Optimal Nutrition and Diet Therapy with the local organic resources to cater to 'Holistic Health'. This newly-evolved discipline is a far more comprehensive version of the conventional Clinical Nutrition in the present-day Health Delivery System. It stipulates providing point-by-point coverage of all the essential needs in different situations like:

(a) Growth needs of the body,

(b) Maintenance requirements,

(c) Total 'wellness' or physical fitness,

(d) Preventive treatment by boosting body resistance through improved immune system,

(e) Curative treatment in the case of some chronic maladies like Vitamin deficiency, etc.

Nutrification may be defined as the addition of nutrients to the commonly used food mixtures, which can lead to an improved intake for greater physiological benefits. Nutrification of the existing foods may take the form of

1. Fortification

2. Enrichment

3. Restoration

4. Supplementation

Nutrification has a long history since Boussingault first proclaimed the virtue of this bold concept by suggesting, in the year 1831, the addition of iodine to the table salt to prevent Goitre. In the present scenario of festering nutrition deficiencies, Nutrification has become the most rapildy applied, the most flexible and universally acceptable method of intervention to help change the nutrient intake of a people. As it is, it can be effected without any extensive education and further, it is something that does not call for any radical change in the consumption pattern of a community.

In the modern era of stress and strain, Bio-Nutrition aims at broadbasing the role of nutrition to cover all the health contingencies and then help build up organically the inner reserves to combat all sort of disease, leading ultimately to 'Assured Good Health'. Unlike the Western systems, Bio-Nutrition calls for greater dependence on the local 'Bio-resources', rather than the synthetic supplements that add to the costs, besides injecting some unwanted liabilities. Rather than resort to the indiscriminate use of pills and potions containing vitamins, iron or iodine etc, Bio-Nutrition relies more on the extracts from agri-horticulture/

forestry sources that systematically add to the present nutritional status of the staple diet used by the not-so-well off majority.

Herein, Vegetable and Fruit Juice Therapy, as personally experienced by this author (67), provides a far more efficacious and speedier curative treatment. Lest it be dismissed as another gimmick for the Ayurvedic or Unani systems, it may be added that Bio-Nutrition visualizes judicious blending some food adjuvants with other herbals having a specified medicinal value, hence it is called Nutrification.

Perforce, these new 'Nutrified Staples' call for low-cost technology that is mass replicable, rather than the high capital, high-tech models of the modern medicine.

THE JUICE MIRACLE

The juice of fresh fruits (+ vegetables) is the richest available source of vitamins, minerals and enzymes, besides some half-known 'Anutrients'. And it is a natural concoction that is digested and assimilated within a span of 20-30 minutes, thus proving to be an instant *Energy Booster*. Fruits differ from other foods in that their nutritive elements exist in the soluble forms of organic sugars, dextrin and fruit acids, which are found almost exclusively in their juices.

An eminent authority, Dr. Joy Kurdich (nicknamed the 'Juiceman') has rightly pontificated:

'All life on earth emanates from the green of the plant'.

Technically speaking, this 'Green' (Chlororphyll) is the most concentrated 'Sun-power'. From the medical angle, chlororphyll boosts the function of heart, effects circulatory system, intestines, uterus and lungs. In practice, chlorophyll, which forms the rock-foundation of Bio-Nutrition, is the *'Greatest Ever Tonic'* that keeps the body and soul going in the top gear all the time.

As such, raw fruits and vegetables are the Nature's way of giving us life. A still more powerful endorsement comes from Dr. Bircher-Benner, the founder of the world-famous Bircher-Benner Clinic at Zurich in Switzerland, who had said:

'Nothing more therapeutic exists on the earth than Green Juice'.

Already, the leading health authorities in the USA, viz. Surgeon General (Report 1989), the Secretary of Health and Human Services (Health America, 2000), the National Cancer Institute, as also the Dietary Goals for United States—all these forcefully recommend:

'Eat more fruits and fresh vegetables'.

That way, juice is a concentrated form of nutrients packaged in the best natural proportion to offer synergistic effect of all the nutrients working in concert to enhance man's health and spirits. In essence, this vitamin and mineral mixture may rightly be called the 'Green or Golden Cocktail' (cf. Poem: Green Gold in the Supplement at the end of this Chapter).

Somehow this truism is bit relegated by the market forces of globalisation and the bane of the 'Pizzas and Pleasure Foods'. And all this costs a fortune in medical bills.

PHYTOCHEMICALS (ANUTRIENTS)

By now, it has been well recognised that the orange-red vegetables offer a high level of carotenes, which have anti-cancer properties. Citrus fruit provides vitamin C and bioflavonoids, the immune-strengthening nutrients. And dark green leafy vegetables are rich in folic acid, a vitamin B complex known for the proper maintenance of red blood cells and the nervous system. In fact, Naturopathy and Bio-Nutrition offer an infinite range of sure-shot and efficacious juice remedies, even for chronic maladies like cancers. This emphasis on fresh produce and *'Diet that is unrefined'* is indeed become the dominant trend in contemporary nutrition and clinical dietetics. In reality, this raw juice healing goes back to the nineteenth century, when the juice making process involved the cumbersome squeezing of crushed vegetables through muslin cloth. So much for its inherent wisdom!

CURING CANCER

Apart from the pioneering work of Dr. Benner, credit must also be given to the eminent cancer specialist, Dr. Max Gerson, who has done very extensive research and successfully cured many terminally-ill cancer parties—all of which has been recorded in his book, *A Cancer Therapy: Results of Fifty Cases (1958)*. He was fully convinced that cancer did not require any specific treatment. The main point is that the whole body must be detoxified with raw fruit and vegetables juices. The much acclaimed β-carotenes apart, new α-carotenes have been discovered which show protective effect against vulvar cancers. And then we have the phytochemicals like phenols, indoles, aromatic isothio-cyanates, terpenes and organo-sulfur compounds, collectively called 'Anutrients', which have specific anti-cancer properties.

A very interesting custom is reported from Europe, *i.e.* Grape Cure. People go all the way and stay to recuperate in grape-growing areas. Once they are there, they eat nothing but grapes for days and days. On the outer coat of the seeds, there is the special layer, Cream of Tartar, which is the greatest thing to cut the mucus and catarrh so that these can be rapidly eliminated from the body.

The alphabeticelly-arranged repertoire of Juicing (cf. Supplement) sums up the beauty and bounty of the Green Gold-Chlorophyll, *the 'Greatest benefactor of the Mankind.'*

As the famed Dietician: Dr. Cherie Calbom says, *'Sickness or Health - the choice is yours'*. The physical condition you have tomorrow starts with what you do for your body today. And today is the time when you begin with the Miracle Formula called Juicing. Let us go back 2400 years to the prophetic words of Hippocrates, the Father of Medicine:

'Let living (natural) food be thy medicine!'

Unlike any of the earlier modes of health delivery, Bio-Nutrition offers limitless socio-economic ramifications, whose area of influence increases with greater innovation and experimentation. The proposed amplification of this new discipline of nutrition has quite a legitimate historic background. To quote H.M. Sinclair:

'Medicine arose from Dietetics'.

The ancient Pythagorians, including the Father of Medicine, Hippocrates, used to prevent and cure diseases through nutritional remedies. They resorted to drugs only when the former modes failed to help. As such, Bio-Nutrition is the latest and the best incarnation of all the principles of health and medicine—be these Ayurvedic, Unani or Tibetan and Chinese, else the ultramodern treatment systems supported by the 'Nutrified Foods' and the 'Enteral Diet' of the West. This system of 'Holistic Health' offers wide ranging benefits than what was purported to be the original definition of nutrition given by the American Medical Association (cited earlier) a few decades back.

Planned judiciously, Bio-Nutrition will ensure far greater spread-effect and also cost effectiveness than any modern method of treatment. That way, it would also ensure greater acceptability by the masses. The new slogan has got to be the Nutrification of the staples like wheat, rice, maize and sorghum with the local organic resources. This concept has been vindicated by J. Christopher Bauernfeind in the book: *Modern Nutrition in Health and Disease* (1996). He too supports that the carrier should be a food ingredient universally consumed by the targeted population. Not burgers, beverages or the bounty of 'Pleasures Foods' of the West, but the major local cereals ought to become the new tools, nay the *Tool nulli secundus* of the modern health therapy. In countries like India and Africa, nutrient-rich protein concentrates and soy products, besides gooseberry (Amla) or Leh-berry extracts, alfalfa seeds, grain amaranth and stable, full fat rice bran should be made the mandatory adjuncts for Nutrified Foods. For the infants and vulnerable women, it could be Nutrified Bakery products, bread and biscuits.

THE ULTIMATE MANTRA

In the developing countries, the major deficiencies that stand out are iodine, iron and vitamins. By evolving scientifically-crafted cereal-plant protein concentrates and 'Designer Organic Supplements', Bio-Nutrition can become the best tool for fighting the age-old 'Protein-Energy Malnutrition (PEM)', as also the 'Hidden Hunger' of about 4000 million destitutes in the Third World countries.

Must not we hark back to the great words of wisdom uttered by Hippocrates way back in the Fifth century:

> *'I MAINTAIN that research on the subject of diet is of all*
> *the objects of medicine most worthy of our closest attention.*
> *It will contribute much, both in re-establishing health and*
> *preserving those who are at present in normal health by*
> *providing them with a sound constitution.'*

Indeed, Bio-Nutrition is the right corollary to this Fifth Century wisdom that holds good even today! Yes, Bio-Nutrition is the *'New Mantra'* that would redeem the present situation! It is the *'Mantra of the Last Resort'* that would overhaul, nay resuscitate and rejuvenate the sagging health of the rich and the poor alike!

Bio-Nutrition is indeed the New Health Revolution in the making. Let us herald

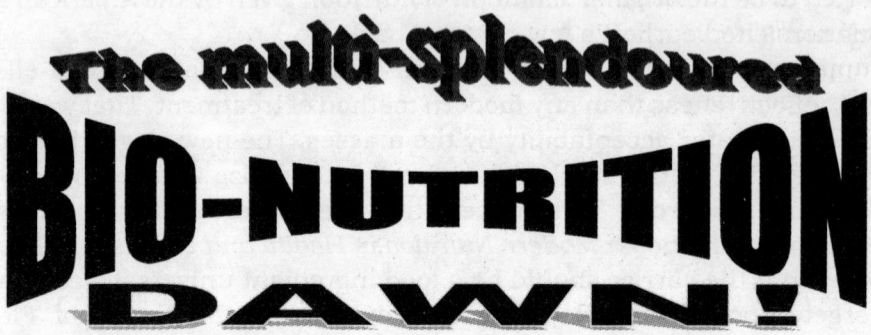
The multi-splendoured BIO-NUTRITION DAWN!

BIOLOGICAL EQUATION

There does exist a perfect equation between man and food. This biological equation was first enunciated by Dr. Francis D. Moore, Professor of Surgery at Harvard in 1963 while addressing the New York Academy of Sciences. He had then stated:

$$MAN = CM + EST + FAT$$

where, **CM** denotes Cell Mass—the active tissue carrying out all the work of the body.

EST denotes Extracellular Supporting Tissue that supports the cell mass. These could be divided into two components:

(a) Extracellular fluids that comprise of blood plasma and lymph, as also the fluid which bathes these cells.

(b) Minerals and protein fibres in skeletal and other supporting tissue.

FAT denotes energy reserves held in the adipose tissue beneath the skin and around internal organs.

As such, this biological equation could be interpreted in a mathematical manner to show that the man's body or his physical being is divided into three compartments of

- Cell mass
- Supporting tissue
- Energy reserves.

And food/nutrition is the basic constituent that supports all these parts of the biological equation.

From Dr. Bernard Jensen's Book: FOODS THAT HEAL

HEALTH COCKTAIL FOR COMMON DISORDERS

No.	Ailments	Recommended Juice Therapy
1.	**Anemia**	Blackberry and Parsley Juice; Parsley and Grape Juice
2.	**Arthritis**	Celery and Parsley Juice
3.	**Asthma**	Celery and Papaya Juice; Celery and Carrot Juice
4.	**Bladder Ailments**	Pomegranate and Celery Juice; Shavegrass Herb Tea
5.	**Blood Ailments**	Blackberry Juice; Black Cherry Juice; Parsley Juice
6.	**High Blood Pressure**	Carrot and Parsley and Celery Juice; Lime Juice and Whey Powder; Grape Juice and Carrot Juice
7.	**Low Blood Pressure**	Parsley Juice; Also Capsicum and Garlic Juice
8.	**Bronchitis**	Lemons (2) Juice with Honey—3 tsp added to one Pint Flaxseed Tea—use one tsp every hour;
		Bake a Lemon, then juice half of it and add to one cup of Oat Straw or Boneset Tea, then retire and perspire
9.	**Sore Throat, Catarrh and Colds**	Watercess and Apple Juice with ¼ Tsp pure Cream of Tartar (from Grape Juice)
10.	**Poor Circulation**	Beet and Blackberry Juice; Parsley and Alfalfa Juice with Pineapple Juice; Grape Juice with one Egg Yolk
11.	**Colds and Sinus Infections**	Celery and Grapefruit Juice; Watercess and Apple Juice with ¼ Tsp pure Cream of Tartar; Also No.1 with ¼ Tsp Cream of Tartar
12.	**Gastritis, Colitis/Gas**	Coconut Milk and Carrot Juice
13.	**Complexion Problems**	Cucumber and Endive and Pineapple Juice; Apple concentrate—1 tsp; Cucumber Juice and Water—half glass each
14.	**Complexion(Yellow)**	Grapefruit Juice
15.	**Constipation, Stomach Ulcers**	Celery Juice with little Sweet Cream; Spinach and Blackberry Juice
16.	**Diarrhoea**	Carrot and Blackberry Juice
17.	**Eczema, Scurvy**	Carrot and Lemon and Celery Juice
18.	**Fever, Gout, Arthritis**	Celery and Parsley Juice
19.	**Gall Bladder Problems**	Radish and Prune and Blackberry and Celery Juice; Carrot and Beetroot and Cucumber Juice
20.	**Gall Stones**	Beetroot and Radish Juice
21.	**Heart Problems**	Carrot and Pineapple Juice with Honey; Alfalfa (Liquid Chlorophyll); Parsley and Alfalfa and Pineapple Juice
22.	**Indigestion, Underweight**	Coconut Milk and Fig Juice; Parsley and Carrot Juice
23.	**Infections**	Carrot and Blackberry Juice

24.	Insomnia	Lettuce and Celery Juice
25.	Jaundice	Tomato and Sauerkraut Juice—1 glass every day for full one week
26.	Kidney Problems	Celery and Parsley and Asparagus Juice; Carrot and Parsley Juice
27.	Urinary Bladder Problems	Black Currant Juice with Juniper Berry Tea; and Goat Whey; Celery and Pomegranate Juice.
28.	Liver Problems	Radish and Pineapple Juice; Blackberry Concentrate and Chlorophyll; Carrot and Beet and Cucumber Juice
29.	Memory-Poor	Celery and Carrot and Prune Juice with Rice Polishing
30.	Nervous Tension	Celery and Carrot and Prune Juice; Lettuce and Tomato Juice
31.	Nervous Disorder	Radish and Prune Juice with Rice Polishing
32.	Neuritis, Neuralgia	Cucumber and Endive and Pineapple Juice; Cucumber and Endive Juice with Goat's Whey
33.	Obesity, Overweight	Green Beets and Parsley and Celery Juice
34.	Perspiration	Celery and Parsley Juice; Cucumber and Pineapple Juice
35.	Rheumatism	Cucumber and Endive Juice and Goat's Whey
36.	Rickets	Dandelion and Orange Juice
37.	Sinus	Sip Lemon Juice with a little Horseradish; Sip mixture of Cayenne Powder in a cup of water
38.	Thyroid Problems	Clam and Celery Juice
39.	General Vitality	Apple Concentrate—one Tsp with Almond Nut Butter—one Tsp and one cup Celery Juice
40.	Reducing Weight	Parsley and Grape and Pineapple Juice
41.	Retaining Youth	Oat Straw Tea 2/3 cup with 1/3 cup Celery and Prune or Fig Juice with ¼ cup
	(Aging)	Powdered Nova Scotia Dulse to each cup; Cucumber and Radish and Pepper Juice—1/3 cup; Pineapple Juice with one Egg Yolk.

N.B.: In the Fourth Part, we have presented a more comprehensive juice regime for all the disease, as being practised by Dr. Cherie Calbom. Besides these, special Diets Charts of Dr. (Mrs) Usha Jain, based solely on fruit and vegetable juice therapy, have been included with individual diseases in Part Three.

The Green Gold

The Green Gold, 'Chlorophyll' is indeed a Boon,
A God-given gift, it acts early morn, late afternoon;
A spark of renewed zeal and instant energy,
Of the Science of Botany and Medicine a 'New Synergy'!

Sun-powered booster this of vigor and potency,
Fights out the microbes, any latent viral militancy;
A 'Miracle' cleanser, it fully eliminates,
Metabolic wastes and toxins in the system checkmates.

A wide array of ailments and the chronic cancer,
A 'Healer Natural' it is a 'Health-dispenser';
Your body ills all it hounds, them systematically rout,
Letting in new spirit, a new health sprout!

Dr. Harry Hoxsey has this experience to say,
Crushed garlic paste, the skin cancer did flay;
Eva Hill, the cancer specialist, her own cured,
Raw fruits and vegetable juice the cancerous face lured.

Dr. Ann Wigmore strongly did comment,
Sprouts and Wheatgrass many a disease prevent;
Delhi's Usha Jain garlic, amla powder and honey recommend.
Heart and blood system it meticulously repairs and all damage mend.

The Father-figure, Hippocrates long ago opined,
'Living foods be thy medicine' his philosophy refined;
Foods cooked may let in growths cancerous and tumours,
Guzzling raw foods, vanished they all as baseless rumours.

This much-wanted and much-flaunted Green Gold,
Since time immemorial, we are told,
Injects health perfect and buoyancy well-rolled,
A 'Fresh New-lease Life' on this strained planet unfold.

Getting the 'Liquid Gold' of fruits into your system,
Revitalizing all parts, a New Spring *ad libitum*;
Chemotherapy and radiation toned down to simple cure,
Wondrous Juice Therapy this one, a panacea so subtle, so sure.

Plants - the spark plug of life do they form,
When the dietary raw fruits and vegetables is the norm;
Cheap sources these of energy, vitamins and minerals,
Enrich your life, obviate an early funeral!

Thanked be the Lord for this 'Miracle of Mother Nature',
A *tool nulli secundus*, a remedy of rare stature;
More the Chlorophyll you eat and drink,
More robust your health, your complexion rosy-pink.

Ah! This Green Gold, Chlorophyll!

September 3, 2002   **Dr. S. Paul**

MALNUTRITION

FAO Reports

Depending upon the extent and magnitude of this problem, one observes two types, viz., the prononced malnutrition and negative spiral, as under:

A: *Pronounced Deterioration*

Afghanistan	Angola	Burundi	Central African Rep.
Congo Dom. Rep.	Eriteria	Ethiopia	Haiti
Kenya	Korea DPR	Liberia	Madagascar
Mongolia	Mozambique	Niger	Rwanda
Tanzania	Zambia		

B: *The Negative Spiral*

Bangladesh	Cuba
Nicaragua	Yemen
Zimbabwe	

UNICEF–2001

Since undernutrition manifests more openly in the low birth weight (LBW, less than 2500 g) and under-5 mortality of the infants, the UNICEF Report:

The State of the World's Children 2001

portrays a more dismal picture of some of the poorer countries (listed here in alphabetic order), as under:

	% of LBW Infants	Under-5 Mortality Rank
Afghanistan	20	4
Bangladesh	30	53
Burkina Faso	21	13
Guinea Bissau	20	12
India	33	49
Malawi	20	7
Myanmar	24	39
Pakistan	25	39
Papua New Guinea	23	39
Solomon Islands	20	112
Togo	20	28

THE SPECTRE OF UNDERNUTRITION

Region/ Country (1)	Total Population 1997 (Mn) (2)	U/N Population 1996-98 (Mn) (3)	U/N Pop. as % of Total Pop.	
			1979-81 (4)	1996-98 (5)
Developing World	4501	792	29	18
Africa	368	36	9	10
A: Sub-Saharan Africa	553	186	38	34
Congo Dom. Rep.	48	29	38	61
Cent. African Rep.	3.4	1.4	22	41
Chad	7	2.7	69	38
B: East Africa	190.4	80	35	42
Somalia	8.8	6.6	55	75
Burundi	6.4	4.3	39	68
Eriteria	3.4	2.2	NA	65
Ethiopia	58	28.4	NA	49
Kenya	28.4	12.2	26	43
Tanzania	31.4	12.7	23	41
C: Southern Africa	82	34.5	33	42
Mozambique	18.4	10.7	54	58
Zambia	8.6	3.9	30	45
Angola	11.7	5	31	43
Madagascar	14.6	5.8	18	40
D: West Africa	204	33	42	16
Liberia	2.4	1.1	22	46
Sierra Leone	4.4	1.9	40	43
Mali	10.4	3.4	60	32
E: North East Africa	232	30	10	13
Afghanistan	21	17	34	70
yemen	16	6	39	35
Iraq	21	3.5	4	17
Asia Region				
A: South Asia	1274	294	38	23
Bangladesh	123	47	42	38

Nepal	22.3	6.2	47	28
Sri Lanka	18.3	4.5	22	25
India	966	208	38	21
Pakistan	144	29	31	20
B: S-E Asia	491	65	26	13
Cambodia	10.5	3.4	61	33
Lao DPR	5	1.5	32	29
C: East Asia	1322	155	29	12
Korea DPR	23	13.2	19	57
Mongolia	2.5	1.1	16	45
Latin America	489	55	13	11
Haiti	7.8	4.8	48	62
Nicaragua	4.7	1.5	26	31
Dominican Rep	8.1	2.2	25	28
Gatemala	10.5	2.5	18	24
Ex-USSR	405	26	NA	6
Azerbaijan	7.6	2.4	NA	32
Tajikstan	5.9	1.9	NA	32
Georgia	5.1	1.2	NA	23
East Europe	121	3.6	NA	3
Bulgaria	8.4	1.1	NA	13
Croatia	4.5	0.5	NA	12
Bosnia and Herzegovina	3.5	0.4	NA	10

Source: Adapted from FAO's Food Insecurity in the World, 1998.

Looking into columns 4 and 5, one finds that in the following countries the situation has gone from bad to worst during the last two decades:

Afghanistan	Angola
Burundi	Central African Rep.
Congo	Haiti
Korea DPR	Madagascar
Zambia	

MALNUTRITION AMONG CHILDREN IN THE INDIAN STATES
(National Family Health Survey (NFHS) Estimates)

	State	Percentage of Malnutrition	
		1993 (Below 4 years)	1998-99 (Below 3 years)
1.	Andhra Pradesh	49.1	37.7
2.	Assam	50.4	36.0
3.	Bihar	62.6	54.4
4.	Gujarat	44.1	45.1
5.	Haryana	37.9	34.6
6.	Himachal Pradesh	47.0	43.6
7.	Jammu & Kashmir	44.5	34.6
8.	Karnataka	NA	43.9
9.	Kerala	28.5	26.0
10.	Madhya Pradesh	57.4	55.1
11.	Maharashtra	52.6	49.6
12.	Orissa	55.3	54.4
13.	Punjab	45.9	28.7
14.	Rajasthan	41.6	50.6
15.	Tamil Nadu	46.6	36.7
16.	Uttar Pradesh	49.8	51.7
17.	West Bengal	56.8	48.7
18.	Arunachal Pradesh	39.7	24.3
19.	Manipur	30.1	27.5
20.	Nagaland	28.7	24.1
21.	Tripura	48.8	NA
22.	Meghalaya	45.5	37.9
23.	Mizoram	28.1	27.7
	All India	**53.4**	**47.0**

Source: International Institute of Population Studies, (NFHS), 1993 and 1998-99.

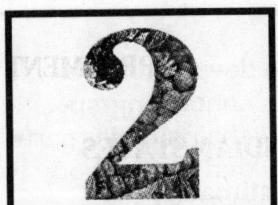

DIGESTION ABSORPTION AND ASSIMILATION (FOOD METABOLISM)

The elaborate phased out process that food undergoes from the time it is taken to its final excretion is known as metabolism of food. This metabolism comprises of two processes that take place in the body viz.,

(1) Anabolism: The process that builds up the body tissues.
(2) Catabolism: The process that breaks down the body substances.

The food consumed normally contains many complex nutrients. These must be broken down into simpler constituents to enable the food to be utilized for various body functions.

To illustrate these processes, proteins are made up of simpler constituents called amino acids that go to build up new body tissue i.e. Anabolism. In catabolism, the tissues break down during an attack of high fever, infections, burns, routine wear and tear as also during the process of energy liberation. All these metabolic process that go on for 24 hours a day require a constant supply of nutrients.

The process of transforming food into simpler substances which could then be taken up by the cells is the complex phenomenon of digestion, absorption and assimilation. It helps the nutrients released from food i.e. intermediate units to be broken down, simplified, re-grouped and re-routed. All this is helped by a well organised chemical environment of the digestive tract, which is further aided by the microflora present in the intestine.

The digestive system of both man and animal is an intricately developed system. It begins at the mouth, followed by esophagus (food pipe), stomach, small intestine and large intestine which ends up at the exit point–anus. Besides, there are other glands like salivary glands, liver, gall bladder and pancreas which secrete special juices or hormones that help in the chemical breakdown of the nutrients. Digestion is the process by which food is broken down chemically in the gastrointestinal tract through the action of secretions containing specific enzymes. Digestion breaks the complex food components into their simpler parts, which are the chemical substances that are ultimately needed by the body to sustain life.

The digestive system begins at the mouth and ends at the exit point, anus. The functions of various parts of the alimentary canal are described in brief, as under:

1. **Mouth:** Mastication or chewing the food and mixing it with saliva coming from the salivary glands.

2. **Oesophagus:** It is the entry point for food into the stomach.

3. **Stomach:** It stores and churns the food, allowing it to mix with the gastric secretions like hydrochloric acid, pepsin and renin, etc.

4. **Small Intestine:** Comprising of three parts, viz. Duodenum, Jejunum and Ileum, it digests the food with the help of pancreatic and bile secretions and then absorbs the finished products through the villi.

5. **Pancreas:** A gland located in the loop of the duodenum, it secretes digestive enzymes and also insulin, the hormone responsible for carbohydrate metabolism.

6. **Liver:** A very large and important gland in the body that secretes bile. Liver also acts as a store-house for sugars (as glycogen) and also the fat-soluble vitamins.

7. **Gall Bladder:** It is the gland that stores bile, secreted earlier by the liver.

8. **Large Intestine:** This is the last portion of GI tract wherein the absorption of water and some B vitamins takes place. And the resultant waste products are passed down into colon and then pass out as feces through the anus.

The whole process of digestion may be divided into three parts, viz.

A: Digestion in the mouth (+ oesophagus)
B: Digestion in the stomach
C: Digestion in the small intestine

All these three phases of digestion have two kinds of action in each part, viz., mechanical digestion and chemical digestion.

Digestion initially prepares the food for our body's use. Herein, two basic types of actions are involved.

(a) Mechanical or muscular activity
(b) Chemical or enzymatic activity.

Gastrointestinal Motility

Mechanical digestion of food is a self-regulated process effected through neuromuscular activity. These actions work in concert to push the food mass along the alimentary tract in a well-streamlined manner that enables optimum digestion and absorption of the nutrient in the body.

There are four types of muscle in the stomach and intestine that contribute to this gastrointestinal motility:

(i) **Contractile Rings:** A layer of circular contractile muscle rings break up, mix and then thoroughly churn the food.

(ii) **Longitudinal Muscles:** These long smooth muscles help propel the food mass along the digestive tract.

(iii) **Sphinctre Muscles:** These muscle rings located in strategic positions act as valves, pyloric, ileo-cecal and anal, to control passage of materials to the next segment of the intestine.

(iv) **Mucosal Muscles:** These are a thin layer of smooth muscles that raise the intestinal folds in order to increase a hundred-fold the absorbing surface area.

The continuous interaction of these four types of muscles yield two distinct movements:

(1) Tonic contractions or a general muscle tone that ensures continuous passage and also valve control.

(2) Peristalsis, periodic rhythmic contractions, control and mix the food ingredients and further propel the food mass.

An intricate network of nerves within the gastrointestinal walls, called as the intramural nerve plexus controls the muscle tone and regulates the rate and intensity of muscle contractions and coordinates various movements.

Gastrointestinal Secretions

The chemical digestion of food is aided by four types of secretions, viz.

(1) **Enzymes:** Select type and quantity that break down specific nutrients.

(2) **Hydrochloric Acid and Buffer Ions:** They regulate the pH for optimum activity of the given enzymes.

(3) **Mucus:** This agent lubricates and protects the inside wall tissue of the digestive tract that facilitates the passage of food mass.

(4) **Water and Electrolytes:** They help provide a balanced solution base in sufficient volume to circulate the released organic substances.

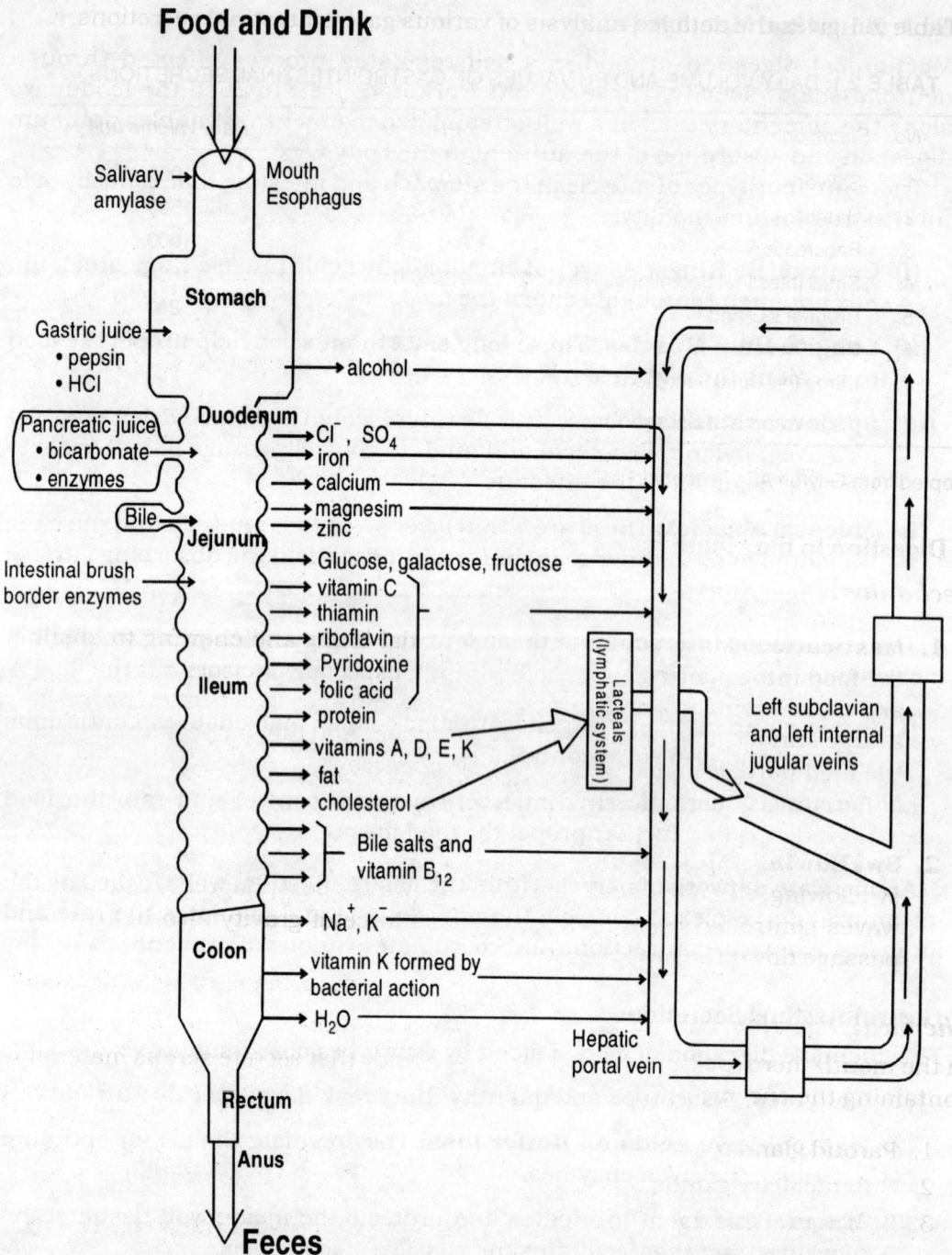

Fig. 2.1: Sites of Secretion and Absorption in the Gastrointestinal Tract

Table 2.1 gives the detailed analysis of various gastrointestinal secretions.

TABLE 2.1: DAILY VOLUME AND PH VALUES OF GASTROINTESTINAL SECRETIONS

No	Secretion	PH	Daily Volume (ml)
1.	Salivary	6.0 - 7.4	1000
2.	Gastric	1.0 - 3.5	1500
3.	Pancreatic	8.0 - 8.3	1000
4.	Small Intestinal Secretions	7.5 - 8.0	1800
5.	Brunner's Gland	8.0 - 8.9	200
6.	Bile	7.5 - 7.8	1000
7.	Large Intestinal Secretions	7.5 - 8.0	200
	Total Volume of Secretions		**6700**

Adopted from Guyton AC: *Textbook of Medical Physiology*, 1991, W. B. Saunders.

A: Digestion in the Mouth

Mechanical Digestion

1. **Mastication:** Mastication means the initial biting and chewing to break the food into smaller particles. The teeth, especially incisors cut the food and molars grind it. This is aided by the jaw muscles. Mastication provides a large surface area of food for enzyme action. And the finer consistency of the food particles facilitates continuous passage of material through the alimentary canal.

2. **Swallowing:** Muscles at the base of the tongue aid the process of swallowing, when the food mass slides down the oesophagus by peristaltic waves controlled by nerve reflexes. The force of gravity also helps this passage down the oesophagus.

Chemical Digestion

In the mouth there are three pairs of salivary glands that secrete serous material containing the enzyme ptyalin. These salivary glands are:

1. Parotid glands
2. Submaxillary glands
3. Sublingual glands

The enzyme ptyalin acts specifically on starches. Mucus is also secreted which lubricates and binds the food particles. The passage of food through mouth is very brief, equally so is the action of ptyalin.

B: Digestion in the Stomach

Mechanical Digestion

Stomach is the multi-function store-house. The muscles of the stomach wall provide three basic motor functions viz.

(1) Storage of food
(2) Mixing of the food mass
(3) Controlled emptying

The stomach wall can stretch them to store as much as one litre of food mass. As the food moves towards the pyloric valve at the distant end of the stomach, the local tonic muscle waves increase the kneading and mixing action. The peristaltic contractions reduce the food mass to semi-fluid chyme. The sphincter muscle constricts and periodically relaxes, then constricts again to control the emptying of the stomach content into the duodenum (small intestine). This control releases the acid chyme slowly enough to be buffered by the alkaline intestinal sections.

Chemical Digestion

There are three stomach secretions viz. acid, mucus and enzyme which aid digestion.

(1) Hydrochloric acid produced in the stomach prepares certain enzymes and materials for digestion and absorption by creating the necessary degree of acidity for enzymes to work upon.

(2) Special mucus secretions protect the stomach lining from the eroding effect of the acid. The mucus also binds and mixes the food mass and then enables it to move along.

(3) The main enzyme in the stomach is pepsin which begins the breakdown of proteins. Incidentally, the inactive form, pepsinogen which is secreted first is activated by hydrochloric acid. A small amount of gastric lipase (Tributyrinase) present there works on the emulsified fats. In children, an enzyme rennin present in the gastric secretions aids in the coagulation of milk. These gastric secretions are activated by two stimuli viz. nerve stimulus and hormonal stimulus. When the pH reaches 2.0, a feedback mechanism stops further secretions of the hormone to prevent excess acid formation. Another hormone: Enterogastrone, produced by glands in the duodenal mucosa, counteracts excessive gastric activity by inhibiting acid and pepsin secretions and gastric motility.

C: Digestion in the Small Intestine

Mechanical Digestion

There are three layers of muscles that aid the digestion process in the small intestine. These muscles are

(1) Mucosa or muscularis mucosa: The thin layers of smooth muscles, with fibres extending up into the villi.

(2) Circular muscle layer.

(3) Longitudinal muscle next to the outer serosa.

These muscles produce five different types of movements to aid digestion. These muscular movements are

(1) **Segmentation Contractions** of circular muscle rings chop the food into boluses, mixing food and secretions.

(2) **Longitudinal Rotation** which rolls the slowly moving food mass in a spiral motion, thus exposing greater surface for absorption.

(3) **Pendular Movements** that sweep back and forth and stir the chyme.

(4) **Peristalsis** produces wave-motions that propel the food mass slowly forward.

(5) **Villi Motions** consistently sweep the mucosal surface with alternating contaction and extension of the muscle fibres, thus helping expose additional nutrient material for absorption.

Chemical Digestion

Of all the alimentary tract, it is the small intestine that carries the major share of process of digestion. It secretes a large number of enzymes, each with a select action, say for fats, carbohydrates or proteins.

Four basic secretions herein that help complete the chemical breakdown in small, intestine are:

(1) **Enzymes** like Amylase, Lactase, Sucrase, Maltase and Lipase act on specific nutrient material, and break it down into easily assimilable forms.

(2) **Mucus:** Glands in the duodenum secrete large quantities of mucus, which protects the mucosa from highly acid gastric juices at this point. These secretions lubricate and protect the tissues.

(3) **Hormone Secretions**, produced by the apex part of small intestine, stimulates pancreas to send alkaline pancreatic juices into the duodenum. These act as buffer to the entering gastric acid chyme. Table 2.2 gives the overview of these hormones.

TABLE 2.2: IMPORTANT FUNCTIONS OF GASTROINTESTINAL HORMONES

Hormone	Site of Release	Stimulants of Release	Organ Affected	Effect on Organ
Gastrin	Antral mucosa of stomach	Polypeptides Amino acids	Esophagus	Increases resting pressure of lower esophageal sphincter
	Duodenum Jejunum	Caffeine Alcohol	Stomach	Stimulates secretion of HCl and Pepsinogen by parietal and chief cells, respectively
		Food extracts		Increases gastric antral motility
		Distention of stomach antrum	Gallbladder	Weakly stimulates contraction of gallbladder
		Vagal nerve	Pancreas	Weakly stimulates pancreatic secretion of bicarbonate
Secretin	Duodenal mucosa	Gut acidity (pH < 4-5)	Esophagus	Reduces resting pressure of lower esophageal sphincter
			Stomach	Reduces gastric and duodenal motility Stimulates pepsinogen secretion Inhibits gastrin-stimulated gastric acid secretion
			Duodenum	Decreases motility Increases mucous output of Brunner's glands
			Pancreas	Increases output of H_2O and bicarbonate Increases some enzyme secretion from the pancreas as well as insulin release
			Liver	Increases volume and electrolyte output of bile
Cholecystokinin Pancreozymin (CCK-PZ)	Proximal small bowel	Amino acids (esp. tryptophan)	Small bowel	Increases motility
			Gallbladder	Causes contraction of gallblad.
		HCl	Pancreas	Stimulates enzyme secretion of pancreas
		Fatty acids (< 9c)		Potentiates effect of secretin on pancreas
		Food		Slows gastric emptying May mediate feeding behaviour
Gastric inhibitory polypeptide (GIP)	Small intestine	Glucose	Stomach	Inhibits gastrin-stimulated gastric acid secretion
		Fat	Pancreas	Stimulates insulin secretion
Enteroglucagon and Glucagon	Duodenum Jejunum	Carbohydrate Long-chain triglycerides	Liver	Stimulates glycogenolysis
			Pancreas	Inhibits pancreatic enzyme secretion
			Small intestine	Inhibits motility

Motilin	Duodenum Jejunum	Alkalinity in the Duodenum	Stomach	Decrease gastric emptying Regulates gut motility
Somatostatin	Antrum of stomach Upper small intestine	Gastric and Duodenal acidity	Pancreas	Inhibits release of insulin and glucagon Decreases pancreatic enzyme production
	Hypothalamus primarily	Amino acids Fat (?)	Stomach	Inhibits gastrin release
			Gallbladder	Inhibits contraction
			Others	Suppress secretion of growth hormone
				Suppress secretion of thyroid-stimulating hormone

(4) **Bile:** This emulsifying agent for fats is produced in the liver, which is then concentrated and stored in the gall bladder. The hormone, 'Cholecystokinin', secreted by the glands in the intestinal muscle, stimulates the gall bladder to contract and release the bile needed for fat digestion. Besides, there are other factors like control by hormones and nerve plexus, stimulated by physical contact with food material, which influences the digestion process in the small intestine.

D: Digestion in Large Intestine

The large intestine is involved in two primary operations. First, it absorbs water and electrolyte from the digested food material entering the proximal half of the intestine. Second, it stores fecal matter till defecation, which occurs in the distal half of large intestine.

Large intestine can absorb 5-7 litres of fluid and electrolyte in a day. The large intestine is inhabited by more than 400 different species of bacteria. Some of these bacteria produce nutrients that can be absorbed. The latter include vitamin K, biotin and short chain fatty acids (SCFA).

The composition of feces, the end product of the digestion and absorption process, is as under:

Bacteria	Approx. 30%
Fat	10-20%
Inorganic matter	10-20%
Proteins	2-3%
Undigested fibre	30%

The coloring of the feces is primarily attributed to stercobilin and urobilin, which are the metabolites of bilirubin. The odor in the feces is due to bacterial byproducts like indoles, skatole, mercaptans and hydrogen sulphide.

Table 2.3 summarizes the overall digestion of the nutrients in the human body.

TABLE 2.3: DIGESTION OF CARBOHYDRATES, FATS AND PROTEINS

	Enzyme	*Substrate*	*Products*
Mouth	Salivary amylase	Starch	→ Dextrins and Maltose
Salivary glands	(Ptyalin)		
Stomach	Gastric protease		
Gastric Mucosa	Pepsin	Proteins	→ Polypeptides
	Renin	Casein	→ Insoluble Casein
	Gastric Lipase	Short- and medium-chain Triglycerides	→ Fatty acids and Glycerol
Small Intestine			
Pancreas	Pancreatic Proteases		
	Trypsin	Proteins and	→ Smaller Polypeptides and Amino
	Chymotrypsin	Polypeptides	acids
	Carboxypeptidases		
	Pancreatic Lipase (Steapsin)	Fats	→ Mono- and Di-glycerides Fatty acids and Glycerol
	Pancreatic Amylase (Amylopsin)	Amylose and Amylopectin	→ Maltose, Maltotriose and α-limit Dextrins
Intestinal Mucosa	Intestinal Peptidases	Polypeptides	→ Smaller Polypeptides and Amino
Brushborder	Aminopeptidases	Dipeptides	acids
	Dipeptidases		
	Intestinal Saccharidases		
	α-Dextrinase (Isomaltase)	α-limit dextrins	→ Glucose
		Sucrose	→ Glucose and Fructose
	Sucrase	Maltose	→ Glucose (2 molecules)
	Maltase	Lactose	→ Glucose and Galactose
	Lactase		

See also the Appendix 1 at the end of the Chapter.

Absorption

Absorption is the process by which food material passes through epithelial cells of the alimentary track into the blood or lymph. The end-products of digestion can be subdivided into three groups:

(a) Monosachharides: glucose, fructose and galactose from carbohydrates,
(b) Fatty acids and glycerides from fats,
(c) Amino acids from proteins.

Small peptides may be absorbed intact and finally broken down to amino acids within the muscle cells. Vitamins and minerals are also liberated. Finally, with a water base for solution and transport, plus necessary electrolytes, the total fluid mass is now got ready for absorption.

(A) *Absorption in the Small Intestine*

Three structures in small intestine help enlarge the surface area for absorption. These are:

(1) Mucosal folds, just like the hills and valleys in a mountain range.

(2) Villi or finger like projections on these folds, seen only under a microscope.

(3) Microvilli or extremely small projections on the villi. These can be seen only with an electronic microscope. These are called 'Brush Border'.

Each villus has a large network of blood capillaries and a central lymph vessel called a 'Lacteal'. These 3 surface structure increase the inner absorbing surface area 600 times over that of the outside serosa. Small intestine or gut is thus the most highly developed, specially designed tissues in the human body that accomplish the final task of absorption of the nutrients. The transport mechanisms involved in absorption are passive diffusion and osmosis, active carrier-mediated diffusion, energy-driven active transport and pinocytosis.

After absorption, the end products of proteins and carbohydrates enter the blood stream directly and are transported to liver and other tissues. Fats are carried by bile and are converted to a complex with protein as a carrier, packaged as lipo-proteins, which flow into the lymph. The initial lipo-proteins, called 'Chylomicrons' are rapidly cleared from the blood by a special fat enzyme 'Lipoprotein lipase.' The lymphatic system provides an essential accessory route by which body fluids from interstitial spaces pass into the blood. As such, lymph has the same composition as the tissue fluid from which it comes.

(B) *Absorption in the Large Intestine (Colon)*

Large intestine is mainly responsible for the absorption of waste. Within a 24-hour period, about 500 ml of the remaining food mass leaves ileum—the portion of small intestine and enters cecum—the pouch at the start of the large intestine. With each peristaltic wave, the ileo-cecal valve squirts a small amount of chyme into cecum. This intricate mechanism permits adequately long stay for the food mass in the small intestine to ensure digestion and absorption of all the vital nutrients.

The watery chyme continues to move slowly through the large intestine, this process being aided by mucous secretions as also muscular contractions. Majority of the water in the chyme (350-400 ml) is absorbed in the first half of the colon. Barely 100-150 ml water remains to form the feces.

Usually a meal, having travelled 21-22 ft of small intestine, starts to enter cecum about 4 hours after it has been eaten. It takes another 8 hours to reach the sigmoid colon from where it descends very slowly towards the anus. Even 72 hours after a meal almost 25% of it may still be retained in the rectum.

(C) *Mineral and Vitamin Absorption*

Intestinal absorption is a major balance control point for most of the minerals. Electrolytes, mainly sodium, are transported into the blood stream from the colon. But most of the dietary intake of minerals remains unabsorbed for elimination through feaces. Thus, 50-70% of calcium and about 80% of the ingested iron is excreted out in the feces.

Many colon bacteria synthesize vitamin K and some vitamins of the B-complex group, which are then absorbed from colon to help meet the body's daily requirements.

Table 2.4 gives an overview of the absorption of nutrients from the gastro-intestinal tract.

TABLE 2.4: SITES OF ABSORPTION OF NUTRIENTS FROM GASTROINTESTINAL TRACT

No.	Nutrients	Site in Small Intestine
1.	Glucose	Lower Duodenum Upper Jejunum
2.	Amino Acids	Lower Duodenum Jejunum
3.	Fats	Lower Duodenum Upper Jejunum
4.	Iron	Duodenum
5.	Calcium	Duodenum
6.	Sucrose	Lower Duodenum Ileum
7.	Lactose	Jejunum Upper Ileum
8.	Maltose	Jejunum Upper Ileum
9.	Vitamin D	Jejunum Ileum
10.	Vitamin B_{12}	Ileum

See also the summary of absorption in Appendix 2 at the end of the Chapter.

Other Bacterial Action

Intestinal bacteria effect the color and odor of the feces. Brown color represents bile pigments formed by the colon bacteria from bilurobin. Clay or white color indicates that bile flow is hindered. The odor results from amines-indole and skatole. Flatus or intestinal gas produced by bacterial action is hydrogen sulphide or methane.

As humans have no microorganisms or enzymes that can break fibre, this remains as residue after absorption, although pectin is degraded in the large intestine. The undigested fibre gives the bulk to the diet and forms stools. The feces normally contain 75% water and 25% solids.

Table 2.5 summarizes the absorption of various nutrients in the body.

TABLE 2.5: DAILY ABSORPTION IN GASTROINTESTINAL TRACT

Intake	Intake (L)	Intestinal Absorption (L)	Elimination (L)
Food Ingested	1.5	--	--
Gastrointestinal secretion	8.5	--	--
Total Food Mass	10.0	--	--
Fluid Absorbed in Small Intestine	--	9.5	--
Fluid Absorbed in Large Intestine	--	0.4	--
Total Absorbed	--	9.9	
Feces	--	--	0.1

METABOLISM

Cell metabolism is a very crucial function that handles all the absorbed nutrients. Metabolism is, in reality, the sum total of all the physical and chemical changes that take place within an organism, by which it maintains itself and also produces energy needed for all other body functions. Technically speaking, it is a dual-phased process:

(1) Anabolism or constructive metabolism, which is concerned with the building up of materials and tissue.

(2) Catabolism or destructive metabolism, which accounts for the breaking down of the materials and tissues.

In the GI tract, there are three specific metabolic process going on:

(A) Carbohydrate metabolism
(B) Fat (Lipids) metabolism
(C) Protein metabolism

A: Carbohydrate Metabolism

Blood Glucose

The end product of carbohydrate metabolism is the sugars, more so the blood sugars. The sources of blood glucose could be either carbohydrates or non-carbohyhdrates:

A: Cabohydrates Sources:

(i) Dietary starches and sugars
(ii) Glycogen stored in liver and muscles (glycogenolysis or glycolysis is the hydrolysis of glycon to glucose)

(*iii*) Lactic acid and Pyruvic acid, the products of intermediary carbohydrate metabolism.

B: Non-Carbohydrate Sources:

Proteins and fat provide the additional sources of glucose. Glycerol from the breakdown of fats, is converted to glycogen in the liver, which is then made available for glucose formation. The production of glucose from the non-carbohydrate sources is called gluconeogenesis.

Uses of Blood Glucose: Blood sugar within a range of 70-120 ml/dl offers three main uses:

(*i*) Energy production to meet the constant demand of body.

(*ii*) Energy storage as glycogen in liver muscles and fat in adipose tissue.

(*iii*) Glucose products like galactose, select amino acids, besides DNA and RNA

Hormonal Control: Some hormones influences the glucose metabolism and so help regulate the blood sugar levels in the body.

1. **Sugar-lowering Hormones:** Insulin, produced by the β cells in pancreas, acts to lower blood glucose level. This is done through:

(a) Glycogensis or conversion of glucose to glycogen in liver to provide for energy reserve.

(b) Lipogenesis or conversion of glucose to fat for storage in adipose tissue.

(c) Cells permeability to glucose is increased, thus allowing it to pass into the cells and supply energy by oxidation.

2. **Sugar-raising Hormones:**

(a) Glucagon acts opposite to insulin and increases breakdown of liver glycogen to glucose.

(b) Somatostatin suppresses insulin and glucagon.

(c) Steroid hormones release glucose-forming carbon units from proteins and act as insulin antagonists.

(d) Epinephrine stimulates breakdown of liver glycogen and instant release of glucose.

(e) Growth hormone and Adreno-corticotropic hormone (ACTH) act as insulin antagonists.

(e) Thyroxine influences the breakdown rate of insulin.

B: Lipid (Fat) Metabolism

Fat Synthesis and Breakdown

Liver and adipose tissue help in fat synthesis and breakdown. Fatty acids released from fat are used by body cells as a concentrated fuel for producing energy.

Lipoproteins

The lipid-protein complexes transport fat in the blood circulation. Excess of these in the blood give rise to a condition known as Hyperlipoproteinemia.

Hormonal Control

As fat and carbohydrate metabolism are very closely inter-related, hence the same hormones as of carbohydrate metabolism also help in fat metabolism.

C: Protein Metabolism

Metabolism of proteins involves two stages:

(1) **Anabolism or Tissue Building:** Protein tissues are built through the synthesis of new proteins, guided by DNA in the cell nucleus. It is also helped by the Growth hormones, gonadotrophins and thyroxin.

(2) **Catabolism or Tissue Breakdown:** Amino acids released in this process are further broken down and utilized for other purposes. These could be nitrogen-containing group, wherein through the process of de-amination, nitrogen is converted to ammonia. Else, the non-nitrogen residues *i.e.* keto acids which are used to form carbohydrates or fats. These are also re-aminated to form a new amino acid.

There are certain cell enzymes and co-enzymes that influence tissue catabolism. In a healthy human being, there is a dynamic equilibrium between these two processes of anabolism and catabolism.

ASSIMILATION

The term 'Assimilation' is coterminous with anabolism. In this process, all the digested foodstuffs are eventually absorbed and utilized by the body tissues.

Table 2.6 shows the assimilation of various nutrients in the human body.

TABLE 2.6: ASSIMILATION OF NUTRIENTS

Nutrients	Digestion	Assimilation
Proteins	As amino acids in the small intestine	If not needed, proteins are de-aminized Nitrogen removed, these are changed into urea and excreted. Converted to glucogenic and ketogenic amino acids, they enter Kreb's cycle to ultimately release energy and form CO_2 and H_2O
Fats	As fatty acids and gly-cerol in small intestine	Oxidized for energy to CO_2 and H_2O; else stored as fatty acids. Some combine with phosphorus to form phospholipids
Carbohy-drates	Absorbed as glucose or monosachharides	These are oxidized for energy to CO_2 and H_2O. Also changed to glycogen and then stored in the liver Also changed to fat and then stored as the fatty tissue

METABOLIC INTER-RELATIONSHIP

Each of the chemical process of body metabolism is charged with a specific task and all the processes of metabolism are interdependent. The whole mechanism subserves two essential needs of the human body:

(a) To produce energy
(b) To grow and maintain healthy tissues.

And all these intricately balanced processes are controlled by a series of cell enzymes, their co-enzymes and special hormones.

In the overall analysis, human metabolism is indeed a very exciting and well-orchestrated Bio-chemical process that sustains and protects life.

APPENDIX 1

Summary of Digestive Processes

Nutrient	Mouth	Stomach	Small Intestine
Carbohydrate	Starch $\xrightarrow{\alpha\text{-amylase}}$ Dextrins		**Pancreas**
			(Disaccharides)
			Starch $\xrightarrow{\text{Amylase}}$ Maltose and sucrose
			Intestine
			(Monosaccharides)
			Lactose $\xrightarrow{\text{Lactase}}$ Glucose and galactose
			Sucrose $\xrightarrow{\text{Sucrase}}$ Glucose and fructose
			Maltose $\xrightarrow{\text{Maltase}}$ Glucose and glucose
Protein		Protein $\xrightarrow{\text{Pepsin HCl}}$ Polypeptides	**Pancreas**
			Protein, Polypeptides $\xrightarrow{\text{Trypsin}}$ Dipeptides
			Protein, Polypeptides $\xrightarrow{\text{Chymotrypsin}}$ Dipeptides
			Polypeptides, Dipeptides $\xrightarrow{\text{Carboxypeptidase}}$ Amino acids
			Intestine
			Polypeptides, Dipeptides $\xrightarrow{\text{Aminopeptidase}}$ Amino acids
			Dipeptides $\xrightarrow{\text{Dipeptidase}}$ Amino acids
Fat		Tributyrin (butterfat) $\xrightarrow{\text{Tributyrinase}}$ Glycerol Fatty acids	**Pancreas**
			Fats $\xrightarrow{\text{Lipase}}$ Glycerol Glycerides (di, mono-) Fatty acids
			Intestine
			Fats $\xrightarrow{\text{Lipase}}$ Glycerol Glycerides (di, mono-) Fatty acids
			Liver and Gallbladder
			Fats $\xrightarrow{\text{Lipase}}$ Emulsified fat

Intestinal Absorption of Some Major Nutrients

Nutrients	Form	Means of Absorption	Control Agent or Required Cofactor	Route
Carbohydrate	Monosaccharides (Glucose and Galactose)	Competitive Selective Active transport via Sodium pump	— — Sodium —	Blood
Protein	Amino acids Some dipeptides	Selective Carrier transport systems	— Pyridoxine (Pyridoxal phosphate)	Blood Blood
	Whole protein (rare)	Pinocytosis	—	Blood
Fat	Fatty acids	Fatty acid-bile complex (Micelles)	Bile	Lymph
	Glycerides (mono, di-) Few Triglycerides (Neutral Fat)	Pinocytosis	— —	Lymph Lymph
Vitamins	B_{12} A K	Carrier transport Bile complex Bile complex	Intrinsic factor (IF) Bile Bile	Blood Blood From large intestine to Blood
Minerals	Sodium	Active transport via Sodium pump	—	Blood
	Calcium Iron	Active transport Active transport	Vitamin D Ferritin mechanism	Blood Blood (as Transferritin)
Water	Water	Osmosis	—	Blood, lymph, Interstitial Fluid

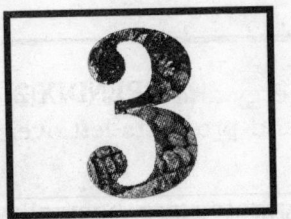

3

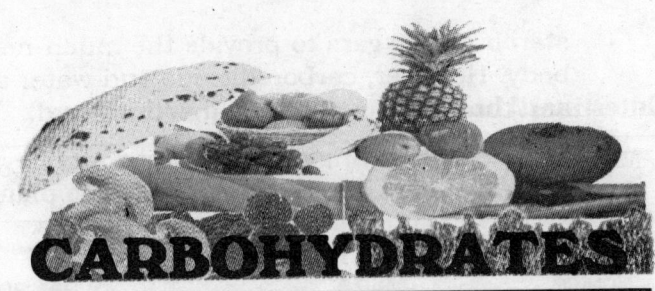

CARBOHYDRATES

Amongst the three principal macro-nutrients, viz., proteins, fats and carbohydrates, carbohydrates are the most popular, as they are most crucial ingredient of the human diet. They form the primary source of energy for the vast majority in the developing countries, apart from the fact that they are also an equally important element in the diet of the rich and the affluent. While in the Western countries, these account for 45-50% of the total calories in the diet, in Asia and Africa, their share goes up to 80% or more of the total calorie intake.

Carbohydrates are the most important food item for three reasons:

1. **Easy Availability:** Carbohydrates are very widely distributed and the most universally cultivated crop source all over the world. Be it the common cereals, fruits, vegetables or tubers, all these are superabundantly rich in carbohydrates. Both genetically and geographically, *i.e.* species-wise, as also space-wise, carbo-hydrates are ubiquitous in nature - to be found everywhere. In large parts of Africa and to a considerable extent in Asia too, they are indeed the principal diet of the people. In terms of biochemistry and also from the genetical viewpoint, carbohydrates or sugars and the chains of sugar units that go to make their end-products, are the most universal component of all the living matter.

2. **Low Costing:** Compared to proteins and fats, carbohydrates are the cheapest source of energy, owing to their prevalence world-wide. In the overall total food budget, their share is the smallest. From the marketing angle, their processing and storage entails not much liability. Further, they have a very long shelf life.

3. **Body Fuel:** Carbohydrates provide a quick and sustained body fuel. The human energy system, so well organized and streamlined, readily oxidizes

starch and sugars to provide the much-needed energy and heat for the body. However, carbon dioxide and water are the end-products left over and these do not pose any health hazard.

From operational angle in human dietetics, carbohydrates are basically starches and sugars supplied mainly by the plant foods. Fig. 3.1 presents the overview of the principal dietary carbohydrates.

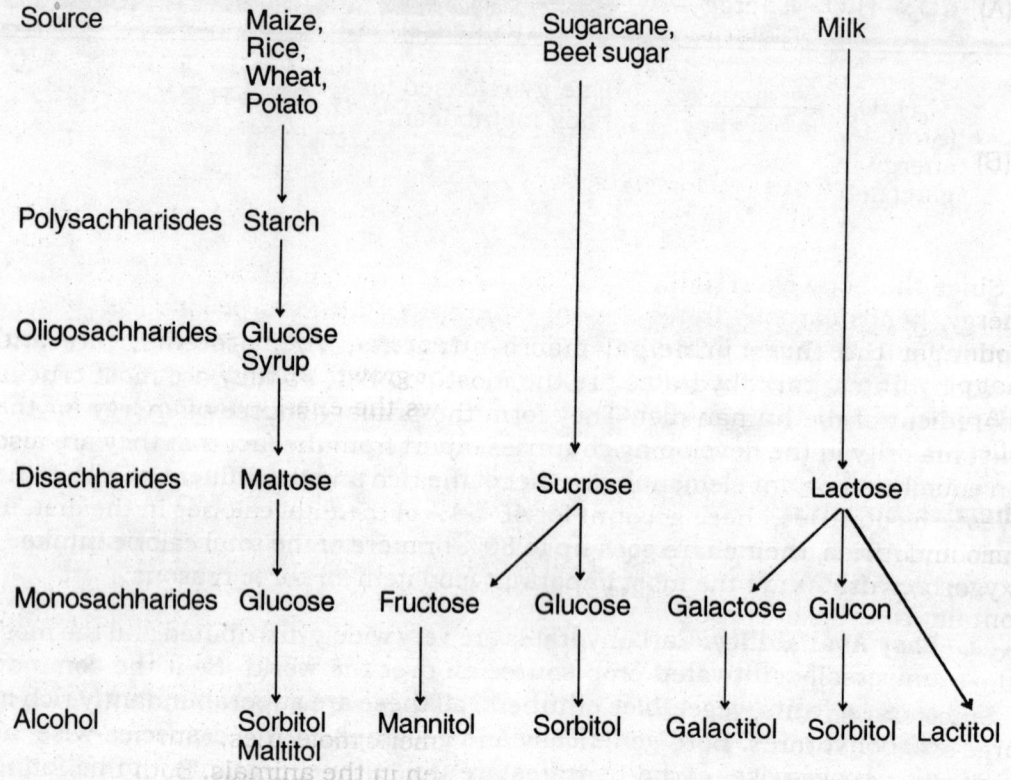

Fig. 3.1: Summary of Principal Dietary Carbohydrates

(Adapted from Ian Macdonald in '*Modern Nutrition in Health and Disease*', Vol. 1)

QUICK ENERGY SOURCE

Energy sustains life! For any system of energy to be functionally successful, there are four stipulations:

1. There must be a basic fuel that is readily available,
2. Mechanism to convert this basic fuel to a refined fuel that could be utilized directly by the system,
3. Means to transport this refined fuel to the site where energy is to be produced,
4. Mechanism to burn the fuel at the site in order to produce the required energy.

Carbohydrates are the ideal basic fuel that could fulfill all these conditions in the human system. The basic form of carbohydrates are starches and sugars found naturally in the foods. It is the solar energy which synthesizes these carbohydrates in the plants with the help of water from the soil, carbon dioxide from the air and green chlorophyll present in the plants, as shown in the figure below:

(A) $CO_2 + H_2O + Energy \xrightarrow{Chlorophyll} C_6H_{12}O_6$
               (Solar)   (Glucose)

(B) $C_6H_{12}O_6 \xrightarrow[\text{Human system}]{\text{Oxidation in the}}$ Energy released for body metabolism $+ CO_2 + H_2O$
      (Stored energy in glucose)

Fig. 3.2: Energy Cycle on Earth

Since the body can readily break up all these starches and sugars to yield energy, hence carbohydrates are also called 'Quick Energy Foods'. Of all the foodstuffs to be found in any milieu, carbohydrates are the one single source that provide the largest proportion of energy for growth and development.

Appendix 1 at the end of the Chapter shows the energy made available by different foodstuffs.

Chemical Structure

Carbohydrate is a chemical compound that is made up of carbon, hydrogen and oxygen atoms. The fundamental unit of carbohydrate is a monosachharide. It contains a series of carbon atoms linked together in a chain and attached with oxygen and hydrogen atoms. Its formula is $C_6H_{12}O_6$. Of all the monosachharides, Glucose is the most common sugar which is used to store and release energy.

Since carbohydrates in the form of glucose cannot be stored in nature on a large scale, they form chain-like complex polymeric molecules, with the removal of water, just like starch in plants and glycogen in the animals. Both these can be broken into simple form, glucose in the presence of water. Glycogen is stored in the liver and muscles, from where it is demobilized the moment glucose level in the blood dips below normal.

CLASSIFICATION OF CARBOHYDRATES

Carbohydrates are usually classified into three sub-groups, depending upon the number of basic sugars or sachharide units that go to make their structure. These are monosachharides, disachharides and polysachharides. The classification of carbohydrates is presented in Table 3.1.

Monosachharides

Monosachharides are the simple sugars composed of one sachharide (sugar) unit. Technically, these are 3, 4, 5 and 6 carbon sugar units, called trioses, tetroses, pentoses and hexoses respectively. The three main monosachharides are glucose, fructose and galactose.

TABLE 3.1: CLASSIFICATION OF CARBOHYDRATES

Carbohydrates	Examples	Source
1. Monosachharides (Simple Sugars which contain a single unit)	(a) Glucose (Dextrose) (b) Fructose (Levulose) (c) Galactose	Corn Syrup, Fruits, Vegetables, Honey Honey, Fruits, Vegetables The digestion of Lactose
2. Disachharides (Double Sugars which contain two monosach- haride units)	(a) Sucrose (1 gluocse +1 fructose) (b) Lactose (1 galactose + 1 glucose) (c) Maltose (2 glucose)	Cane, Beet, Fruits, Vegetables Milk Starch in sprouting grains and the digestion of starch
3. Polysachharides (complex compounds which contain many monosachharide units)	(A) Digestible (a) Starch (many units of glucose) (b) Dextrins (c) Glycogen (animal starch) (B) Indigestible (a) Cellulose (b) Hemicellulose 1. Pectin 2. Agar-agar commonly used in food as China grass	 Grain products, Legumes and Root Vegetables Results from first chemical change in digestion of starch Animal body converts glucose into glycogen, which can readily be converted back to glucose Structural parts of Fruits, Vegetables, Whole Grains Cereals, Seeds and Nuts Fruits like Guava, Apples Gelatinous product obtained from Sea-weeds

1. Glucose

A moderately sweet sugar, glucose is found naturally 'preformed' in only a few foods. In the human system, it is mainly generated by the digestion of starch. All other starches are metabolized and eventually converted into glucose. It is in the form of dextrose that sugar circulates in the bloodstream. It is glucose which is the ultimate common refined body fuel that is oxidized in the cells and provides the much-needed energy.

The normal blood sugar level ranges from 70-100 mg/dL. When this sugar level goes down, the condition is called 'Hypoglycemia'. But when the blood sugar rises beyond the normal level, it is called 'Hyperglycemia'.

2. Fructose (Fruit Sugar or Levulose)

Fructose is the sweetest of all the sugars. It is found in most of the fruits and honey. In the process of metabolism, fructose is converted into glucose to be utilized as a source of energy. Being very sweet, only small amounts of fructose are needed for preparing the foods.

3. Galactose

Galactose is a sugar that is normally not found in the human body, but is produced in the process of digestion from lactose (milk sugars), which is then converted into glucose for energy. This reaction being positively reversible, it helps to reconvert glucose into galactose for use in milk production. However, in the disease condition of 'Galactosemia', the enzyme for this change to glucose is missing and the galactose accumulates in the system. Table 3.2 depicts the physiologic significance of select monosachharides.

Besides these three, there are a few additional monosachharide compounds which do play an important role in clinical care. These monosachharides are glycosides, doxy sugars and amino sugars.

TABLE 3.2: PHYSIOLOGIC AND NUTRITIONAL SIGNIFICANCE OF MONOSACHHARIDES

Monosachharides	Source	Significance
Pentose		
D-Ribose	Formed through metabolic processes	Component element of nucleic acids and coenzyme, RNA; ATP; NAD, NADP (DPN and TPN) and flavoproteines
Hexose		
D-Glucose	Fruit Juices, Hydrolysis of starch, Cane Sugar, Maltose and Lactose	Body sugar, Blood and Tissue Fluids, Cell fuel
D-Fractose	Fruit Juices, Honey, Hydrolysis of sucrose from cane sugar	Changed to glucose in the liver and intestine to serve as basic body fuel
D-Glactase	Hydrolysis of lactose (Milk sugar)	Change to Glucose in liver; cell fuel, synthesized in mammary glands to make lactose of milk; constituent of glycolipids and glycoproteins.
D-Mannose	Hydrolysis of Plants Mannosans and Gums	Component of Polysachharides of albumins, Globulins, Mucoproteins and Glycoproteins

Disachharides

When two molecules of monosachharides combine with the removal of one molecule of water, Disachharides are formed, as shown in the following reaction:

$$\underset{\text{(Glucose)}}{C_6H_{12}O_6} + \underset{\text{(Fructose)}}{C_6H_{12}O_6} \xrightarrow[\text{Enzyme}]{\text{Energy}} \underset{\text{(Sucrose)}}{C_{12}H_{22}O_{11}} + H_2O$$

Three major disachharides of physiologic significance are sucrose, lactose and maltose. Their respective monosachharide components are shown hereunder:

Sucrose = Glucose + Fructose
Lactose = Glucose + Galactose
Maltose = Glucose + Glucose

1. *Sucrose*

Sucrose is the common table sugar. It is the most widely prevalent disachharide found in fruits and vegetables, sugarcane and sugarbeet. Sucrose contributes over 30% of the total energy budget (kcal) in an average adult's diet.

2. *Lactose*

Lactose is a sugar found in milk. It is the least sweet of all the disachharides - being one-sixth as sweet as sucrose. In the body, it is formed from glucose to supply the much-needed sugar during lactation period. Lactose increases absorption of calcium from the intestinal tract and provides a medium for the growth of favourable microflora in the intestines.

3. *Maltose*

Maltose is a sugar that is found in commercial malt products obtained from the hydrolysis of starch. It is also found in germinating cereal grains. Though present in very small amounts, it is a highly significant metabolic carbohydrate as an intermediate product of starch digestion. Table 3.3 sums up the physiologic importance of the Disaccharides.

TABLE 3.3: PYSIOLOGIC SIGNIFICANCE OF DISACHHARIDES

Disachharides	Source	Significance
Maltose	Starch digestion by Amylase, commercial hydrolysis, malt and germinating cereals	Hydrolyzed to D-glucose, basic body fuel and metabolite, fermentable
Sucrose	Cane and beetsugar, sorghum cane, carrots and pineapple	Hydrolized to Glucose and fructose, body fuel
Lactose	Milk	Hydrolized to Glucose and Galactose, body fuel, constituent for milk production during lactation

Polysachharides

Polysachharides are complex compounds with heavy molecular weight. They are made up of many single sugar (sachharide) units. Their structural formula is $(C_6H_{10}O_5)_n$, where n is more than two. The polysachharides are the least sweet of all the sugars, while disachharides are moderately sweet and monosachharides are the sweetest of all.

The most important polysachharide in nutrition is starch; others in this group are glycogen and dextrins. Besides, there are non-digestible polysachharides, which provide the much-needed bulk to the diet.

1. *Starch*

In the human nutrition, starch is the most important polysachharide. It is a relatively large complex compound made up of many branching chains of simple sugar (glucose) units, which yield glucose on digestion. The cooking of starch not only improves its flavour, but also softens and ruptures the starch cells, which makes digestion easier.

Starch is the storage form of carbohydrates in plants and constitutes the primary source of energy in diet. Cereal grains, roots and tubers like potatoes contain large amount of starch. While in the West, starches form 50 -60% of the total diet energy, in the developing countries, this share goes up to 80% or more. Rather, starch becomes the staple diet of the poorer sections of society.

2. *Glycogen*

Glycogen is the starch stored in the animal body—liver and muscles, as compared to the starch stored in plants. Fresh Oysters is another rich source of glycogen. These stored polysachharides help sustain the normal blood glucose levels during fasting periods and provide immediate fuel for the body needs. However, dietary carbohydrates are essential to maintain these needed glycogen stores and prevent the symptoms of low carbohydrate intake, which manifests in the form of fatigue, dehydration and loss of energy and other syndromes like *Ketoacidosis*.

In the sports field, athletes resort to '*Glycogen loading*' to provide added fuel stores, but this practice may cause complications later on (More details in Chapter 15 on Athletics).

3. *Dextrins*

Dextrins are the polysachharide compounds formed as intermediate products in the breakdown of starch, as shown below. This breakdown of starch is a regular phenomenon in the process of digestion.

Starch	+	H_2O	→ Soluble Starch + Maltose
Soluble Starch	+	H_2O	→ Dextrin + Maltose
Dextrin	+	H_2O	→ Maltose
Maltose	+	H_2O	→ Glucose + Glucose

4. *Dietary Fibre*

This component, Dietary Fibre is the non-digestive or non-nutritive carbohydrate, like cellulose, hemicllulose, gums, pectins and lignins. Being not digested, dietary fibres form the bulk in the intestines and by stimulating peristaltic movements, they aid in the evacuation of bowels. Dietary fibre thus helps counter the tendency of constipation. The lack of fibre in the diet can eventually lead to cancer of the colon.

(a) **Cellulose:** Cellulose makes the principal structure of the plant cell walls and provides most of the crude fibre. Its main sources are stems and leaves of vegetables, seeds and grain covering and hulls.
Although indigestible, dietary fibres help increase the bulk in the diet. This bulk moves the food mass along and stimulates bowel movements.

(b) **Non-Cellulose:** This group of dietary fibre polysachharides comprises of hemicellulose, pectins, gums, mucilages and algal substances. They help absorb water and slow the gastric emptying time. They also prevent the pressure being built up in the colon by providing the bulk for the movements of the intestinal muscles.

(c) **Lignins:** Lignins are the only non-carbohydrate dietary fibre which forms the woody part of the plants. They combine with bile acids in the intestine to form insoluble compounds, which prevent their absorption.

Table 3.4 shows the food sources of dietary fibre.

TABLE 3.4: FOOD SOURCES OF DIETARY FIBRES

Dietary Fibre Class	Grains	Fruits	Vegetables
Cellulose	Bran, Whole Wheat, Whole Rye	Apples Peers	Beans, Peas, Cabbages, Root Vegetables and Tomatoes
Non-cellulose Polysachharides			
Hemicellulose	Bran, Cereals, Whole Grains	—	—
Pectins	—	Apples, Citrus fruits, Berries	Green beans, Carrots
Gums	Oatmeal	Food products, Thickener, Stabilizer,	Dried Beans, Other Legumes, Vegetable Gums used in Food processing
Mucilages	—	Food products, Thickener, Stabilizer,	—
Algal Substances	—	Food products, Thickener, Stabilizer	
Non-carbohydrate			
Lignins	Whole Wheat, Whole Rye	Strawberries, Peaches, Peas, Plums	Ripe Vegetables

Some of these dietary fibres like mucilages and gums in our diet have been shown to lower blood cholesterol in hypocholestrolemic patients and blood glucose levels in the diabetics.

Table 3.5 categorically lists the function of different components of dietary fibre and the manner in which they can influence man's health.

TABLE 3.5: FUNCTIONS OF DIETARY FIBRE

Dietary Fibre	Source	Function
Cellulose	Main cell wall constituent of plants	Holds water; reduces elevated colonic intraluminal pressure; binds zinc
Non-cellulose Polysaccharides Gums Algal polysaccharides Pectin substances	Secretions of plants Plant secretions and seeds Algae, seaweed Intercellular cement plant material	Slows gastric emptying; provides fermentable material for colonic bacteria with production of gas and volatile fatty acids; binds bile acids and cholesterol
Hemicellulose	Cell wall plant material	Holds water and increases stool bulk; reduces elevated colonic pressure; binds bile acids
Lignin	Woody part of plants	Antioxidant; binds bile acids, cholesterol, and metals

The ongoing study and research of the clinical role of dietary fibre in disease prevention and management of health problems like heart diseases, diabetes, colon cancer and obesity are summarized in Table 3.6.

The term dietary fibre was initially applied to the total amount of all the natural, non-digestible material found in the plants. Crude fibre, on the other hand, is the material remaining after vigorous treatment of the foodstuffs with acid and alkaline agents in the laboratory. Hence, the term Crude fibre is not of great relevance in the day-to-day health matters.

Appendix 1 at the end of the Chapter gives the composition of dietary fibre of the select food plants.

FUNCTIONS OF CARBOHYDRATES

1. Energy Intake

The foremost function of carbohydrates in human nutrition is to provide fuel for energy. When carbohydrates are burnt in the body as fuel, they provide 4 kcal per gm of energy. This is called '*Fuel Factor*'. Hence, the fuel factor of carbohydrates is four.

Usually, there is no recommended dietary allowance for carbohydrates. A minimum of 100 g per day is required to prevent proteins and fats breakdown to supply energy needs of the body. About twice the amount (200 g) is needed for normal energy balance in the body.

2. Energy Reserve

The amount of carbohydrates in the body, though small and constantly turning over, enters into daily energy resources and is important in maintaining 'Energy reserves'. Normally, in an adult male, about 300 g are stored in liver and muscle tissue as glycogen, which is being constantly synthesized from glucose. Another 10 grams are present in the circulating blood. Now the total available amount of body glycogen provides energy sufficient for only half a day in case of modest level of activity. It thus calls for more frequent ingestion of carbohydrates at regular intervals to meet the constant energy demand of the body.

TABLE 3.6: RELATIONSHIP BETWEEN FIBER AND VARIOUS HEALTH PROBLEMS

Problem	Effect of Fiber	Possible Mode of Action
Diabetes Mellitus	Reduces fasting blood sugar levels Reduces Glycosuria Reduces Insulin requirements Increases Insulin sensitivity	Slows carbohydrate absorption by: 1. Delaying gastric emptying time 2. Forming gels with pectin or guar gum in the intestine, thus impending carbohydrate absorption 3. 'Protecting' carbohydrates from enzymatic activity with a fibrous coat 4. Allowing 'protected' carbohydrates to escape into large colon where they are digested by bacteria
	Inhibits postrandial (after meals) Hyperglycemia	Alters gut hormones (for example, glucagons) to enhance glucose metabolism in the liver
Obesity	Increases satiety rate	Prolongs chewing and swallowing movements
	Reduces nutrient bio-availability	Increases fecal fat content
	Reduces energy density	1. Inhibits absorption of carbohydrates in high-fiber foods 2. Decrease transit time
	Alters hormonal response	Alters action of insulin, gut glucagons, and other intestinal hormones
	Alters Thermogenesis	
Coronary Heart Disease	Inhibits recirculation of bile acids	1. Alters bacterial metabolism of bile acids 2. Alters bacterial flora, resulting in a change inmetabolic activity forms gels that bind bile acids 3. Alters the function of pancreatic and intestinal enzymes
	Reduces triglyceride and cholesterol level	1. Reduces insulin levels Binds cholesterol, preventing absorption 2. Slows fat absorption by forming gel matrices in the intestine
Colon Cancer	Reduces incidence of disease	Bile acids or their bacterial metabolites may affect the structure of the colon, its cell turnover rate, and function
Other Gastrointestinal Disorders	Reduces pressure from within the intestinal lumen	Decreases transit time
Diverticular Disease -Constipation -Hiatal Hernia -Hemorrhoids	Increases diameter of the intestinal lumen, thus allowing intestinal tract to contract more, propelling contents more rapidly and inhibiting segmentation	Increases water absorption resulting in a larger, softer stool.

Adapted from *Nutrition and Diet Therapy* by S. R. Williams (Mosby Pub.) 1990.

3. Protein-sparing Action

Another important function of carbohydrates is to help regulate the metabolism of proteins in the body, by preventing too much proteins being utilized for energy production. A minimum of 100 g/day glucose is required to spare and save the protein breakdown to serve the glucose needs of the brain. The portein-sparing action of carbohydrates allows most of the protein being used for tissue building.

4. Anti-ketogenic Effect

As in the case of Number 3, similar is the use of carbohydrates in the case of of fats. It helps prevent their breakdown to supply a back up source of energy.

5. Energy for Heart

Regular and proper heart action is maintained through muscular exercise. While the fatty acids are the regular fuel of heart, it is glycogen present in cardiac muscles that provides an additional source of contractile energy. If a heart is damaged, angina symptoms go to show the poor stored glycogen or the low intake of carbohydrates by the patients.

6. Energy for Central Nervous System

The brain does not have any stored supply of glucose. That way, it depends on the minute-by-minute supply of glucose from the blood. Sustained shock from lack of constant glucose to supply brain function needs may cause irreversible brain damage. As such, carbohydrates are indispensable for maintaining a healthy nervous system.

Carbohydrates, in combination with proteins, form several compounds that play an important role in the body. Mucopolysachharides (Hoxamine derivatives), such as hyaluronic acid are invaluable as lubricants in the joints. Other mucopolysaccharides and mucoproteins in body form vital components of nail, bone, cartilage and skin.

EFFICIENCY FACTOR IN CARBOHYDRATES

Another point in favour of carbohydrates (sugars) is that it is the most efficient source of calories. To produce one million Kcal of energy from any crop, one would need:

— 0.15 acres land under sugarbeet/sugarcane
— 0.40 acres land under rice
— 1.0 acres land under wheat
— 2–17 acres land for animal products.

As such, carbohydrates are not only the most efficient source of energy, they are indeed the most valuable macro-nutrient for growth, health and maintenance.

DIGESTION OF CARBOHYDRATES

Mouth

Small particles of food broken down during mastication are mixed with saliva. The salivary amylase secreted by the parotid glands acts on the starch, which then breaks down into dextrins and maltose.

Stomach

The peristaltic movements of stomach muscles help mix further the gastric secretions. The salivary amylase is not active at an acid pH. Before the complete mixing of food with gastric secretions, bout 30% of the starches may have been changed into maltose. This thick creamy chyme is then emptied into the duodenum.

Small Intestine

While peristalsis aids in the digestion in small intestines by mixing and moving the chyme, chemical digestion is completed in the small intestines by two enzymes, *viz.*, pancreatic amylase and intestinal secretions. The digested product in the form of monosachharides are absorbed into the portal blood circulation. Table 3.7 summarises the digestion of carbohydrates.

Large Intestine

All carbohydrates that reach the large intestine may be fermented by the colonic microflora, with the production of short chain fatty acids (SCFA) and gas, as shown in Fig. 3.3.

TABLE 3.7: DIGESTION OF CARBOHYDRATES

	Site	Substrate	Enzyme	Digestion Product
1.	Mouth	Food	Food	Small Food Particles (Bolus)
2.	Mouth	Starch	Ptyalin (Salivary amylase)	Shorter chain Dextrins
3.	Esophagus	Starch	Ptyalin	Shorter chain Dextrins, possibly maltose
4.	Stomach	Sucrose	—	Glucose and Fructose (through HCL)
5.	Small Intestines			
		(a) Starch and Dextrins	Pancreatic Amylase	Maltose
		(b) Maltose	Maltase	Glucose
		(c) Sucrose	Sucrase	Glucose and Sucrose
		(d) Lactose	Lactase	Glucose and Galactose

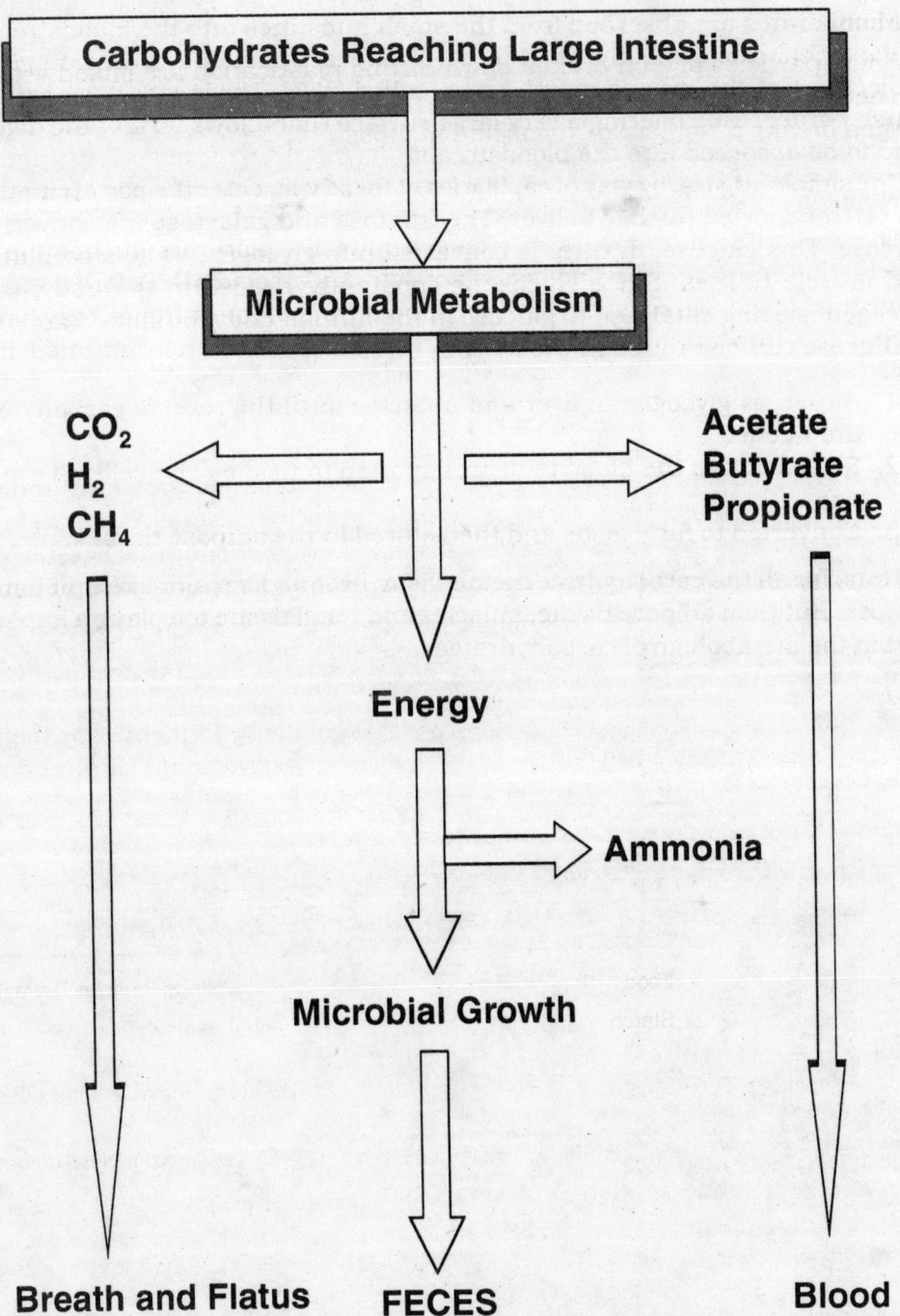

Fig. 3.3: Fermentation of Carbohydrates in Large Intestine

ABSORPTION OF CARBOHYDRATES

Carbohydrates are absorbed from the small intestines into the bloodstream as monosachharides, mostly as glucose. There are millions of tiny finger-like projections of the mucus membranes, called 'Villi'. These villi have extended brush border, thus offering a very large surface that allows 90% of the digested food to be absorbed into the bloodstream.

The simple sugars, by way of capillaries of these villi, enter the portal circulation -to be transported further to liver. The fructose and galactose are converted to glucose. This glucose, in turn, is converted into glycogen, to be stored in liver and muscle tissues. Since glucose is constantly needed in the body, so the glycogen is being catalysed to glucose in the human body for immediate needs.

Glucose can be utilized in the body in three ways:

1. Stored as glycogen in liver and muscles until the reserve carbohydrates are needed.
2. Released into the blood to be transported to tissues and cells all over the body.
3. Converted to fatty acids and then stored in the adipose tissues.

Thus, for all the carbohydrate metabolism, liver is the major site that handles glucose. But then adipose tissue, muscles and renal tissue too play an important part in the metabolism of carbohydrates.

Dietary Fiber and Kcalorie Values for Selected Foods

Foods	Serving	Dietary Fiber (g)	Kcal
Breads and cereals			
All Bran	⅓ cup	8.5	70
Bran (100%)	½ cup	8.4	75
Corn Bran	⅔ cup	5.4	100
Oat Bran	⅓ cup	4.3	110
Bran Flakes	¾ cup	4.0	90
Air-popped Popcorn	1 cup	2.5	25
Oatmeal	1 cup	2.2	144
Whole Wheat bread	1 slice	1.4	60
Legumes, cooked			
Kidney beans	½ cup	7.3	110
Lima beans	½ cup	4.5	130
Vegetables, cooked			
Green Peas	½ cup	3.6	55
Corn	½ cup	2.9	70
Parsnip	½ cup	2.7	50
Potato, with skin	1 medium	2.5	95
Brussels sprouts	½ cup	2.3	30
Carrots	½ cup	2.3	25
Broccoli	½ cup	2.2	20
Beans, green	½ cup	1.6	15
Tomato, chopped	½ cup	1.5	17
Cabbage, red and white	½ cup	1.4	15
Kale	½ cup	1.4	20
Cauliflower	½ cup	1.1	15
Lettuce, fresh	1 cup	0.8	7
Fruits			
Apple	1 medium	3.5	80
Raisins	¼ cup	3.1	110
Prunes, dried	3	3.0	60
Strawberries	1 cup	3.0	45
Orange	1 medium	2.6	60
Banana	1 medium	2.4	105
Blueberries	½ cup	2.0	40
Dates, dried	3	1.9	70
Peach	1 medium	1.9	35
Apricot, fresh	3 medium	1.8	50
Grapefruit	½ cup	1.6	40
Apricot, dried	5 halves	1.4	40
Cherries	10	1.2	50
Pineapple	½ cup	1.1	40

Adapted from Lanza, E., Butrum, R. R.: A critical review of food fiber analysis and data. *J. Am. Diet Assoc.*, **86**: 732, 1986.

Dietary Fiber in Select Plant Foods

Food	Amount	Weight (g)	Total Dietary Fiber (g)	Non-Cellulose Polysaccharides (g)	Cellulose (g)	Lignin (g)
Apple	1 med					
Flesh		138	1.96	1.29	0.66	0.01
Skin		100	3.71	2.21	1.01	0.49
Banana	1 small	119	2.08	1.33	0.44	0.31
Beans						
Baked	1 cup	255	18.53	14.45	3.59	0.48
Green, cooked	1 cup	125	4.19	2.31	1.61	0.26
Bread						
White	1 slice	25	0.68	0.50	0.18	Trace
Whole meal	1 slice	25	2.13	1.49	0.33	0.31
Broccoli, cooked	1 cup	155	6.36	4.53	1.78	0.05
Brussels sprouts, cooked	1 cup	155	4.43	3.08	1.24	0.11
Cabbage, cooked	1 cup	145	4.10	2.55	1.00	0.55
Carrots, cooked	1 cup	155	5.74	3.44	2.29	Trace
Cauliflower, cooked	1 cup	125	2.25	0.84	1.41	Trace
Cereals						
All-Bran	1 oz	30	8.01	5.35	1.80	0.86
Corn Flakes	1 cup	25	2.75	1.82	0.61	0.33
Puffed Wheat	1 cup	15	2.31	1.55	0.39	0.37
Rice Krispies	1 cup	30	1.34	1.04	0.23	0.07
shredded Wheat	1 biscuit	25	3.07	2.20	0.66	0.21
Cherries	10 cherries	68	0.84	0.63	0.17	0.05
Corn	1 cup	165	7.82	7.11	0.51	0.20
Canned	1 cup	165	9.39	8.20	1.06	0.13
Flour						
Bran	1 cup	100	44.00	32.70	8.05	3.23
White	1 cup	115	3.62	2.90	0.69	0.03
Whole meal	1 cup	120	11.41	7.50	2.95	0.96
Grapefruit	½ cup	100	0.44	0.34	0.04	0.06
Jam, Strawberry	1 tbsp	20	0.22	0.17	0.02	0.03
Lettuce	⅛ head	100	1.53	0.47	1.06	Trace
Onions, raw, sliced	1 cup	100	2.10	1.55	0.55	Trace
Orange	1 cup	200	0.58	0.44	0.08	0.06

Table (*contd.* on page 63)

Table (*contd.* from page 62)

Parsnips, raw, diced	1 cup	100	4.90	3.77	1.13	Trace
Peach, flesh and skin	1 med.	100	2.28	1.46	0.20	0.62
Peanuts	1 oz	30	2.79	1.92	0.51	0.36
Peanut butter	1 tbsp	16	1.21	0.90	0.31	Trace
Pear	1 med.					
Flesh		164	4.00	2.16	1.10	0.74
Skin		100	8.59	3.72	2.18	2.67
Peas, canned	1 cup	170	13.35	8.85	3.91	0.60
Peas, raw or frozen	1 cup	100	7.75	5.48	2.09	0.18
Plums	1 plum	66	1.00	0.65	0.15	0.20
Potato, raw	1 med.	135	4.73	3.36	1.38	Trace
Raisins	1 oz	30	1.32	0.72	0.25	0.35
Strawberries	1 cup	149	2.65	1.39	1.04	0.22
Tomato						
Raw	1 med.	135	1.89	0.88	0.61	0.41
Canned, drained	1 cup	240	2.04	1.08	0.89	0.07
Turnips, raw	1 med.	100	2.20	1.50	0.70	Trace

Adapted from Southgate, D. A. T., *et al.*: A guide to calculating Intakes of Dietary Fiber. *J. Hum. Nutr.*, **30**: 303, 1976.

Share of Carbohydrates in Common Foods

Category	Foodstuffs	Starch %
A: Starches		
	Barley—pearled	79
	Bread—all types	52-58
	Cassava, meal and flour	85
	Cornmeal and grits	74-78
	Crackers	71-74
	Noodles, Spaghetti and Marconi	73-77
	Oatmeal and Oat Cereals	70
	Potatoes, cooked	19
	Rice or Rice Cereal	79
	Rye Flour	68-78
	Wheat Flour	69-79
	Wheat Cereal	72-80
B: Sugars		
	Cake	52-62
	Candies	56-99
	Cookies	60-80
	Dried Fruits	75-88
	Honey	80
	Jam/Jelly	65-71
	Syrups	74
	Cane/Beet Sugar	100

Types, Sources and End Products of Carbohydrates

Carbohydrates	Food Sources	End Products	Remarks
Polysaccharides			
Indigestible			
1. Cellulose	Stalks and leaves of vege-	—	May be partially split to glucose by bacterial action in large bowel
2. Hemicelluloses	tables; outer covering of seeds		
3. Pectins	Fruits	—	These substances have an affinity for water, form bulk, slow gastric emptying time, and may bind bile acids
4. Gums and Mucilages	Plant secretions and seeds		
5. Algal Substances	Seaweeds and Algae	—	
Partially Digestible			
1. Inulin	Jerusalem artichokes, Onion, Garlic and Mushrooms	Fructose	Digestion is incomplete; further splitting by bacteria may occur in the large bowel; may be production of flatus from Raffinose and Stachyose
2. Galactogens	Snails	Galactose	
3. Mannosans	Legumes	Mannose	
4. Raffinose	Sugar beets, Kidney beans, Lentils and Navy beans	Glucose, Fructose, and Galactose	
5. Stachyose	Beans	Pentoses	
6. Pentosans	Fruits and Gums		
Digestible			
1. Starch and Dextrins	Grains, Vegetables (esp. Tubers and Legumes)	Glucose	The most important group quantitatively; usually accompanied by some maltose
2. Glycogen	Meat products and Seafood	Glucose	
Disaccharides and Oligosaccharides			
1. Sucrose	Cane and Beet sugars, Molasses and Maple syrup	Glucose and Fructose	
2. Lactose	Milk and Milk products	Glucose and Galactose	
3. Lactulose	Synthetic products	Not metabolised	Does not appear in foods; is synthetic, not digested; and is used as a laxative
4. Maltose and Maltotriose	Malt products, some Break-fast Cereals	Glucose	
5. Trehalose	Mushrooms, Insects, Yeast	Glucose	

Table (*contd.* on page 66)

Table (*contd.* from page 65)

Monosaccharides			
Hexoses			
1. Glucose	Fruits, Honey, Corn syrup	Glucose	In fruits and vegetables the contents of Glucose and Fructose depend on species, ripeness, and state of preservation
Sorbitol	Fruits, Vegetables, Dietetic products		
2. Fructose	Fruits, Honey	Fructose ⎤	These monosaccharides do not occur in free form in foods
3. Galactose		Galactose ⎬	
4. Mannose		Mannose ⎦	
Mannitol	Pineapples, Olives, Asparagus, Sweet Potatoes, Carrots, and Dietetic products		
Pentoses			
1. Ribose	—	Ribose ⎤	Ribose, Xylose and Arabinose do not occur in free form in foods. They are derived from pentosans of fruits and from the nucleic acids of meat products and seafood
2. Xylose	Fruits, Vegetables, Cereals, Mushrooms, Seaweed, Dietetic Chewing gum, and other Dietetic products	Xylose ⎬	
Xylitol			
3. Arabinose	—	Arabinose ⎦	
Carbohydrate Derivatives			
1. Ethyl alcohol	Fermented Liquors		These substances are the products of natural or induced carbohydrate breakdown
2. Lactic acid	Milk and Milk products	Absorbed as same	
3. Malic acid	Fruits		

APPENDIX 5

Dietary Fiber Content of Foods in Commonly Served Portions

Food Group	<1 g	1-1.9 g	2-2.9 g	3-3.9 g	4-4.9 g	5-5.9 g	>6 g
Breads (1 slice)	Bagel White French	Whole Wheat	Bran muffin (1)	NA	NA	NA	NA
Cereals (1 oz)	Rice Krispies Special K Cornflakes	Oatmeal Nutri-Grain Cheerios	Wheaties Shredded Wheat	Most Honey Bran	Bran Chex 40% Bran Flakes Raisin Bran	Corn Bran	All-Bran Bran Buds 100% Bran
Pasta (1 cup)	NA	Macaroni Spaghetti	NA	Whole Wheat Spaghetti	NA	NA	NA
Rice (½ cup)	White	Brown	NA	NA	NA	NA	NA
Legumes cooked (½ cup)	NA	NA	NA	Lentils	Lima Beans Dried Peas	NA NA	Kidney Beans Baked Beans Navy Beans
Vegetables (½ cup unless stated)	Cucumber Lettuce (1 cup) Green pepper	Asparagus Green Beans Cabbage Cauliflower Potato with/ without skin (1) Celery	Broccoli Brussels sprouts Carrots Corn Potato with skin (1) Spinach	Peas	NA	NA	
Fruits (1 medium fruit unless stated)	Grapes (20) Watermelon (1 cup)	Apricots (3) Grapefruit (½) Peach with skin Pineapple (½ cup)	Apple, with/without skin Banana Orange	Apple, with skin Pear, with skin Raspberries (½ cup)	NA	NA	NA

Source: Slavin, J. L., Dietary fiber: Classification, chemical analysis and food sources. *J. Am. Diet Assoc.*, **87**: 1164, 1987.

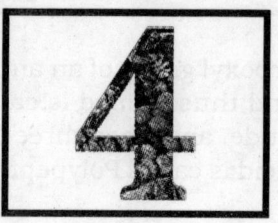

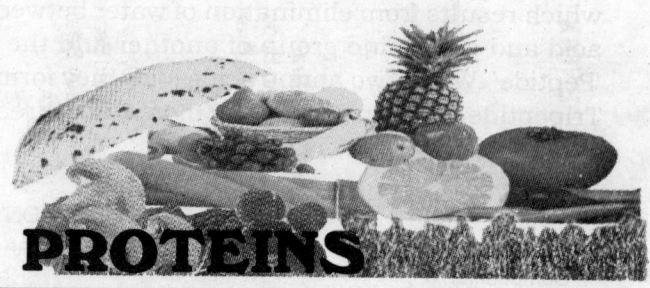

PROTEINS

The term protein comes from a Greek word that means 'Primary' in 'Holding First Place'—indeed an appropriate name for the most crucial life-sustaining and life-forming substances of all the fauna and flora.

Proteins may be defined as organic substances which yield, on digestion, the building block or amino acids. It is these amino acids which form the complex molecule of a protein.

Proteins generally provide 10-15% of the total dietary energy. More than a source of energy (their main job is to supply nitrogen to build body tissue), greater significance lies in the fact that they are the major structural and functional component of all the cells of body.

Physically speaking, proteins are ubiquitous in nature, being found throughout in all the life forms. All the enzymes, membrane carriers, blood transport molecules, intracellular matrix and even the hair and the finger nails are proteins, as are many hormones and a large part of the membranes. Moreover, their constituent amino acids act as precursors of many co-enzymes, hormones, nucleic acids and many other molecules essential for life.

CHEMICAL COMPOSITION

Proteins are complex organic compounds containing the same three elements, viz., carbon, hydrogen and oxygen. But unlike fats and carbohydrates, protein contain in addition, nitrogen, besides sulfur and sometimes iron, phosphorus, iodine and copper.

Proteins are classified according to their composition, nutritional quality, structure as also their solubility, as shown in Table 4.1.

Proteins are macromolecules consisting of large chains of amino acid sub-units. In the protein molecule, amino acids are joined together by 'Peptide bond', which results from elimination of water between the carboxyl group of an amino acid and the amino group of another and the compound thus formed is called 'Peptide'. When two amino acids join, they form a Dipeptide, and when three it is Tripeptide. A chain containing more than three amino acid is called Polypeptide, which ultimately forms the protein.

TABLE 4.1: CLASSIFICATION OF PROTEINS

Composition & Properties	Nutritional Quality	Structure	Solubility
1. Conjugated or Compound	1. Complete 2. Partially complete	1. Globular or Fibrous	1. Acid 2. Water
2. Divided	3. Incomplete		3. Alcohol

Each amino acid has an acidic (COOH) carboxyl group and a basic (NH$_2$) group. By varying the grouping attached to the carbon containing the amino group, many different amino acids are formed, as shown below:

CH$_2$(NH$_2$)·COOH	— Glycine
CH$_3$CH(NH$_2$)·CPPH	— Alanine
CH$_2$CH$_2$CH$_2$CH(NH$_2$)COOH	— Lysine

Amino Acids

The 22 amino acids are classified as essential and non-essential, as shown in Table 4.2. They are called 'essential', because they cannot be synthesized by the body. Arginine is a semi-essential amino acid because its rate of synthesis in the body is inadequate. The remaining 12 are non-essential amino acids, because the human body can synthesize these from simple precursors.

Valine, Leucine and Isoleucine

These three essential amino acids are called 'Branched Chain amino acids' (BCAA), since they have branching side-chain. These BCAA are used in special amino acid products for the treatment of liver and kidney failure. They also help reduce the muscle-protein breakdown and speed up the recovery process in the patients hospitalized for severe illness and injury.

Threonine and Lysine

Threonine has got an attached hydroxyl (OH) group, just as in H$_2$O. Lysine has an extra nitrogen atom in the additional nitrogenous group (NH$_2$) at the end of the long carbon chain. Lysine is also a precursor of the lesser known but important amino acid, carnitine.

TABLE 4.2: AMINO ACID CLASSIFICATION

Essential Amino Acids	Semi-essential * Amino Acids	Non-essential Amino Acids
Histadine	Arginine	Alanine
Isoleucine		Asparagine
Leucine		Aspartic acid
Lysine		Cystine (Cysteine)
Methionine		Glutamic Acid
Phenylalanine		Glutamine
Threonine		Glycine
Tryptophan		Hydroxylysine
Valine		Hydroxyproline
		Proline
		Serine
		Tyrosine

Phenylalnine and Methionine

Both these essential amino acids are of great significance in genetic and metabolic conditions. Phenylalanine is involved in the genetic diseases of the New-born, *viz.*, Phenylketonuria (PKU). It is also a precursor of non-essential amino acid, tyrosine. Methionine is a major source of dietary sulfur and is involved in renal calculi, cystine stones, as methionine is the precursor of non-essential amino acid, cystine. Alongwith one of its metabolites, cysteine, it contributes to the synthesis of amino acid, taurine.

Tryptophan

This essential amino acid has a side-chain that contains a double ring. Tryptophan has the unique capacity of being able to produce vitamin B, *viz.*, niacin.

Histadine

Earlier considered as semi-essential, histadine has a ring in its side-chain that contributes more nitrogen.

The essential amino acid, methionine can be converted into cystine, but cystine cannot be converted to methionine. Similarly, phenylalanine can be converted to tyrosine, but not vice versa. Hence, cystine and even tyrosine are classified as semi-essential amino acids.

---

*They are considered 'Semi-essential' owing to their inadequate production in the body, which is not enough to support growth. As such, they may be reckoned as 'Essential' for children. Some researchers have pointed out that some Histadine may be required by the adults also.

As stated earlier, the amino acids have a '*Buffer*' capacity, since they ionize in solution to behave either as an acid or as a base, depending upon the pH of the solution.

Table 4.3 gives the requirements of essential amino acids for different age groups.

TABLE 4.3: ESSENTIAL AMINO ACID REQUIREMENTS FOR CHILDREN AND ADULTS

Amino Acid	Children (2-5 years) mg/kg/day	Children (10-12 years) mg/kg/day	Adults (18 years and over) mg/kg/day	Adults (Revised estimates) mg/kg/day
Isoleucine	31.0	28.0	10.0	23.0
Leucine	73.0	44.0	14.0	39.0
Lysine	64.0	44.0	12.0	30.0
Methionine/Cystine	27.0	22.0	13.0	15.0
Phenylalanine/Tyrosine	69.0	22.0	14.0	39.0
Threonine	37.0	28.0	7.0	15.0
Tryptophan	12.5	3.3	3.5	6.0
Valine	38.0	25.0	10.0	20.0
TOTAL	**351.5**	**216.3**	**83.5**	**187.0**

TYPES OF PROTEINS

From the nutrition angle, proteins may be divided into two groups *viz.*, complete proteins and incomplete proteins.

Complete Proteins

This group of proteins contains all the essential amino acids in sufficient quantity and in a proper ratio to meet all the needs of human body. Even if they happen to be the exclusive source of proteins, they can fully sustain life processes. These complete proteins are, *prima facie*, of animal origin. i.e. milk, meat, fish and poultry products. Qualitatively, these proteins are far more superior than the incomplete proteins.

Incomplete Proteins

These proteins are usually deficient in one or more of the essential amino acids. The deficiency on this count in the vegetable proteins is shown hereunder:

Foodstuffs	Limiting Amino Acids
Cereals	Lysine and Threonine
Maize	Lysine and Tryptophan
Pulses	Methionine and Tryptophan
Groundnut	Lysine, Methionine and Threonine
Soyabean	Methionine
Coconut	Lysine and Methionine.

As such, on their own they cannot support life. These are mostly the proteins derived from plant sources, such as fruits and vegetables, cereals, pulses, nuts and oilseeds. In the Indian dietary, it is a common practice to combine two or three different sources in one meal, thus resulting in almost fuller supplies of protein constituents. This is called Supplementary Value of Foods. This supplementation may be as under:

1. Wheat/Maida with Animal Foods
2. Maize with Milk, Cereals and Legumes
3. Legumes with Animal Foods
4. Soya with Sesame.

In the protein group, only gelatin is the one derived from animal sources. It lacks three amino acids, viz. tryptophan, valine and isoleucine, with a relatively small share of leucine. Proteins may be simple proteins when they contain an amino acid. Others are complex proteins when other non-proteins groups are there along with simple proteins. These include

(1) Nucleoproteins
(2) Glycoproteins and Mucroproteins
(3) Phosphoproteins
(4) Chromoproteins
(5) Lipoproteins
(6) Metalloproteins

Table 4.4 gives the FAO/WHO norms of protein intake for different age groups.

TABLE 4.4: SAFE LEVELS OF PROTEIN INTAKE AS PROPOSED BY THE FAO/WHO/UNU

Age group		Male g/kg/day	Female g/kg/day
3-6	months	1.85	1.85
6-9	months	1.65	1.65
9-12	months	1.50	1.50
1-2	years	1.20	1.20
2-3	years	1.15	1.15
3-5	years	1.10	1.10
5-7	years	1.00	1.00
7-10	years	1.00	1.00
10-12	years	1.00	1.00
12-14	years	1.00	0.95
14-16	years	0.94	0.90
16-18	years	0.88	0.80
Adults		0.75	0.75
During Pregnancy			Add 6.0 g to total
Lactation: 0-6 months			Add 17.5 g to total
Lactation: older than 6 months			Add 13.0 g to total

TYPES OF VEGETARIAN DIETS

Vegetarian diets differ according to the beliefs of persons following these food patterns. In general, there are three basic types as mentioned below.

Lacto-ovo Vegetarians

Lacto-ovo vegetarians follow a food pattern that allows dairy products and eggs. Some may even accept fish and perhaps occasional poultry. Their mixed diet of both plant and animal food sources, excluding only meat, especially red meats, poses no nutritional problems.

Lacto-vegetarians

Lacto-vegetarians accept only dairy products from animal sources to complement their basic diet of plant foods. The use of milk and milk products such as chese with a varied mixed diet of whole or enriched grains, legumes, nuts, seeds, fruits and vegetables in sufficient quantities to meet energy needs provides a balanced intake.

Vegands

Vegands follow a strictly vegetarian diet and use no animal foods. Their food pattern is composed entirely of plant foods, whole or enriched grains, legumes, nuts, seeds, fruits and vegetables. The use of soybeans, soy milk, soybean curd (tofu), and processed soy products is specially recommended.

FUNCTIONS OF PROTEINS

The role and functions of proteins in the human body are of three types viz. building tissues, performing special regulatory or physiologic functions and occasionally providing energy to the body.

Growth and Maintenance

The primary function of dietary proteins is to supply building material for growth and proper maintenance of all the body tissues. This job is done by furnishing the proper type and numbers of amino acids for efficient synthesis of particular cellular proteins. Proteins also supply amino acids for other essential nitrogen-containing substances, such as enzymes and hormones.

Special Physiologic Role

Proteins are needed for the regulation of highly specialized or physiologic functions in the human body like

(i) Immune Proteins

For providing immunity to the body against various infections, antibodies are needed. Further, plasma proteins guard water balance in the body. All these antibodies are basically proteins in nature.

(ii) Hormones

All the hormones, like insulin or adrenocorticotrophic hormones are proteins.

(iii) Enzymes

The process of digestion, absorption and mobilization calls for enzymes to be present in the system. And these enzymes are proteins.

(iv) Nucleoproteins

These control and govern the synthesis of all the body proteins.

(v) Contractile Proteins

Herein, actin and myosin are responsible for the action of the body muscles.

(vi) Blood Proteins

The most familiar hemoglobin constituent of blood is the protein that carries oxygen.

Mentions needs be made of other proteins found in blood, viz. lipoproteins, transferrin, retinol-binding protein, immunoglobulins and serum-albumins. The last one is responsible for regulating osmotic pressure and proper maintenance of the fluid balance of the body.

Other Specific Functions

Some amino acids have very specific functions, to perform in the systems, such as:

(i) Tryptophan, precursor of vitamin B, niacin and neuro-transmitter serotonin.
(ii) Methionine supplies the methyl group for synthesizing choline which, in turn, prevents accumulation of fat in liver. Choline is also a precursor of acetylcholine, a major neurotransmitter in the brain. Methionine is also the precursor of cystine, carnitine and taurine.
(iii) Glycine is needed for the formation of the porphyrin ring of haemoglobin. It also forms an important constituent of nucleic acids
(iv) Phenylalanine is the precursor of the non-essential amino acid tyrosine, which leads to formation of hormones—thyroxine and epinephrine.

Non-Protein Pathway

Amino acids are also involved in the synthesis of other nitrogenous compounds important to physiological viability. Some pathways have the potential for exerting substantial impact on utilization of certain amino acid. As shown in Table 4.5, glycine is involved in five significant pathways in the synthesis of creatine (muscle functions), haematine (oxygen transport), glutathione (protective reaction).

TABLE 4.5: NON-PROTEIN PATHWAY OF AMINO ACID UTILIZATION

End-Product	Precursor Amino Acid
Serotonin	Tryptophan
Nicotinic Acid	Tryptophan
Catecholamine	Tryptophan
Thyroid Hormone	Tryptophan
Melanin	Tryptophan
Carnatine	Lysine
Taurine	Cysteine
Glutathione	Glutamine, Cysteine, Glycine
Nuc. Acid Basis	Glutamine, Aspartate, Glycine
Haematine	Glycine
Creatine	Glycine, Arginine, Methionine
Methyl Group	
Metabolism	Methionine, Glycine, Serine
Bile Acids	Glycine, Taurine

Source: *Human Nutrition and Dietetics*—J. S. Garrow *et al.*

Available Energy

Proteins have a fuel factor of 4, *i.e.* they yield 4 kcal/g energy. However, it is not metabolized for energy except in emergency situation like fasting and extended physical exercises and marathon races. After the removal of nitrogenous portion of the constituent amino acid, the amino acids residue, its carbon skeleton, called 'keto acid', may be converted into glucose or fat. However, the aromatic amino acids, phenylalanine and tyrosine are catabolized to fumerate. Both phenylalanine and tyrosine are also metabolised to acetoacetate which, in turn, may be either ketogenic or be metabolized via acetyl-CoA in the citric acid cycle. Lucine is the only purely ketogenic amino acid. All others are glycogenic.

On an average, 58% of the total dietary proteins may become available as glucose according to the need and may be oxidized as such to yield available energy. Thus, sufficient amounts of non-protein kilocalories from carbohydrates are always needed to save the proteins for the primary building activities and to prevent unnecessary protein breakdown in providing energy.

DIGESTION OF PROTEINS

1. Mouth

Only mechanical breaking up of the proteins into smaller particles takes place in the mouth. It is then mixed with saliva, to be passed onto stomach as a semi-solid mass.

2. Stomach

It needs a series of enzymes to break the complex mass of protein finally to amino acids. The three enzymes in the gastric secretions that help in this task are: pepsin, hydrochloric acid and rennin.

1 Pepsin, the main gastric juice, is first produced as an inactive pro-enzyme called pepsinogen from the mucosal cells of stomach walls. Pepsinogen, in the presence of HCl, gets activated to the enzyme pepsin. The latter starts splitting the peptide linkages between the protein amino acids to yield smaller peptides.

2 The gastric HCl acts as an important catalyst. It provides the acid medium necessary to convert pepsinogen into pepsin.

3 This gastric enzyme is present only in early infancy and disappears in adult life. It is particularly important in infants' digestion of milk. By coagulating milk, rennin prevents too rapid a change of food from the child's stomach.

3. Small Intestine

These pancreatic enzymes continue breaking down the proteins into simpler susbtances.

1 Trypsin, secreted as inactive trypsinogen, it is activated by the hormone, Enterokinase produced by glands in the duodenal wall. It acts on large, polypeptide fragments, breaking them into smaller dipeptides.

2 Chymotrypsin, produced in the pancreas as chymotrypsinogen, which is then activated by trypsin already present. Thus, the protein-splitting action goes on.

3 Carboxypeptidase attacks the carboxyl end (COOH) of the peptide chain, thus providing smaller peptides and free amino acids.

Besides, there are 2 more enzymes in the peptide group viz. Aminopeptidase and dipeptidase, which help break the remaining material into free amino acids. Table 4.6 summarises the protein digestion

ABSORPTION

A few larger peptides or smaller intact proteins are absorbed as such and thus, hydrolized within the absorbing cells into their amino acids. In the human nutrition, amino acids are the Metabolic currency of the proteins. After absorption, the amino acids are taken up by blood capillaries of the mucosa and transported through the plasma and erythrocytes to liver and other tissues for metabolic utilization. Some of the remainder pass through into the systemic circulation and are then transported into the cells of the tissues.

TABLE 4.6: SUMMARY OF PROTEIN DIGESTION

Organ	Enzyme			Digestive Action
	Inactive Precursor	Activator	Active Enzyme	
Mouth			None	Mechanical only
Stomach (acid)	Pepsinogen	Hydrochloric acid	Pepsin	Protein → Polypeptides
			Rennin (infants) (Calcium necessary for activity)	Casein → Coagulated Curd
Intestine (alkaline)				
Pancreas	Trypsinogen	Enterokinase	Trypsin	Protein. Polypeptides → polypeptides, dipeptides
	Chymotripsinogen	Active Trypsin	Chymotrypsin	Protein Polypeptides → polypetidies, dipeptides
			Carboxyspeptidase	Polypeptides → simpler peptides, dipeptides, amino acids
Intestine			Aminopeptidase	Polypeptides → peptides, dipeptides, amino acids
			Dipeptidase	Dipeptides → Amino acids

HOMEOSTASIS (BALANCE CONCEPT)

Homeostasis is a state of dynamic equilibrium. There are many an interdependent checks and balances that exist in the body that help to keep the whole system as a fine-tuned orchestra. There is an endless process of building up and breaking down of some tissues or parts and depositing of some components as reserves in the body. It is this highly, nay critically sensitive balance between body parts and functioning that eventually sustains a healthy disease-free life.

PROTEIN COMPARTMENTS

There exists a very subtle balance between two compartments, viz., Tissue proteins and Plasma proteins. On an interchangeable basis, proteins from one compartment may be drawn to supplement those of the other, e.g during fasting, the reserves of the body protein may be called upon for tissue synthesis. As such, the body's state of stability is the result of a protein balance between the rate of breakdown and re-synthesis.

Equally so is the case with amino acid reserves, or what may apply to called the 'Metabolic Pool' of amino acids. In the case of starvation, wasting diseases and geriatrics, the tissue breakdown exceeds that of synthesis. Hence, the body goes on steadily deteriorating. If a negative Nitrogen balance occurs, then the muscle tissues are usually broken down to supply the essential amino acids. A person in this state would lose muscle mass. On the other hand, a positive Nitrogen balance means that Nitrogen is being incorporated into the body by the growth of new tissues. One finds this is the case in the growing children. It also happens in the tumerous growths or cancer.

Fig. 4.1 shows the balance between protein components and the amino acid pool available in the body.

On the other hand, the high-value diet of the Americans contributes to much of the adverse effects like obesity or cardiovascular problems. Whether it is the proverbial Protein-Energy Malnutrition of the poor, else the habitual excess intake of the rich, both have to be studied, scrutinized and then kept under control (i.e. equilibrium). This calls for special indices to measure the protein quality.

Nitrogen Balance

Nitrogen is lost from the body through urine, feces, perspiration, as also through functions like desquamation of epithelium, growth of hair and nails, besides other excretions like nasal mucus and dietary tears. Nitrogen balance indicates the net outcome of dietary nitrogen intake and the excretion (output) through urine and feces. A man is said to be in Nitrogen balance, i.e. equilibrium, when the intake and output of Nitrogen are equal. In the case of growing child, pregnant women and convalescents, it is a positive Nitrogen balance.

PROTEIN QUALITY INDICES

Biological Value (B.V.)

Biological Value is the index that shows the percentage of absorbed Nitrogen from dietary proteins actually retained by the body. This is calculated as under:

$$B.V. = \frac{Nitrogen\ retained}{Nitrogen\ absorbed} \times 100$$

From practical considerations, the above equation may be written more explicitly in the following step-by-step reaction,

$$B.V. = \frac{Dietary\ Nitrogen - (Urinary\ N + Fecal\ N)}{Dietary\ Nitrogen - Fecal\ Nitrogen} \times 100$$

Higher the amount of Nitrogen retained, greater is the B.V. of that foodstuff, as shown by a few illustrations:

B.V. of Egg   = 87-97
B.V. of Cow's milk   = 85-90
B.V. of Rice and Tofu = 75

Net Protein Utilization (NPU)

NPU reflects the relative digestibility of different proteins. It can be represented by the equation:

$$NPU = \frac{Dietary\ N - (Urinary\ N + Fecal\ N)}{Dietary\ N} \times 100$$

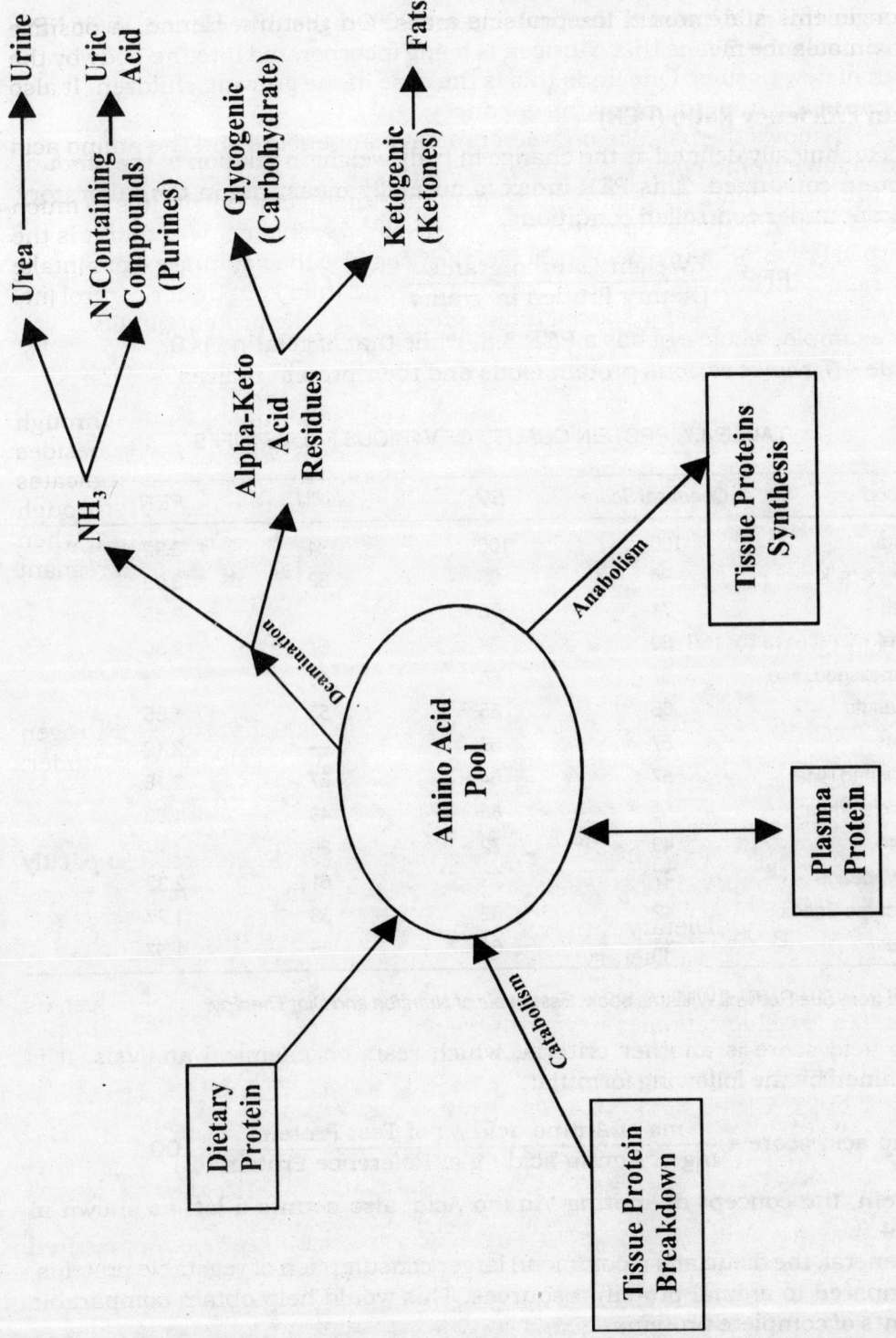

Fig. 4.1: Balance Between Protein Components and Amino Acid Pool

As a general rule, most of the proteins are 90% digestible. Hence, their NPU approximates the BV.

Protein Efficiency Ratio (PER)

PER is technically defined as the change in body weight in relation to the amount of protein consumed. This PER index is normally measured in the laboratory rats, kept under controlled conditions.

$$PER = \frac{\text{Weight Gain in grams}}{\text{Dietary Protien in grams}}$$

For example, whole egg has a PER 3.8, while that of gelatine is 0. Table 4.7 shows various protein foods and their protein indices.

TABLE 4.7: PROTEIN QUALITY OF VARIOUS FOODSTUFFS

Food	Chemical Score	BV	NPU	PER
Eggs	100	100	94	3.92
Cow's milk	95	93	82	3.09
Fish	71	76	—	3.55
Beef	69	74	67	2.30
Unpolished Rice	67	86	59	—
Peanuts	65	55	55	1.65
Oats	57	65	—	2.19
Polished Rice	57	64	57	2.18
Whole Wheat	53	65	49	1.53
Corn	49	72	36	—
Soyabeans	47	73	61	2.32
Sesame Seeds	42	62	53	1.77
Peas	37	64	55	1.57

Adapted from Sue Rodwell Williams book: *Essentials of Nutrition and Diet Therapy.*

Amino acid score is another criteria, which rests on chemical analysis. It is determined by the following formula:

$$\text{Amino acid score} = \frac{\text{mg of Amino acid / g of Test Protein}}{\text{mg of Amino acid / g of Reference Protein}} \times 100$$

Herein, the concept of limiting 'Amino Acid' also counts a lot, as shown in Table 4.8.

In general, the dieticians recommend larger consumption of vegetable proteins, as compared to animal protein resources. This would help obtain comparable amounts of complete proteins.

TABLE 4.8: LIMITING AMINO ACIDS AND VEGETABLE (PROTEIN) FOODS

	Category of Foods/ Vegetables	Limiting Amino Acids
1.	Cereal Grain Products	Lysine, Threonine
2.	Legumes and Pulses	Methionine, Tryptophan
3.	Green Leafy Vegetables	Methionine
4.	Leaves and Grasses	Methionine
5.	Nuts and Oilseeds	Lysine

Essential Amino Acid Composition of Different Foodstuffs

(mg amino acid/g protein)

EFA	Hen's Eggs	Cow's Milk	Beef Muscles	Wheat Flour
Isoleucine	54	47	53	42
Leucine	86	95	82	71
Lysine	70	78	87	20
Methionine and Cystine	57	33	38	31
Phenylalanine and Tyrosine	93	102	75	79
Threonine	47	44	43	28
Tryptophan	17	14	12	11
Valine	66	64	55	42

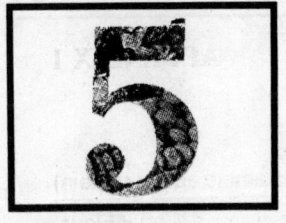

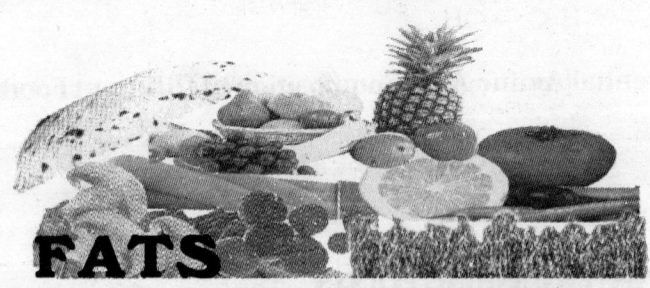

FATS

FATS (LIPIDS)

An important major nutrient, fats have been mired in many a controversy owing to the name being associated with a number of current health problems, particularly heart diseases. The blame however rests not upon fats *per se*, but on the man's natural hankering for higher intake of dietary fat.

In the Western countries, fats contribute over 45% of the total caloric intake, though in the Third World, this proportion comes down to 20-30 % (or even less). Energy apart, fat plays an important role in human diet.

LIPIDS

Fats are members of a class of compounds called 'Lipids'. The lipids in food and in the human body include triglycerides (fats and oils), phospholipids and sterols. Chemically, fats are organic substances consisting of the basic element carbon with attached hydrogen and oxygen atoms and other radicals. The basic structural elements of fats are the same as those of carbohydrates. Though they differ in many ways, fats contain more carbon and hydrogen and less oxygen. Fats are more complex in nature, with fatty acids as the common structural unit. Chemical name of fats is triglyceride-esters of glycerol and 3 molecules of fatty acids. These are called 'Endogenous Fats', since they form a part of internal body tissues. When they are part of the diet from outside plant/animal sources, they are called 'Exogenous Fats'.

A typical fat molecule consists of glycerol combined with 3 fatty acids. Glycerol and butyric acid, common fatty acids found in the butter have the following formula:

$$H_2C - OH$$
$$|$$
$$HC - OH \qquad HOOC - CH_2 - CH_2 - CH_3$$
$$| \qquad\qquad\qquad\qquad (Butyric\ Acid)$$
$$H_2C - OH$$
(Glycerol)

DISTINGUISHING POINTS

Fats differ very significantly from the other macronutrients like proteins and carbohydrates in following respects:

1. Fats are a dense energy source. Their energy efficiency lies in the fact that they provide 9 kcal/g energy, as against 4 kcal/g of proteins and carbohydrates.
2. Fats in the natural foods have other important macronutrients as important components associated with them, like

   (a) Vitamins A, D, E and K
   (b) Sterols—Cholesterols in vegetable fats
   (c) Natural lipid emulsifier—Phospholipids.

3. Fats do not form long molecular chains.
4. Fats do not contribute to any structural strength to animal or plant issue.
5. Fats are not the polymers of repeating molecular units.
6. Fats have special properties like shortening, lubricating, emulsifying and whipping, thus facilitating wider usage in the food industry.
7. Fats, as a raw material, are a versatile group of natural fats with varying properties. They can be blended with various natural hydrogenated or crystallized fats to yield an endless number of permutations and combinations i.e., Fats can be tailor-made for diverse usage.

DIETARY FATS

To keep healthy, a man needs fats in the food, as also in his body. Both the food fats and the body fats perform important functions in nutrition, as listed below.

A: Food Fats

1. **Fuel Source:** For supplying basic fuel for energy (9 kcal/g).
2. **Essential Nutrients:** Food fats provide essential fatty acids, particularly Linoleic acid and Arachidonic acid, both needed to supplement the endogenous supply.
3. **Satiety:** Fats impart a special aroma or flavour to the food that leads to greater satisfaction or satiety that lasts long. This satiety is enhanced by the full texture and body that fat lends to the food and also to the slowing down of the gastric emptying time.

Body Fats

1. Energy: The most important function of fats is to supply an efficient fuel to the body tissue, except for the central nervous system which depends upon glucose.
2. Insulation: The fat layer under the skin provides thermal insulation by controlling the body temperature.
3. Protection: The adipose fat surrounding the organs acts as a protection pad against shocks to sensitive organs like kidneys.
4. Fat is a constituent of cell membranes that helps in the transport of nutrients and other metabolites in the system.
5. Impulse Transmission: The fat surrounding the nerve fibres provides electrical insulation and transmits nerve impulses.
6. Metabolism: By combining with proteins, it forms 'Lipoproteins', which carry fat in the blood to the cells all over the body.
7. Precursors: By providing fatty acids and cholesterol, it helps in the synthesis of many more compounds required for the body metabolism.

CLASSIFICATION OF FATS (LIPIDS)

Fats are classified into three main groups:

Simple Lipids

These are the neutral fats, chemically made up of triglycerides. A triglycaride contains a glycerol base with 3 fatty acids as shown below:

$$C_3H_5(OH_2C—OHH)_3 + 3 \text{ molecules Fatty acids} \rightarrow \text{Neutral Fat.}$$

These neutral fats account for almost 99% of food and body fats.

Compound Lipids

The compound lipids are made of simple lipids containing phosphorous, carbon and proteins. Such compounds are known as phospholipids, glycolipids and lipoproteins. However, it is the lipoproteins which are the most important, as they act as carriers of lipids in blood and also form cell membranes. On the other hand, phospholipids are usually associated with the nerves and the nervous system.

Derived Lipids

They are the fat-like substances obtained from fats and fatty compounds. Glycerol and fatty acids are the two important derived lipids. Glycerols make up about 10% of the body fat. It is the water-soluble base of triglycerides or neutral fats. In the process of digestion, glycerol is removed and made available for conversion to glucose.

Unsaponifiable Lipids

This group of unsaponifiable lipids includes steroids and terpenoids substances that contain sterols—cholesterol being the most important member of this group.

FATTY ACIDS

Fatty acids are the key refined fuels of fat that the cells burn for securing energy. They are the structural part of fats and may be saturated or unsaturated fatty acids depending upon the double bond between the carbon atoms in their molecules. Important fatty acids are oleic acid, linoleic acid, linolenic acid, arachidonic acid, palmitic acid, myristic acid and stearic acid.

The food fats are a mixture of both saturated and unsaturated fatty acids. The saturated fatty acids in a fat make it solid at room temperature, whereas the unsaturated ones keep it as a liquid.

As a rule, most of the animal fats are saturated, while those of plant origin are unsaturated fatty acids. Table 5.1 gives the composition of different oils.

TABLE 5.1: FATTY ACID COMPOSITION OF COMMON OILS

	Oil		Saturated Fatty Acid	Mono-unsaturated Fatty Acid	Poly-unsaturated Fatty Acid
1.	Coconut Oil	- Cocus mucifera	91	8	1
2.	Cottonseed Oil	- Gossypum	34	26	40
3.	Groundnut Oil	- Arachis hypogaea	20	54	26
4.	Mustard Oil	- Brassica compes	6	73	21
5.	Niger Oil	- Guizotia abyssinica	10	35	55
6.	Palm Oil	- Elaeis guinensis	80	13	7
7.	Safflower Oil	- Carthamus tinctorious	11	13	76
8.	Sesame Oil	- Sesamum indicum	14	46	40
9.	Soyabean Oil	- Glycine max	15	25	60
10.	Sunflower Oil	- Helianthus annus	8	34	58

Source: Central Food Technological Research Institute, Mysore.

If a fat is filled with hydrogen, it is called saturated fat. But if it not so saturated with hydrogen, then it is called unsaturated fat.

Cis-Fatty Acids

Cis-fatty acids refers to the structural configuration of the fatty acid molecule, where the hydrogens next to carbon-to-carbon double bonds are on the same side, assuming a U-shape. This Cis-configuration occurs naturally in foods, but becomes trans-fatty acids when the foods are processed.

Essential Fatty Acids (EFAs)

The type of fatty acids present in the fat may be essential or non-essential. The body cannot synthesize essential fatty acids. As such, they have got to be supplied through diet. The three fatty acids considered physiologically essential are:

Linoleic Acid
Linolenic Acid
Arachidonic Acid.

On the other hand, non-essential fatty acids synthesized in the body are:

Palmitic Acid
Oleic Acid
Butyric Acid.

Of the EFAs, linoleic acid and linolenic acid must be present in the diet. Linoleic acid serves as a precursor for the biosynthesis of arachidonic acid. These essential fatty acids play a very important role in the body, as under:

1. Membrane Structures: Linoleic acid, by preventing an excessive increase in skin and membrane permeability, strengthens cell membranes. The lack of linoleic acid in body results in a breakdown of skin integrity and causes eczema and skin lesions. Many other tissue membranes show similar effect.

2. Transporting Cholesterol: Linoleic and other fatty acids combine with cholesterol to form cholesterol esters, which can be transported by blood.

3. Serum-Cholesterol: The EFAs help lower the serum-cholesterol levels. They thus help in the transport of cholesterol and also its proper metabolism in the body.

4. Blood Clotting: The metabolic products of the EFAs help prolong the blood clotting time. They also result in increased fibrinolytic activity.

5. Local Hormone-like Action: Linoleic acid is an important precursor of eicosanoids. These physiologically active compounds are prostacyclins, prostaglandis, thromboxanes and leukonutrienes. All of these are long 20-carbon chain polyunsaturated fatty acids and have got a profound hormone-like effect. Their compounds are synthesized from arachidonic acid in the body.

However, a more comprehensive spectrum of these food fats and their physiologic action is given in Fig. 5.1.

Free Fatty Acids (FFA)

Free fatty acids are non-esterified fatty acids. Plasma free fatty acids like oleic acid, palmitic acid, stearic acid and linolenic acid are bound to serum albumin as a part of the lipoproteins. They help in the transport of fat, both from alimentary sources and from fat depots to be oxidized in various tissues. During periods of fasting, there is an increase of EFAs from depot fat, while glucose and insulin administration decreases the movement of depot fatty acids to plasma FFA.

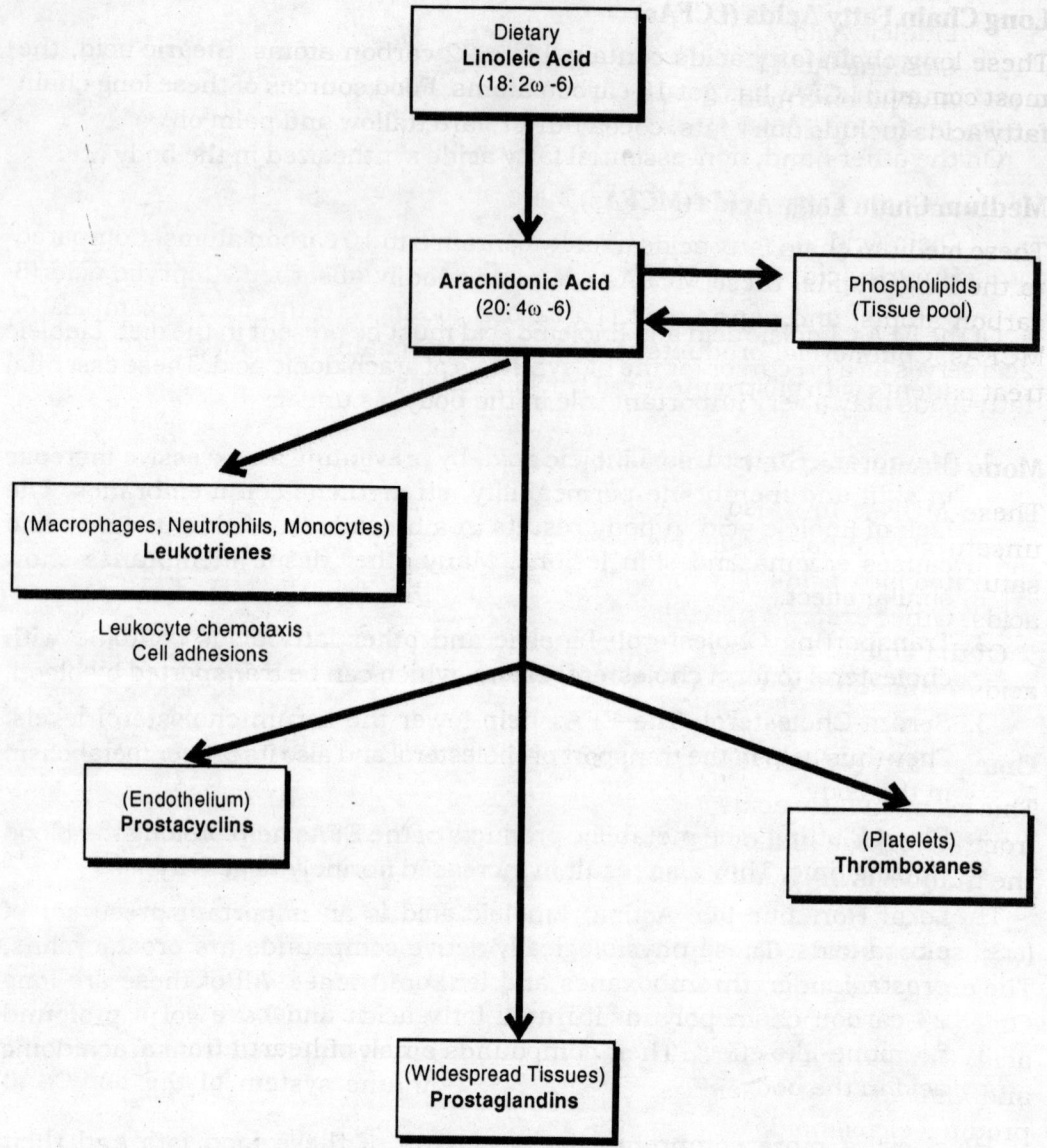

Fig. 5.1: Spectrum of Food Fats according to Degree of Saturation of Component Fatty Acid

Long Chain Fatty Acids (LCFAs)

These long chain fatty acids contain 12 to 22 carbon atoms. Stearic acid, the most common LCFA, has got 18 carbon atoms. Food sources of these long chain fatty acids include dairy fats, cocoa butter, lard, tallow and palm oil.

Medium Chain Fatty Acids (MCFAs)

These medium chain fatty acids usually contain 8 to 10 carbon atoms. Compared to the long chains, these MCFAs are more readily absorbed. Caprylic acid (8 carbon atoms) and capric acid (10 carbon atoms) are the main examples of MCFAs. Commercial products of these medium-chain triglycerides are used to treat patients with gastrointestinal tract infections.

Mono Unsaturated Fatty Acids (MUFAs)

These MUFAs are also called monoenoic fatty acids—those with only one unsaturated linkage or double bond, having two hydrogen atoms fewer than the saturated fatty acids. The most abundant MUFAs are oleic acid and palmitoleic acids. Other examples are olive oil and canola oil.

Of the animal fats, lard, suet and chicken fat have 40-50% of the total fatty acids as monounsaturated fatty acids.

Omega Fatty Acids (OFAs)

This group of fatty acids is designated by the position of double bonds starting from the omega end or the methyl (CH_3) carbon. The symbol ω is followed by the number, which indicates the location of the nearest double bond.

The three examples of OFAs of greater dietary significance are the Omega-3 (ω3), such as linolenic acid, eicosapentaenoic acid, and docosahexaenoic acid. The omega-6 (ω6) group includes linoleic acid and arachidonic acid, while the Omega-9 (ω9) group includes oleic acid. Omega-9 is a monounsaturated fatty acid. Omega-3 is reported to help reduce the risk of heart attacks. Omega-3 and Omega-9 fatty acids strengthen the immune system of the body and produce eicosanoids.

Prostaglandins

Prostaglandin is the most important omega-3 long chain fatty acid. Though initially thought to originate from prostrate glands, these eicosanoids exist in all the body tissues. Prostaglandins play the role of local hormones by directing and coordinating important biologic functions. These Prostaglandins are powerful modulators of vascular smooth muscle tone and platelet aggregation. That way, this group of eicosanoids plays a very crucial role in cardiovascular disease.

Food Sources of Omega Fatty Acids

Omega-3	Very abundant in Fish Oils, viz., salmon, mackerel, tuna and anchovy.
Fatty Acids	Limited amounts in plant sources, like linseed, rapeseed (Canola), walnut and wheat germ.
Omega-6 Fatty Acids	Plant sources: corn, cottonseed, saffron and soyabeans and sunflowers oil.
	Animal sources: Dairy products and Organ meats.

Polyunsaturated Fatty Acids (PUFAs)

The polyunsaturated fatty acids have two or more unsaturated linkages or double bonds and they are categorized as dienoic, trienoic and tetraenoic acids. The most significant members of PUFA group are:

Linoleic Acid	-	(Two double bonds)
Linolenic Acid	-	(Three double bonds)
Arachidonic Acid	-	(Four double bonds)

The polyunsaturated fatty acids play an important role in immune function, fat transport and metabolism, as also in the maintenance of the integrity of cell membranes.

| Fat sources very rich in PUFAs: | Corn, cottonseed, safflower, sesame, soyabeans and safflower oil. |

Saturated Fatty Acids (SFAs)

These fatty acids have all the carbon atoms of the molecule linked to hydrogen, so that only one single bond exists. These saturated fatty acids impart firmness to fats at room temperature. Herein, the important SFAs are palmitic acid and stearic acid.

| Primary Animal food sources: | Butter, bacon, cream, lard, pork, meat and poultry. |
| Plant sources: | Palm oil and coconut oil. |

Table 5.2 gives the fatty acids contents of fats of animal and plants origin.

Short Chain Fatty Acid (SCFAs)

These fatty acids have less than 6 carbon atoms. Though these short chains are very abundant in food fats, yet their energy value is low about 5 kcal/g versus 9 kcal of long chain fatty acids. Also called 'Volatile Fatty Acids', this group includes caproic acid (6 carbon atoms) and butyric acid (4 carbon atoms). The SCFAs are basically the products of bacterial fermentation of indigestible carbohydrates and fibre polysaccharides.

TABLE 5.2: FATTY ACID CONTENT OF FATS OF ANIMAL AND PLANT ORIGIN

| | Saturated Fats | | | Unsaturated Fats | | |
Animal Fats	Palmitic	Stearic	Others	Oleic	Linoleic	Others
Lard	29.8	12.7	1.0	47.8	3.1	5.6
Chicken	25.6	7.0	0.3	39.4	21.8	5.9
Butterfat	25.2	9.2	25.6	29.5	3.6	7.2
Beef fat	29.2	21.0	3.4	41.1	1.8	3.5
Vegetable Oils						
Corn	8.1	2.5	0.1	30.1	56.3	2.9
Peanut	6.3	4.9	5.9	61.1	21.8	—
Cottonseed	23.4	1.1	2.7	22.9	47.8	2.1
Soyabean	9.8	2.4	1.2	28.9	50.7	7.0@
Olive	10.0	3.3	0.6	77.5	8.6	—
Coconut	10.5	2.3	78.4	7.5	Traces	1.3

(*Source*: NRC Pub. No. 575: The Role of Dietary Fat in Human Health)
    @ - Mostly Linolenic acid.

Energy apart these short chain fatty acids promote sodium and water absorption in the colon. They also stimulate pancreatic enzyme secretion, besides helping in the proliferation of gut mucosa. They promote wound healing after bowel resection. The short-chain fatty acids play a very beneficial role in conditions like short bowel syndrome, ulcerative colitis and disuse atrophy.

Trans-Fatty Acids (TFAs)

Herein, the hydrogen atoms, next to the carbon-to-carbon double bonds, are on the opposite side, assuming a linear form. These trans-fatty acids raise the plasma levels of LDL-cholesterol and lower the HDL-cholesterol. The process of hydrogenation in Vanaspati making converts some Cis-fatty acids into trans-fatty acids.

Unsaturated Fatty Acids (UFAs)

These are the fatty acids which contain one or more double bonds between one or more of the carbon atoms in the chain. All the unsaturated fatty acids are liquid at room temperatures. Vegetable oils like olive oil, corn oil, cottonseed oil and soyabean oil are the rich food source of the UFAs.

Very Long Chain Fatty Acids (VLFAs)

Herein, the carbon chain comprises of 24 or more carbon atoms. The best example of the group is hexacosanoic acid (C 26 : 0). This VLFA group is associated with the condition, Adrenoleukodystrophy (ALD).

SPECIAL COMPOUND LIPIDS

Lipoproteins

Lipoproteins are the compounds of fats with proteins which play a very significant role in human nutrition. Lipoproteins are the complexes of lipids and apoproteins which provide the main vehicle for the transport of fat in the blood stream. Since fat is insoluble in water, the lipoproteins provide packages of fat wrapped in water-soluble proteins. These plasma lipoproteins contain fatty acids and other important compounds like triglycerides, cholesterols and phospholipids, besides traces of fat-soluble vitamins and steroid hormones. It is the relative share of fat and proteins which helps determine the high or low density of lipids, the higher density accounting for greater proportion of proteins.

There are 5 subgroups of Lipoproteins:

1. **Chylomicrons:** Their special role is to deliver diet fat to liver cells so that it could be converted to other lipids. Chylomicrons are formed in the intestinal wall following a meal. They have a very high proportion of fat (90%) but the protein share is very small. As such they have a low density.

2. **Very Low-Density Lipoproteins (VLDLs):** These lipoproteins help transport triglycerides to the tissue cells in the body.

3. **Intermediate Low-Density Lipids (ILDLs):** Their role is the same as of the lipoproteins in number 2.

4. **Low-Density Lipoproteins (LDLs):** These LDLs help transport cholesterol to the peripheral tissue cells.

5. **High-Density Lipoproteins: (HDLs):** This high-density group helps in the transfer of free cholesterols from body tissues to lever for catabolism and excretion.

Phospholipids

These are compounds of triglycerides, phosphoric acid and a nitrogenous base. A phospholipid is similar in structure to the triglycerides but has a phosphorous containing acid, such as colin attached to the glycerol base, taking the place of fatty acids. The largest group of phospholipids are the 'Lecithins'. The lecithins are not dietary essential, but they certainly are essential tissue component. They also help coat fat droplets for transport within the body, acting as detergent to keep the fat particles finely dispersed. This detergent action is essential for normal functioning of the lungs.

Glycolipids

The Glycolipids are similar compound lipids with two fatty acids attached to two of the glycerol-base carbon atoms, but with a different radical attached to the

3rd carbon atom. The simple glycolipids contain galactose as the carbohydrate with sphingosine, a long chain monounsaturated amino alcohol, supplying the nitrogen. Because they are found solely in the brain tissue, so they are also called 'Cerebrosides'.

Sterols
Cholesterol

Though associated with fats and lipids, in reality cholesterol is not a fat. It is only a fat-related compound that is quite distinct in structure from triglycerides. Cholesterol usually travels in blood attached to long chain fatty acids in the form of cholesterol esters. Cholesterol plays a crucial role in metabolism in the body and is a precursor to the all the steroid hormones.

A compound, 7-dehydrocholesterol which is a derivative of cholesterol, is irradiated by ultraviolet rays to produce a vitamin D hormone. Cholesterol is also essential for the formation of bile acids, which emulsify fats by enzymatic digestion. It then serves as a carrier for fat absorption. Besides being present in large amount in brain and nerve tissues, cholesterol is found in all the cells of body and is indeed an essential component of cell membranes. Even if the diet contains no cholesterol, the body is able to synthesize the required amount on its own.

Cholesterol, *prima facie*, occurs in animal foods, but none in the plants. The main food sources of cholesterol are egg yolk, liver and kidney muscles.

From the health angle, cholesterol is the main culprit in the development of atherosclerosis, which leads to many coronary heart diseases. The high serum cholesterol levels leads to the formation of fatty plaques in the blood vessels. As such, it is advisable to reduce the dietary cholesterol intake to 300 mg/day. Probably the most effective preventive measure is to increase the amount of soluble diet fibre in the food. These fibres bind the bile acids and dietary cholesterol, thus helping remove extra cholesterol from the body.

DIGESTION OF FATS

The process of digestion helps break the food fats into the refined body fuel of fatty acids, as under:

Mouth

The fats are broken down in the mouth into small particles through mastication. These are then moistened for smooth passage into the stomach.

Stomach

The peristaltic movements help mix fats with stomach secretions. There is not much of an enzymatic action, except that of gastric lipase, which acts on emulsified butter fat. Thus, fat is separated from other nutrients and is made readily available for further action in the small intestine.

Small Intestine

It is only in the small intestines that the fats are chemically broken down. Herein, the secretions from liver and gall bladder and others from pancreas and small intestine do the formal breaking of the fat particles. Cholecystokin hormone from intestinal walls helps lower the surface tension of the suspended fat globules and thus allows the enzyme to penetrate more easily. The bile also provides an alkaline medium for the action of fat enzyme, Lipase.

Pancreatic Lipase, a powerful fat enzyme, breaks off one fatty acid at a time from the glycerol base of fats. The final product of fat digestion to be absorbed in the body are fatty acids, viz., diglycerides, monoglycerides and glycerol. The enzyme cholesterol enterase acts on free cholesterol to form cholesterol esters by combining free cholesterol and fatty acids for final absorption. Another enzyme in the small intestine, lecithinase acts on lecithins to break them down into smaller particles for absorption. Table 5.3 gives the summary of fat digestion.

TABLE 5.3: SUMMARY OF FAT DIGESTION

Organ	Enzyme	Activity
Mouth	–	Mechanical breakdown through mastication
	Gastric Lipase (small amount)	Converts butter fat to fatty acids and glycerol.
Small Intestines		
	Gall Bladder Bile salts	Emulsification of Fats
	Pancreatic Lipase	Converts triglycerides to diglycerides and monoglycerides and finally to fatty acids and glycerol.

ABSORPTION OF FATS

The final breakdown products—triglycerides and other fat materials are wrapped in proteins to form lipoproteins, called Chylomicrons. These are then carried into a milk-like liquid, Chyle. These then cross the cell membrane into lymphatic system and are carried into portal blood. Here, the enzyme, Lipoprotein lipase helps clear the large mass of dietary fat from blood circulation. The liver converts the fat to other lipoproteins, which are then transported to the body cells all over for energy and other structural functions.

FATS AND HEALTH

The overall health implication of the fats may be summarized as under:

1. Saturated fatty acids elevate blood cholesterol and are the main dietary determinants of blood cholesterol levels. Diets low in saturated fatty acids helped lower blood cholesterol levels.
2. Adding polyunsaturated fatty acids to the diet lowered blood cholesterol levels still further.

3. The omega-3 fatty acids appear to reduce blood cholesterol. Herein, the most conclusive evidence came from the Inuit people of Alaska and Greenland, who otherwise consumed high-energy, high-fat, high cholesterol diets. Their marine food were rich in omega-3 fatty acids, particularly EPA and DHA—hence the recommendations of the American Heart Association to use 2-3 fish meals per week.

4. Omega-3 fatty acids also help prevent cancer. It is reported that polyunsaturated fats and fish oils may delay cancer development, slow tumour growth rates and reduce the size of tumour.

5. Mono-unsaturated fatty acids seems to have cholesterol, although it is less so than polyunsaturated fatty acids. This fact is noticed when olive oil or canula oil replace beef fat in the diet.

Diet Recommendations

The dietary guidelines recommend that total fat intake should not be more than 30% of the total energy consumed; it should preferably be brought down to 20%. As such, saturated fats should not exceed 10% and further that the remaining 10% may be provided through monounsaturated fats. For cholesterol intake, the recommended guideline is 300 mg per day.

FAT REPLACERS

The Western markets offer fat-free bakery products, frozen desserts and a variety of cheese that taste rich, but offer less than half a gram of fat in each serving. Many of the products use traditional ingredients like sugar, starch, non-fat milk, soluble fibre and egg white in place of fat.

Other products use designated fat-replaces. These fall into 3 categories:

1. Carbohydrate-based replacers
2. Protein-based replacers
3. Fat-based replacers.

1. **Carbohydrate-based Fat Replacers:** The US Deparment of Agriculture has developed Oatrim, which is derived from oat fibre. Not only that it lowers cholesterol, it also provides dietary fibre. Oatrim is used in frozen desserts, salad dressings and bakery products. Another item is Z-trim prepared from seed hulls of oats, peas, soyabeans, rice or from the bran of corn and wheat. Z-trim provides no calories, nor does it lend any flavour to the foods. It can be used in baked goods, cheese and meat products.

2. **Protein-based Fat Replacers:** 'Simplesse' has been approved by the FDA for use in ice creams and frozen desserts. It is made from proteins of egg white or milk. Simplesse cuts down the calorie content by 80% and imparts rich taste and texture to the foods. It is used in ice creams, yogurts, salad dressings, butter and mayonnaise.

3. **Fat-based Replacers:** These replacers use triglycerides that have been altered to contain the desired level of fatty acids. Salatrim and Olestra are the examples of this category of fat-replacers. Olestra is the only synthetic product approved officially. It is a combination of sucrose and fatty aids that looks, feels and tastes like food fats.

Of all the fat replacers in the market, olestra is the product most widely in demand. Olestra is fortified with vitamins A, D, E and K for any possible loss of nutrients in the new combination of foods.

Common Fatty Acids

Common Name	Systematic Name	No. of Carbon Atoms	No. of Double Bonds	Typical Fat Source
Saturated Fatty Acids				
Butyric	Butanoic	4	0	Butterfat
Caproic	Hexanoic	6	0	Butterfat
Caprylic	Octanolic	8	0	Coconut oil
Capric	Decanoic	10	0	Coconut oil
Lauric	Dodecanoic	12	0	Coconut oil, Palm kernel oil
Myristic	Tetradecanoic	14	0	Butterfat, Coconut oil
Palmitic	Hexadecanoic	16	0	Palm oil, Animal fat
Stearic	Octadecanoic	18	0	Cocoa butter, Animal fat
Arochidic	Elcosanoic	20	0	Peanut oil
Behenic	Docosanoic	22	0	Peanut oil
Unsaturated Fatty Acids				
Caproleic	9-Decenoic	10	1	Butterfat
Lauroleic	9-Dodecenoic	12	1	Butterfat
Myristoleic	9-Tetradecenoic	14	1	Butterfat
Palmitoleic	9-Hexadecenoic	16	1	Some Fish oil, Beef fat
Oleic	9-Octadecenoic	18	1	Olive oil, Canola oil
Elaidic	9-Octadecenoic	18	1	Butterfat
Vacceric	11-Octadecenoic	18	1	Butterfat
Linoleic	9, 12-Octadecadienoic	18	2	Most vegetables oils esp. Safflower, Corn, Soyabean, Cottonseed
Linolenic	9, 12, 15-Octadecatrienoic	18	3	Soyabean oil, Canola oil, Walnuts, Wheat Germ
Gadoleic	9-Eicosenoic	20	1	Some Fish oils
Arachidonic	5, 8, 11, 14-Eicosatetra-enoic	20	4	Lard Meats
—	5, 8, 11, 14, 17-Eicosa-pentaenoic (EPA)	20	5	Some Fish oils, Shelfish
Erucic	13-Docosenoic	22	1	Canola oil
—	4, 7, 10, 13, 16, 19-Do-cosahexaenoic (DHA)	22	6	Some Fish oils, Shellfish

Adapted from *ISEO: Food Fats and Oils*, 6th ed. Washington DC, Institute of Shortening and Edible Oils, 1998.

APPENDIX 2

Fat Content of Some Common Foods

0 gram Fat	1-3 grams Fat	4-6 grams Fat	7-10 grams Fat	15 grams Fat	20 grams Fat	25+ grams Fat
Most fruits and Vegetables	Popcorn, oil-popped, unbuttered, 1 cup	Low-fat yogurt, 1 cup	Cheese, cheddar, 1 oz	Hot Dog, Beef, 2 oz	Cheese cake, 1/12 cake	Polish Sausage, 3 oz
Nonfat Milk	Low-calorie Salad dressing, 1 tsp	Cheese, Mozarella, part-skin, 1 oz	Milk, whole, 1 cup	McDonald's Chicken Mcnuggets, 6 pieces	Losagna with Meat, 1 medium piece	Cheeseburger, large
Nonfat Yogurt	Baked Beans, ½ cup	Chicken, roasted with skin, 3 oz	Bologna, Beef, 1 oz	Peanut Butter, 1 tsp	Macaroni and Cheese, homemade, 1 cup	Pie, pecan, 1/8th of 9"
Plain pasta and Rice	Soup, Chiken noodle, canned, 1 cup	Egg, scrambled, 1	Sausage, 1 patty	Pork chop, broiled, 3 oz	Peanuts, dry roasted, ¼ cup	Chicken pot pie, frozen, baked, 1 pie
Angel food cake	Whole Wheat bread, 1 slice	Turkey, roasted, 3 oz	Steak, sirloin, broiled, 3 oz	Sunflower seeds, dry roasted, ¼ cup	Ground Beef, broiled, 3 oz	Quiche, Bacon, 1/8 pie
Popcorn, air-popped, unbuttered	Dinner roll, 1	Granola, 1 cup	Potatoes, French fried, 10	Avocado, ½ meium		
Soft Drinks	Waffle, frozen, 4", 1	Muffin, Bran, 1 small	Chow mein, Chicken, 1 small	Chop suey, Beef and Pork, 1 cup		
Jam, Jelly	Coleslaw, ½ cup	Pizza, Cheese, ¼ of 12"	Corn chips, 1 oz	Cinnamon roll, 1		
	Flounder or sole, baked, 3 oz	Burrito, Bean, 1	Doughnut, cake			
	Chicken, without skin, roasted, 3 oz	Browine, with nuts, 1 small	Mayonnaise, 1 tsp			
	Tuna, canned in water, 3 oz	Margarine or Butter, type, plain, 1 tsp	Chocolate candy bar, 1 oz			
	Cheese, cottage, 2 % fat, ½ cup	Popcorn, Oil popped, buttered, 1 cup				
	Ice Milk, soft serve, ½ cup	French Dressing, regular, 1 tsp				

Source: Data from Healthy Dividends, Rosemont, 14 National Dairy Council, 1990.

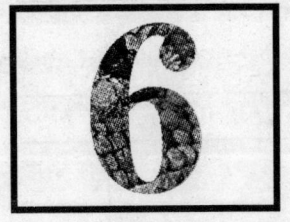

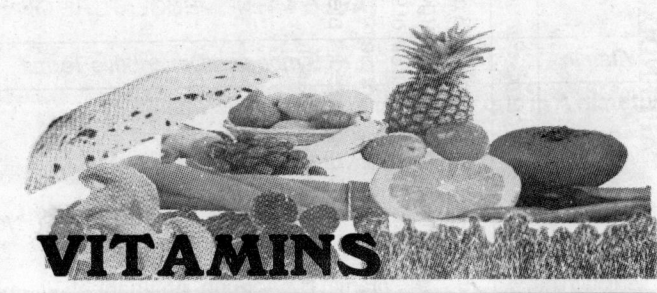

VITAMINS

Vitamins are organic compounds, which are needed, in very small amounts to regulate some body functions. Vitamins are not energy-providing carbohydrates, fats or proteins but they are meant to perform specific metabolic functions of growth, maintenance and reproduction or to prevent an associated deficiency disease. They function in enzyme systems, which facilitate the metabolism of proteins, fats and carbohydrates. Most of the vitamins are not synthesized by the body and hence these must be supplied through the diet.

Vitamins are divided into two categories, depending upon their solubility:

(a) Fat-soluble Vitamins   –   Vitamins A, D, E and K
(b) Water-soluble Vitamins   –   Vitamins B group and Vitamin C.

Provitamins are the substances which the human body can convert into vitamins like:

(1) β-Carotene, the precursor of vitamin A, also called Provitamin A
(2) Dehydrocholesterol and Ergesterol, the precursors of Vitamin D.

The fat soluble vitamins show the following characteristics:

1. Not easily destroyed by fats/cooking oils.
2. Being stored in the body, they cause toxicity when supplied in excess.
3. If mineral oil is present in the intestine, it hampers their absorption.
4. Destroyed by rancidity

Unlike the past, when the vitamins were known by alphabet letters, nowadays all the vitamins are known by their chemical nature/functions, as shown in Table 6.1

TABLE 6.1: NOMENCLATURE OF VITAMINS

Vitamin	Synonyms/Descriptive Terms
Vitamin A group	Antixerophthalmic Vitamin
A_1	Retinol
A_2	Dehydroretinol
A acid	Retinoic acid (Tretinoin)
Provitamin A	Carotene (α and β), Cryptoxanthin (Hydroxyl β carotene)
Vitamin B group	Formerly Vitamin B complex
Thiamine	Vitamin B_1, Aneurin, Anti-beriberi Vitamin, Antineuritic Factor
Riboflavin	Vitamin B_2, Lactoflavin, Ovoflavin, Yellow Enzyme
Niacin	Nicotinic acid and Nicotinamide, Pellagra-preventive Factor, Anti Black Tongue Factor
Pantothenic acid	Formerly Vitamin B_3, Chick Antidermatitis Factor, Anti-Grey Hair Factor
B_6	Pyrodoxine, Pyridoxal, Pyrodoxamine, Rat Acrodynia Factor
Biotin	Co-enzyme R
Folacin	Folic acid (Pteroylglutamic acid, PGA) and Polyglutamates, Tetrahydrofolic acid, Folinic acid (formerly Citroverum factor)
B_{12}	Anti-Pernicious Anaemia Vitamin, Cyanocobalamin, Hydroxocobalamin (formerly Vitamin B_{12a}), Aquocobalamin (formerly Vitamin B_{12b}) and Nitrocobalamin (formerly Vitamin B_{12c})
Vitamin C	L-ascorbic acid, L-dehydroascorbic acid, Antiscorbutic Vitamin
Vitamin D group	Antirachitic Vitamin
D_2	Ergocalciferol (formerly calciferol), Activated Ergosterol.
D_3	Cholecaliferol, Activated 7-dehydrocholesterol
Vitamin E group	
α-Tocopherols	Possess Vitamin E activity in varying degrees.
β-Tocopherols and	They occur as fatty acid esters
Tocotrienols -	
Gamma (γ) Delta (δ)	
Vitamin K group	Antihaemorrhagic Vitamin
K_1	Phylloquinone } Naturally
K_2	Farmoquinone } occuring
K_3	Menadione, Menaquinone
$K_4 - K_7$	Biologically-active analogues of Menadione (synthetic)

The water-soluble vitamins B and C show the following characteristics:

1. Very unstable, since they are easily affected by heat, light, radiation and oxidation.
2. Affected by culinary practices, if the water in which cooked is thrown away.
3. Excessive intake results in urinary excretion of the surplus vitamins.
4. All are synthesized by the plants and supplied in the diet by plant foods (also animal foods), except for cobalamin (vitamin B_{12}).
5. Storage: All the water-soluble vitamins have no stable storage form. These must therefore be provided regularly in the diet, save for cobalamin (vitamin B_{12}).
6. Function: All serve as co-enzyme factors in cell enzyme reactions.

FAT–SOLUBLE VITAMINS

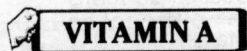 **VITAMIN A**

Vitamin A is a generic term for three compound viz., Retinol, Retinal and Retinoic acid having similar biologic activity. Because of its specific function in the retina (eye) and its being an alcohol, vitamin A has been given the chemical name Retinol. It is soluble in fat and ordinary fat solvents. Being insoluble in water, vitamin A is quite stable in cooking.

There are two dietary forms of vitamin A. One is the performed vitamin A or Retinol. This is the natural vitamin found in animal sources—dairy products, egg yolk and organ meat like liver. The second form is provitamin A, the β carotene. The original source of retinol is this pigment, β carotene which animals eat and then convert to retinol for being stored. It was first called carotene, because it was mainly derived from carrots. It is the most common precursor of vitamin A and supplies nearly two-thirds of vitamin A supply in human nutrition. It is found in all the yellow and orange colored vegetables, as well as green leafy vegetables.

The δ carotene and crytoxanthin also exhibit provitamin A activity, but it is less than that of β carotene.

Digestion and Absorption

The pancreatic and intestinal enzymes hydrolyze Retinyl esters. After absorption, retinol is re-esterified, which is then transported to blood. In the intestine, carotenes are split to form retinaldehyde, which is later reduced to retinol. Some carotenes are absorbed as such and then converted to vitamin A in the liver and kidneys. Bile is necessary for the absorption of vitamin A and carotene. Vitamin E in the intestine helps prevent oxidation of this vitamin. Some fats in the food mix, get simultaneously absorbed and stimulate the release of bile for effective absorption. However, mineral oils hinder their absorption, since they dissolve vitamin A.

Functions

Apart from the main function of vision, vitamin A is associated with epithelial tissue integrity, growth and reproductive functions, as shown below:

1. **Vision:** The eye's ability to adapt to change in light depends on a light-sensitive pigment, rhodopsin, also called visual purple. Rhodopsin is composed of vitamin A substance, retinal and the protein, opsin. In case of vitamin A deficiency, rhodopsin cannot be made and the rods and cons of the retina become very sensitive to light changes, which causes night blindness. But this condition, night blindness can be cured in half an hour by an injection of Vitamin A (retinol), which is readily converted into retinal and further into rhodopsin.

2. **Epithelial Tissue:** Vitamin A is very essential to build and maintain epithelial tissue, which provides the primary barrier to infection. The epithelium includes both the outer skin and the inner mucous membranes. In vitamin A deficiency, the epithelial cells become dry and flat, hardening gradually to form keratin, a process called 'keratinisation'. When the body is deficient in vitamin A, many abnormalities occur, as under:

(i) **Eye:** The cornea dries up and hardens, a condition called as xeropthalmia. In acute cases, it leads to blindness. This is a very serious problem affecting millions of the children in poorer countries.

(ii) **Respiratory Tract:** The ciliated epithelium in the nasal passage dries up, thus removing a barrier to the entry of infection. The salivary glands dry up and the mouth becomes dry and cracked.

(iii) **Gastrointestinal Tract:** Mucosal membrane secretions decrease, resulting in the tissues dying up and sloughing off, which ultimately affects both digestion and absorption.

(iv) **Genito-urinary Tract:** The breaking down of epithelial tissue leads to problems like urinary tract infections, calculi and vaginal infections.

(v) **Skin:** Skin becomes dry and scaly, small pustules and pigmented papular eruptions come up around hair follicles, a condition called as 'follicular hyperkeratosis'.

3. **Growth:** Vitamin A is a very essential pre-requisite for the growth of skeletal and soft tissues. This effect is caused by the vitamin's influence on protein synthesis, mitosis (cell division) or stability of cell membranes.

4. **Reproduction:** In both males and females, the retinoids are necessary to support normal reproductive functions. The deficiency of vitamin A produces sterility, testicular degeneration in the males and malformed or aborted offspring in the females.

Unit of Measurement

The earlier measure of International Unit (IU) has now been universally replaced by 'Retinol' Equivalents' (RE). One RE equals 1 μg retinol or 6 μg of β-carotene. It is also equal to 3.33 IU of vitamin activity from retinol and 10 IU of vitamin A activity from β carotene. The recommended allowance for an adult male in USA is 1000 retinol equivalents. It is 80% in the case of women, which allowance goes up during lactation period.

Toxicity

Longer and prolonged ingestion of vitamin A can lead to Hypervitaminosis A. This manifests in the form of joint pains, loss of hair, thickening of long bones and jaundice. Vitamin A toxicity may also cause liver damage that could lead to portal hypertension and ascites.

Sources of Vitamin A

Yellow and green leafy vegetable and yellow orange colored fruits are the richest source of vitamin A. These include carrots, sweet potatoes, apricots, cantaloupe, spinach, broccoli and cabbage. Preformed vitamin A is supplied by dairy products, egg yolk, liver, kidney and fish. In countries like India, Vanaspati (cooking medium) and margarine have got to be mandatorily fortified with vitamins A and D.

Table 6.2 gives the vitamin A contents of important foods.

TABLE 6.2: FOOD SOURCES OF VITAMIN A

(RDA Women 800 µg RE; Men 1000 µg RE)

	Quantity	Vitamin A Allowance (µg RE)
Bread, Cereals, Rice and Pasta		
This group is not an important source of vitamin A		
Vegetables		
Asparagus	½ cup	196
Beet greens	½ cup	1110
Cabbage	½ cup	790
Broccoli (frozen)	½ cup (chopped)	721
Brussels Sprouts	½ cup (4 sprouts)	121
Carrots (raw)	½ cup (1 med.)	2379
Collard greens	½ cup	2223
Corn	1 small cob	93
Dandelion greens	½ cup	1843
Green Beans	½ cup	102
Green Peas	½ cup	144
Kale	½ cup	1369
Lima Beans	½ cup	60
Mustard greens	½ cup	1218
Pumpkin (canned)	½ cup	2353
Lettuce	½ cup (chopped)	157
Spinach	½ cup	2187
Summer Squash	½ cup	123
Sweet Potato (Baked, in skin)	1 med.	2769
Tomato (cooked)	½ cup	325
Winter Squash	½ cup	1021
Fruits		
Apricot (dried)	4 halves	490
Apricot (fresh)	3 med.	867
Avocado	1 med.	189

Table (*contd.* on page 104)

Table (*contd.* from page 103)

Banana	1 med.	69
Cantaloupe	¼ med.	1386
Grapefruit (pink)	¼ med.	162
Orange juice	½ cup	75
Papaya	1 cup (cubes)	735
Peach	1 med.	399
Prunes (dried)	4 prunes	207
Watermelon	1 wedge (4 x 8 in)	753
Meat, Poultry, Fish, Dry Beans, Eggs and Nuts		
Clams (canned)	2 oz	144
Egg Whole	1 large	78
Liver, Beef	3.5 oz	10,831
Liver, Chicken	3.5 oz	4912
Salmon, pink(raw)	3.5 oz	30
Milk and Dairy Products		
Cheddar Cheese	1 oz	90
Milk, low fat 2% (fortified)	8 oz	150
Milk, Skimmed (fortified)	8 oz	150
Milk, Whole (unfortified)	8 oz	101
Ricotta Cheese (Whole milk)	½ cup	182
Swiss Cheese	8 oz	72
Yogurt, Whole	8 fl oz	84
Fats, Oils and Sugar		
Butter	1 tbsp	138
Margarine	1 tbsp	141

Source: Modern Nutrition in Health and Disease. Vol. 1, Pub. Lea and Febiger.

However, a more categorical distinction aout the pre-formed vitamin A, *i.e.,* Retinol is shown in Table 6.3. The composition of provitamin A, *i.e.* carotenoids, which is of far greater significance in the developing countries, is shown in Table 6.4. It shows their α-carotene, β-carotene and cryptoxanthin contents in a more elaborate manner. Both these tables show the composition per 100 gm of food, which is a better analysis than Table 6.2.

The carotenoid content of vegetables will vary, depending particularly on the variety and the maturity of the vegetable. The dark green outer leaves of a cabbage will have a higher carotenoid content than the pale green heart, for example, and the number of outer leaves discarded will influence the carotenoid content of the cooked cabbage portion. Foods such as sweet potato can vary in colour from white to deep orange depending on the variety, and the total carotenoid content can range from less than 100 µg, to more than 1600 µg per 100 g. Similarly, lettuce varieties with darker green leaves will contain substantially more carotenoids than paler varieties and white cassava will contain no carotenoids, while yellow varieties will contain approximately 760 µg/100 g. In ripening fruit, the decrease in chlorophyll is often accompanied by an increase in carotenoid content thus making mature fruit a better source.

TABLE 6.3: RETINOID CONTENT OF COMMON FOODS

Food	Retinol Activity (µg/100 g)
Milk, Whole, pasteurised	38 - 55
Milk, semi-skimmed, pasteurised	21 - 25
Milk, skimmed, pasteurised	traces
Cream, double	455 - 600
Butter	674 - 1062
Cheese, cheddar	260 - 440
Cheese, cottage	45
Eggs, Whole	159 - 210
Beef, lean	10
Kidney, Pig	63 - 265
Liver, Pig	560 - 14,200
Liver, Calf	8,300 - 31,700
Herring	39 - 46
Mackerel	37 - 55
Sardines, canned in oil, fish only	5 - 11
Salmon, Atlantic	7 - 22
Cod Liver Oil	18,000

Source: The Technology of Vitamins in Food, Ed. Berry Ottaway.

TABLE 6.4: CONTENTS OF CAROTENOIDS IN COMMON FOODS (µg/100 g)

Food	α-carotene	β-carotene	α-crypto-xanthin	β-carotene Equivalent	Retinol Equivalent
Milk, Whole	12	–	–	12	2
Cream, double	238	–	–	238	40
Cheese, cheddar	126	–	–	126	21
Oil, Palm	–	500	–	500	83
Broad Beans	9	165	0	170	28
Green Beans	39	310	0	315	53
Peas	19	290	0	300	50
Asparagus	10	310	0	315	53
Beetroot	20	10	0	20	3
Broccoli	0	675	15	685	114
Carrot, old	2425	6905	0	8115	1355
Carrot, new	1765	4355	190	5330	890
Curly kale	0	3130	32	3145	525

Table (*contd.* on page 106)

Table (*contd.* from page 105)

Pepper, green	9	260	0	265	44
red	135	3165	1220	3840	640
yellow	55	135	0	185	31
Pumpkin	29	940	0	955	160
Spinach	0	3515	35	3535	589
Sweetcorn	Traces	19	155	97	16
Tomato	0	620	35	640	105
Apple	0	12	0	12	2
Apricot	0	560	0	560	93
Pear	0	17	0	17	3
Orange	19	38	0	48	8
Grapefruit	0	2	3	4	Traces
Peach	0	86	51	115	19
Banana	12	14	0	20	3
Kiwi	0	43	4	45	8
Grapes	0	33	0	33	6
Plum	0	430	0	430	72
Strawberry	0	9	0	9	2

Source: The Technology of Vitamins in Food, Ed. Berry Ottaway.

Table 6.5 gives the carotene composition, both total carotenes and β-carotenes of vitamin rich foods on the Indian subcontinent.

TABLE 6.5: FOOD SOURCE OF β-CAROTENES

(mg/100 g Edible Stuff)

Food Source	Total Carotenes	β-Carotenes
Agathi (*Sesbania*)	45,000	15,440
Drumstick, Leaves	42,000	19,690
Amaranthus gangeticus	20,160	8,340 (Some varieties recorded 14,190)
Colocasia, Leaves	15,700	5,920
Mint	18,950	5,480
Ponnarganti	24,000	5,440
Radish, Leaves	13,000	2,200
Fenugreak, Leaves	11,800	9,100
Gogu	17,700	6,970
Spinach	9,440	2,740
Carrots	8,840	6,460
Sweet Potato (Yellow)	2,200	1,810
Pumpkin	2,100	1,160
Chillies, green	2,430	1,007
Orange	2,240	190
Mango, ripe	2,210	1,990
Papaya, ripe	2,740	880
Tomato, ripe	3,010	590
Jack Fruit	510	130

Source: Nutritive Value of Indian Foods, National Institute of Nutrition, Hyderabad.

VITAMIN D

Vitamin D is the anti-rachitic vitamin responsible for calcification of structures. Vitamin D is actually a prohormone, activated in our bodies to its full hormone form, caltiriol. It is as this active hormone that vitamin D builds bones by absorbing and depositing calcium. In regular hormone behaviour, it works in balance with parathyroid hormone, which withdraws bone calcium and thyroid hormone calcitonin, which decreases the formation of new bone-eating cells, the osteoclasts.

There are two compounds with vitamin D activity involved in human nutrition: Ergocalciferol (vitamin D_2) and cholecalciferol (vitamin D_3). Since it is of much greater significance, hence cholecalciferol is the chemical name given to vitamin D in common parlance. It is formed by the sun's ultraviolet irradiation of 7-dehydrocholesterol in the skin. Vitamin D_3 is also found in fish oil. Vitamin D is heat-stable and it is not easily oxidized.

Absorption, Transport and Storage

The absorption of dietary vitamin D_3 takes place in the small intestine with the aid of bile. It mixes with the intestinal bile fat complex and is readily absorbed in their fat pockets. It is then transported to the lymph system, where the excess vitamin is stored.

Active Hormone Synthesis

The synthesis of the active hormonal form of 1, 25-dihydroxycholecalciferol is accomplished by the combined action of skin, liver and kidneys—an overall process that is now called the Vitamin D Endocrine System. In the skin, 7-dehydrocholesterol, the precursor cholesterol compound, is irradiated by the sun's ultraviolet rays to produce vitamin D_3. After synthesis in the skin, vitamin D_3 is transported to the liver. Here, a special liver enzyme converts D_3 to the intermediate product, 25-hydroxycholecalciferol, which is carried to the kidneys. It is in the kidney that the physiologically active vitamin D hormone 1, 25-dihydroxycholecalciferol is formed.

Function of Vitamin D

1. *Calcium and Phosphorus:* In balance with parathyroid hormone and the thyroid hormone calcitonin, the vitamin D hormone stimulates the active transport of calcium and phosphorus from the small intestine.

2. *Bone Mineralisation:* After absorption of calcium and phosphorus, vitamin D hormone continues to work with their minerals to form bone tissue. It directly increases the rate of mineral deposits and their resorption in bones—the process by which bone tissue is built and maintained.

Deficiency of vitamin D causes rickets, characterized by the malformation of skeletal tissue in the growing children.

3. **Basic Cell Processes:** Vitamin D hormone is also involved in widespread basic cell processes in a number of organs like brain, kidney, liver, skin, reproductive tissue and certain cells of the immune system. This offers the possibility of vitamin analogs for the treatment of certain leukemias and skin problems like psoriasis.

Measure and Requirement

Vitamin D is measured in terms of IU of cholecalciferol (vitamin D_3). One IU equals 0.025 mg of pure crystalline vitamin D_3.

The recommended daily allowance (RDA) is 10 µg of cholecalciferol (400 IU) for growing children and pregnant/lactating women. For the young people, it is 10 µg and for adults 5 µg.

Deficiency of Vitamin D

When the body does not have enough vitamin D, it cannot build normal bones, in children, this deficiency results in 'Rickets', the malformation of the skeletal tissues. In the adults, it is called Osteomalacia—occurring mostly in women, during child-bearing age. When rickets occurs, the renal threshold for phosphate excretion is lowered through the influence of parathyroid hormone. As a result, kidneys excrete more phosphate than normal. Vitamin D therapy causes the kidneys to reabsorb more phosphate and excrete less, thus helping maintain the plasma phosphate level.

Toxicity

An intake of 1,000-3,000 IU/kg body weight, *i.e.* about 80-100 times the RDA, can lead to hypercalcemia and other complications, like metastatic calcification and renal calculi in the adults. In the case of children, a dose of 2000 IU can inhibit their linear growth. In advanced case, demineralization of bones occurs, resulting in multiple fractures.

Sources

The conventional foods have very little vitamin D to offer. However, it is the egg yolk, which is the best source. Dairy products contain some vitamin D. Livers of fish and oils extracted therefrom are very rich source of vitamin D. Vitamin D is added to fortify the commercial hydrogenated oils.

Total vitamin D activity in eggs is the sum of cholecalciferol and any 25-hydroxycholecalciferol or other metabolites which may be present. Dietary supplements given to hens can increase the vitamin D content of eggs considerably. Levels of vitamin D in battery eggs in Britain have been shown to vary from 0.5-2.1 µg/100 g depending on the season, with the lowest values in June, and the highest values in July and August.

Table 6.6 shows the vitamin D content of some common foods.

TABLE 6.6: COMMON SOURCES OF VITAMIN D

Food	Vitamin D (µg/100 g)
Milk, Whole, pasteurised	0.03
Milk, semi-skimmed, pasteurised	0.01
Milk, skimmed, pasteurised	0
Cream, double	0.27
Butter	0.8
Cheese, cheddar	0.3
Cheese, cottage	0.03
Cheese, Brie, Camembert	0.2
Cheese, Roquefort	0
Eggs	1.5 (0.5–2.1)
Herring	7.5 – 42.5
Mackerel	2.5 – 25
Salmon, canned	5 – 20
Sardines, canned in oil, fish only	6
Cod Liver Oil	210
Herring Liver Oil	3180

Source: The Technology of Vitamins in Food, Ed. Berry Ottaway.

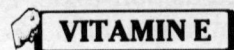 **VITAMIN E**

Named as Tocopherol from a Greek work '*tokos*', which means child birth or to bring forth, it had been known for it reproductive capabilities in rats. But this anti-sterility name has not been scientifically validated so for.

Vitamin E is a generic name for four compounds with similar tocopherol activity α, β, χ and δ tocopherols. Of these, α tocopherol is the most important because of its biologic activity and occurrence. It oxidizes very slowly, which gives it an important role as an anti-oxidant with widespread clinical applications. However, it is δ tocopherols, which shows the highest antioxidant power.

Absorption

Vitamin E is absorbed with the aid of fats and bile salts in the intestine. Along with other lipids in the chylomicrons, it is transported out of intestinal wall into body circulation in blood plasma lipoproteins. It is then stored in different body tissues, especially in fat tissue.

Functions of Vitamin E

1. *As an Antioxidant:* Anti-oxidant vitamin E acts as the nature's most potent fat-soluble anti-oxidant. Its nutritional interaction is seen with a wide

variety of nutrients like vitamin A, selenium, sulfur, amino acids, polyunsaturated fatty acids (PUFA) and possibly vitamin C also.

2. *Cell Membranes:* Vitamin E is known for its most critical interaction with the membranous part of the cells. Here, it integrates with phospholipids, cholesterol and triglycerides which form the main structure of the membranes.

3. *Selenium Relationship:* The trace element selenium spares vitamin E by reducing the vitamin requirement. In a reciprocal manner, vitamin E also helps reduce the selenium requirements. Thus, it provides a second line of defence through the enzyme system, glutathione peroxidase, of which selenium is an integral component.

Deficiency Symptoms

Till so far, no categorical vitamin E deficiency disease has been discovered. However, severe vitamin deficiency may lead to increased haemolysis of the red blood cells, creatinuria, pigmentation of muscles and possibly muscular dystrophy.

Toxicity

Normally, vitamin E is considered as non-toxic. The toxicity symptoms include an increase in serum lipids, impaired blood coagulation and considerable reduction in serum thyroid hormone levels.

Requirement and RDA

Vitamin E is measured in terms of mg of DL-α-tocopherols acetate or as tocopherol equivalent (TE).

Vitamin E requirements vary with the amount of polyunsaturated fatty acids in the diet. The RDA for adults, in α-tocopherol equivalents (α TE), is 10 mg for men and 8 mg for women. For the growing children, it ranges from 3-10 mg TE.

Special Clinical Needs

Vitamin E is a special nutrient in the diet of pregnant and lactating women and also the newborn infants, the old adults and the aged require more vitamin E. A high serum α Tocopherol level was associated with a reduced risk of cancer.

Sources

The richest source vitamin E are the vegetables, which also abound in polyunsaturated fatty acids. Vitamin E is found in a wide range of animal products like dairy products, eggs, meat, besides cereals, nuts, leafy and yellow vegetables.

Table 6.7 gives the vitamin E contents of different food items.

TABLE 6.7: FOOD SOURCES OF VITAMIN E

(RDA for Adult Women 800 mg; Men 100 mg)

	Quantity	Vitamin E (mg α-TE)
1. **Bread, Cereal, Rice and Pasta**		
This food groups is not an important source of vitamin A.		
2. **Vegetables**		
Asparagus (raw)	4 spears / 58g	1.15
Avocado (raw)	1 med./ 173 g	2.32
Brussels Sprouts (boiled)	½ cup (4 sprouts) / 78 g	0.66
Cabbage, green (raw)	½ cup shredded/ / 35 g	0.58
Carrot (raw)	1 med. 72 g	0.32
Lettuce, Iceberg (raw)	¼ head/ 135 g	0.54
Spinach (raw)	½ cup chopped / 28 g	0.53
Sweet Potato (raw)	1 med. / 130 g	5.93
3. **Fruits**		
Apple (raw, with skin)	1 med. / 138 g	0.81
Apricot (canned)	4 halves / 90 g	0.80
Banana (raw)	1 med. / 114 g	0.31
Mango (raw)	1 med. / 207 g	2.32
Pear (raw)	1 med. / 166 g	0.83
4. **Meat, Poultry, fish, Dry Beans and Eggs**		
This food groups is not an important source of vitamin E		
5. **Nuts**		
Almonds (dried)	1 oz / 28 g (24 nuts)	6.72
Hazelnuts (dried)	1 oz / 28 g	6.70
Peanut Butter	1 tbsp / 16 g	3.00
Walnut (dried)	1 oz / 28 g (14 halves)	0.73
6. **Milk and Dairy Products**		
This food group is not an important source of vitamin E		
7. **Fats, Oils and Sugar**		
Corn oil	1 tbsp / 14 g	1.90
Cottonseed oil	1 tbsp / 14 g	4.80
Olive Oil	1 tbsp / 14 g	1.60
Palm Oil	1 tbsp / 14 g	2.60
Peanut Oil	1 tbsp / 14 g	1.60
Safflower Oil	1 tbsp / 14 g	4.60
Soyabean Oil	1 tbsp / 14 g	1.50

Source: *Modern Nutrition in Health and Disease*, Vol. 1.

The total vitamin E activity of foods is primarily due to the presence of α-Tocopherol, although other biologically active tocopherols have been defined. This α-Tocopherol has the greatest biological activity of all the tocopherols, with β-tocopherol having an activity of 40%, and α-tocotrienol having an activity of about 30% of α-tocopherol. γ-Tocopherol has about 10% of the activity of the α form, and the other forms have activities of 5% or less. Vegetable oils are generally the richest source of vitamin E, and wheatgerm oil has the highest content of α-tocopherol, containing 0.85-1.25 mg/g. Some oils such as palm oil contain significant amounts of α- and γ-tocotrienol, as well as α-tocopherol, although some vegetable oils are poor sources of vitamin E, coconut and linseed oils for example.

Table 6.8 outlines the tocopherol contents of a number of different vegetable oils.

TABLE 6.8: TOCOPHEROL CONTENT OF REFINED VEGETABLE OILS, (mg/100 g oil)

Oil	α-T	β-T	γ-T	δ-T	α-T-3	β-T-3	γ-T-3	Vit. E activity
Coconut	0.35	0	0.17	0.35	1.29	0.10	1.32	0.78
Corn	14.26	0.38	64.9	2.75	0.58	0	0	21.1
Cotton seed	35.26	0	29.98	0	0	0	0	38.26
Olive	11.92	0	0.72	0	0	0	0	11.99
Palm	18.32	0	0	0	11.46	0	5.75	21.82
Peanut	11.62	0	12.98	0.33	0	0	0	12.92
Rapeseed	17.65	0	27.04	0.04	0	0	0	20.35
Safflower seed	34.05	0	3.5	0.49	0	0	0	34.4
Soyabean	10.99	0	62.4	20.4	0	0	0	17.43
Sunflower seed	59.5	0	3.54	0	0	0	0	59.85
Wheatgerm	149.44	81.19	0	0	0	0	0	183.0

α-T = α-tocopherol; β-T = β-tocopherol; γ-T = γ-tocopherol; δ-T = δ-tocopherol.
α-T-3 = α-tocotrienol; β-T-3 = β-tocotrienol; γ-T-3 = γ-tocotrienol.
Source: The Technology of Vitamins in Food, Ed. Berry Ottaway.

Non-α-tocopherols are found mainly in non-green tissues such as nuts, fungi and cereal grains, and tocotrienols have been isolated in carrots, kale, broccoli and mushrooms. Tocopherols are more concentrated in the leaves of plants than the roots, and more prevalent in dark green mature leaves than pale or immature leaves, with the lowest amount in the roots and in colourless fruits.

Table 6.9 outlines the α-tocopherol content of some common foodstuffs.

VITAMIN K

Because of its blood clotting function, vitamin K, also called 'Koagulation vitamin' hence the name 'K' taken from this swedish word for its physiologic action.

There are three main groups of Vitamin K:

1. Vitamin K (Phylloquinone), which is the major type found in plants and initially isolated from alfalfa.
2. Vitamin K_2 (Menaquinone), which is synthesized by the intestinal bacteria so that it is not directly needed in the diet.

TABLE 6.9: α-TOCOPHEROL CONTENT OF SOME COMMON FOODS (mg/100 g)

Food	α-tocopherol
Milk, Whole, pasteurised	0.09
Milk, semi-skimmed, pasteurised	0.03
Milk, skimmed, pasteurised	0
Double cream	1.1
Butter	0.5-5.0
Cheese, cheddar	0.6
Eggs	1.1
Beef, average	0.2-0.5
Pork, average	0.1-0.5
Chicken	0.3
Cod	0.2
Herring	0.2-1.1
Prawn	0.9-2.9
Broad Bean	0.05-0.5
Green Bean	0.02-0.2
Peas	0.13-0.21
Asparagus	1.5
Brussels sprouts	0.9
Carrot	0.5
Lettuce	0.5
Parsley	1.7-3.6
Potato	0.06
Spinach	1.75
Watercress	1.3
Apple	0.4
Banana	0.25
Mango	1.1
Orange	0.3
Wheat, Whole grain	0.58-5.2
Oats, Whole grain	1.1
Rice, polished	0.11
Almonds	23-96
Brazil Nuts	6.5
Peanuts	8.3
Sunflower Seeds	50

Source: The Technology of Vitamins in Food, Ed. Berry Ottaway.

3. Vitamin K_3 is a water-soluble analog which does not need bile absorption and goes directly into the portal blood stream.

Absorption, Transport and Storage

More than 50 of the requirement of vitamin K is met by the synthesis by symbiotic bacteria in the lower intestine. After digestion, it is packaged in intestinal chylomicrons and is transported to the lymphatic stream and then into the portal blood for being transported to the liver. It is stored in small amounts in the liver. When administered in therapeutic doses, a large amount of vitamin K is excreted out of the system.

It has been isolated form alfalfa. The major form of this vitamin found in the plants has been named as 'Plylloquinone' for its chemical structure.

Function of Vitamin K

1. **Blood Clotting:** The basic function of vitamin K is to catalyze the synthesis of blood clotting factors in the liver. It produces the active form of several precursors, viz, prothrombin, which combines with calcium to help produce the clotting effect. Vitamin K becomes ineffective if the liver is damaged.

2. **Bone Development:** Osteocalcin, the bone Gla protein, as also the bone matrix Gla protein (MGP) are vitamin K-dependent proteins synthesized by bone and involved with calcium in bone development. These proteins bind calcium but function in bone development to form bone crystals.

Clinical Problems

Clinical problems that relate to vitamin K are:

1. **Malabsorption Disease:** Any defect in fat absorption causes failure of vitamin K absorption, which results in prolonged blood clotting time. Similarly, after cholecystectomy which hinders bile release, it is not readily absorbed. In such cases, the water-soluble analog, K_3, menadione is recommended.

2. **Drug Therapy:** Anti-clotting drug like Dicumerol acts as an antagonist, which inhibits the action of vitamin K. In such like medication, vitamin K is used as 'Balancing Antidote' to the drug in management of blood clotting time.

3. **General Coagulopathy:** In case of malabsorption, antibiotic therapy, hepatic dysfunction or major surgery, vitamin K prevents deficiency problems in patients with very poor appetite.

4. **Neonatology:** The new born's intestinal tract can supply no vitamin K during the first few days. To prevent any haemorrhagic disease in the immediate post-natal period, a prophylactic dose of vitamin K is usually given to the infants soon after birth.

Measure and Requirements

It is usually measured as mg or mg of Menadione activity.

The new RDA standard has been stated as 80 µg/day for men and 65 µg for women, with relatively smaller doses for the children.

Deficiency

The main effect of Vitamin K deficiency is a haemorrhagic diathesis - seen in the infants in early days. This deficiency interferes with the formation of porthrombinogen, thus prolonging the blood clotting time. This condition is called, Hypoprothrombinemia. Internal or external hemorrhages may ensue spontaneously in such cases.

Toxicity

Normally, toxicity from vitamin K has not been observed. Very larger intake may show the toxicity in the form of 'Hyperbilrubinemia'. In the infants, toxicity shows up as jaundice, kernicterus, hemolytic anemia and brain damage.

Sources

The form of the vitamin isolated from plants is generally called phylloquinone, and those forms synthesised by bacteria and in animal products are members of the menaquinone series. Relatively few values for the vitamin content of foods are available since dietary deficiency is not observed, and values for the vitamin K content of foods do not generally appear in all food tables. Table 6.10 gives the vitamin K content of common foods.

TABLE 6.10: VITAMIN K CONTENT OF SOME COMMON FOODS (µg/100 g)

Food	Vitamin K
Milk, whole, pasteurised	4
Milk, skimmed, pasteurised	4
Butter	10-50
Cheese, average	10-50
Egg, whole	50
Egg, yolk	147
Corn oil	60
Soyabean oil	540
Meat, average	4
Liver, average	80-104
Wheat bran	83
Flour, wholemeal	30
Wheatgerm	39
Oats	63
Chick peas	264
Green beans	28
Lentils	223
Mung beans	170
Peas	81
Soya beans	190
Potato	16
Broccoli	132
Cabbage, green	149
Carrot	13
Seaweed, dried	17,000
Spinach	266
Tomato	23
Watercress	57
Tea, green, dry	712

Source: Parrish, 1980; Haroon *et al.*, 1982 and USDA, 1986.

Table 6.11 presents a panoramic summary of the Fat-soluble vitamin group.

TABLE 6.11: SUMMARY OF FAT-SOLUBLE VITAMINS

Vitamin	Physiol. Functions	Deficiency	Requirements	Food Sources
VITAMIN A Provitamin: β carotene Vitamin: Retinol	Production of Rhodopsin and other light-receptor pigments	Poor dark adaptation, nigh blindness, xerosis, xerophthalmia	Adult male : 1000 µg RE. Adult female: 800µg RE.	Liver, cream, butter, whole milk, egg yolk Green and yellow fruits
	Formation and maintenance of epithelial tissue	Keratinization of epithelium, Growth failure	Pregnancy: 800 µg RE.	
	Growth	Reproductive Failure	Lactation: 1300 µg RE. Children: 400-1000 µg RE.	Fortified margarine
	Reproduction, Toxic in large amount	Reproductive failure	Children: 400 - 1000 µg RE.	
Vitamin D Provitamins: ergosterol (plants); 7-dehdrochol-esterol (skin)	1,25 dihydroxy-cholecalciferol, a major hormone regulator of bone mineral (calcium and phosphorus) metabolism	Faulty bone growth: rickets, osteomalacia	Adult 5-10 µg cholecalciferol Pregnancy and Lactation: 10 µg Children: 10 µg	Fortified milk Fortified margarine Fish oils Sunlight on skin
Vitamin: D₂ (ergocholecalci-ferol) and D₃ (cholecalciferol)	Calcium and phosphorus absorption. Toxic in large amounts	–		
Vitamin E Tocopherols	Antioxidation Hemopoiesis Related to action of selenium	Anemia in premature infants	Adults 8-10 µg α TE Pregnancy and Lactation : 10-12 µg α TE. Children: 3-10 µg α TE.	Vegetable oils
Vitamin K K1 (Phylloquinone)	Activation of blood-clotting factors (e.g. prothrombin) by α-carboxylating glutamic acid residues	hemorrhagic disease of the Newborn	Adult: 65-80 µg Children 15-65 µg Infants: 5-10 µg	Cheese, egg yolk, liver
K₂ (Menaquinone)	Toxicity can be induced by water-soluble analogs	Defective blood clotting Deficiency produced by coumarin anticoagu-lants and antibiotics.		GLV synthe-sized by intestinal bacteria

Source: Essential of Nutrition and Diet Therapy, S.R. Williams, Pub. Mosby.

WATER-SOLUBLE VITAMINS

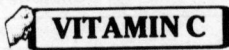 **VITAMIN C**

Vitamin C is also called Ascorbic acid because of its anti-scobutic or anti-scurvy properties. Chemically, its structure is like that of glucose—its metabolic precursor. Save for man and monkey, all animals can synthesize vitamin C from glucose. It exists in nature both as reduced and oxidized forms called dehydroascorbic acid.

Ascorbic acid is a very unstable, easily oxidized compound which can be easily destroyed by oxygen, alkalies and high temperature. As such foods should be cooked for the least period of time and then kept covered. To curtail surface exposure and wastage, the vegetables should not be cut into small piece, until the time of use. Use of pressure cooker saves a large amount of vitamin C.

Digestion and Absorption

Vitamin C is easily absorbed from the small intestine. But lack of hydrochloric acid or bleeding from gastrointestinal tract hampers its absorption. Vitamin C is distributed and stored in almost all the body tissues. Any excess level is excreted through urine.

Cow's milk contains very little vitamin C, hence infant feed formulas made from cows milk are supplemented with ascorbic acid.

Function of Vitamin C

1. ***Intercellular Cement Substance:*** Vitamin C is needed to build and maintain body tissue in general, including cartilages, bone matrix, dentin, collagen and connective tissue. In case of vitamin C deficiency, the important ground substance does not develop into collagen. But the formation of cartilaginous tissue follows quickly after the administration of vitamin C.

2. ***Body Metabolism:*** Metabolically more active tissues like kidney, brain, liver, pancreas and adrenal glands contain more vitamin C. It is closely associated with proteins in tissue growth, tissue building and in cell metabolic processes. As such, one needs larger doses of vitamin C during stress.

3. ***Red Blood Cells:*** Vitamin C helps the formation of hemoglobin and development of red blood cells by influencing the absorption of iron.

4. ***Wounds:*** Vitamin C helps in the speedy healing of wounds and fractures of bones. Larger doses of vitamin are needed in severe burns.

5. **Fevers and Infections:** Proper doses of vitamin C help build resistance to infections.

6. **Stress:** In both emotional strain and general body stress, adrenal tissue requires large doses of vitamin C. So also in the case of pregnancy.

7. **Metabolism of Tyrosine:** Vitamin C is needed for the metabolism of tyrosine and other enzymes.

Deficiency Symptoms

Lack of vitamin C results in defective formation of intercellular cementing substances. Retardation of growth in infants, anemias, poor wound healing, joint pains, breathing difficulties and increased susceptibility to infections are covered by deficiency of vitamin C. Scurvy is the main deficiency syndrome which shows up in the form of black and blue spots on the skin, swelling, infection and bleeding of gums and anaemia. Even a small injury causes bleeding.

Measure and Requirement

Vitamin C is measured in terms of milligrams.

Normally, an intake of 30-40 mg/day is sufficient to maintain a proper body pool of vitamin C in adults. The recommended daily allowance is 60 mg/day for an optimal margin to cover all the contingencies.

Food Sources

Ascorbic acid is found in all fresh fruits and vegetables. Citrus fruits like lemon, oranges and pineapple are the richest source, as is gooseberry (amla). A small intake of amla (8-10 g) can meet the daily requirement of vitamin C of an average adult. Other sources of vitamin C are tomatoes, sweet potatoes, cabbage, lettuce, green peppers and guavas, besides many green and yellow vegetables.

Being very unstable and easily oxidized, it calls for careful evaluation of nutritional contribution of vitamin C in foods during processing and cooking.

Table 6.12 gives the vitamin C contents of different foods.

GROUP B VITAMINS

Starting with the Anti-Beri-beri vitamin, this group of B vitamins have now graduated into eleven distinct chemical entities. As vital control agents, many of these B group vitamins serve as co-enzymes, when they collaborate with key cell enzymes in performing energy metabolism and tissue building jobs. Of these, eight member of vitamin B group are required by the human body. These are further divided in 3 subgroups.

TABLE 6.12: FOOD SOURCES OF VITAMIN C

(RDA for adults: 60 mg)

	Quantity	Vitamin E (mg α-TE)
1. Bread, Cereal, Rice and Pasta		
This food groups is not an important source of vitamin C.		
2. Vegetables		
Asparagus (raw)	½ cup (6 spears)	18
Avocado (raw)	1 medium	14
Broccoli (raw)	½ cup	41
Brussels Sprouts (boiled)	½ cup (4 sprouts)	48
Cauliflower (raw)	½ cup, pieces	36
Green Pepper (raw)	½ cup (chopped)	64
Kale (boiled)	½ cup	27
Potato (baked, with skin)	1 medium	26
Sweet Potato (baked)	1 medium	28
Tomato (raw)	1 medium	22
3. Fruits		
Cantaloupe (raw)	½ cup, pieces	34
Grapefruit, white	½ medium	39
Kiwi (raw)	1 medium	75
Lemon	1 medium	31
Lemon Juice (fruit)	8 oz	112
Orange Juice (fresh)	8 oz	124
Orange naval	1 medium	80
Papaya (raw)	1 medium	188
Pineapple (raw)	1 medium	12
Raspberries (raw)	½ cup	15
Strawberries (raw)	½ cup	44
Tangerine (raw)	1 medium	26
4. Meat, Poultry, Fish, Dry Beans and Eggs		
Beef Liver (fried)	3.5 oz	23
Ham, lean (canned; vitamin C added)	3.5 oz	27
Lentils (boiled)	1 cup	3
Soyabeans (boiled)	1 cup	3
6. Milk and Dairy Products		
Milk, skim	8 oz	2
Mild, Whole	8 oz	4
7. Fats, Oils and Sugar		
This food group is not an important source of vitamin C.		

Source: Modern Nutrition in Health and Disease, Vol. I.

Group A: Classic Deficiency/Disease Factors

    1. Vitamin B_1 - Thiamine

    2. Vitamin B_2 - Ribofavin

    3. Vitamin B_3 - Niacin

Group B: Recently discovered Co-enzyme Factors

    4. Vitamin B_6 - Pyridoxine

    5.   - Pantothenic acid

    6.   - Biotin

Group C: Blood forming Factors

    7.   - Folic Acid

    8. Vitamin B_{12} - Cyanocobalamine

☞ THIAMINE—VITAMIN B_1

Thiamine or vitamin B_1 is the Beri-beri- preventing factor, first isolated from rice polishing. The name Thiamine comes from its chemical ring-like structure—one of its major constituents is a thiazole ring: thi (O + Vit) amin.

Thiamine is a water-soluble fairly stable vitamin. It has got faint yeast-like odor and a salty nut-like taste. Though it is stable in dry form, as also in acid medium, yet it gets easily destroyed in a neutral or alkaline medium in the process of cooking. However, it is not soluble in fat solvents.

Absorption and Storage

Thiamine, consumed in diet, is available both in free form or bound as Thiamine pyrophosphate or as a protein phosphate. However, all the bound forms are split, before being absorbed in the duodenum, whose acid medium activates absorption, Thiamine is not stored in large quantities in the tissues. The tissue content is highly relevant to the increased metabolic demand, as happens in fevers, increased muscular activity, pregnancy and location. The storage functions of Thiamine is also affected by the composition of diet. For example, carbohydrates increase the need for Thiamine vitamin, whereas fats and proteins spare Thiamine. Any excess Thiamine is excreted in urine.

Functions of Thiamine

1. **Co-enzyme Role:** Its main function is that of metabolic control agent in energy metabolism. It is the coenzyme Thiamine pyrophosphate (TPP) in key reaction that produces energy from glucose, or else converts it to fat

for tissue energy storage. Thus, the symptoms of muscle weakness, gastrointestinal disturbance and neuritis associated with Beri-beri can be controlled by Thiamine administration.

2. *Keto Acids*: The pyrophosphate of Thiamine also acts as a co-enzyme in Transketolase. The latter is an enzyme that is required in the production of keto acids.

Deficiency

1. *Gastrotestinal System*: Thimine deficiency leads to anoxeria, indigestion, constipation, gastric atony and deficient hydrochloric acid secretions.

2. *Nervous System*: The central nervous system depends upon glucose to carry on its normal work. Thiamine deficiency leads to impairment of neuronal activity, which results in diminished reflex response and fatigue. It may also lead to peripheral neuritis, which is characterized by weakness of legs, tenderness and cramping of calf muscles and burning or numbness of feet. Even paralysis results, as seen in deficiency disease, Beri-beri.

3. *Cardiovascular System*: Prolonged deficiency leads to weakening of the heart muscles, which may result in cardiac failure. When smooth muscles of the vascular system are involved, it causes dilatation of peripheral blood vessels, which results in edema of the lower legs.

4. *Musculo-Skeletal System*: A chronic painful musculo-skeletal condition, primary fibromyalgia, results from inadequate amount of TPP in the muscle tissue.

Thiamine Requirement

Thiamine requirement is linked to calorific needs. The average adult requires from 0.3-0.5 mg/1000 kcal.

The RDA standard is 0.5 mg/1000 kcal, with a minimum intake level of 1.1 mg to 1.5 mg/day.

Alcoholism, chronic illness and geriatric conditions influence Thiamine requirement. Pregnancy and lactation demand 50% extra Thiamine supplies.

Food Sources

Good sources of Thiamine are the foods rich in proteins like beef, liver, lean pork and nuts. Besides, whole and enriched grains (flour, bread, cereals) and legumes also provide a fair amount of this vitamin. Since processing results in destruction of vitamins, hence enrichment of flours with Thiamine is essential.

TABLE 6.13: FOOD SOURCES OF THIAMINE (VITAMIN B₁) (mg/100 g Edible stuff)

Food	Vitamin B
Milk and Milk Products	
Skimmed Milk Powder	
(Cow's Milk)	0.45
Whole Milk Powder	
(Cow's Milk)	0.31
Khoa	
(Whole Cow's Milk)	0.23
Meat or Poultry	
Pork	0.54
Liver, Sheep	0.36
Mutton	0.18
Nuts and Oil Seeds	
Gingelly (Sesame Seeds)	1.01
Groundnut	0.90
Sunflower Seeds	0.86
Pistachio Nut	0.67
Cashew Nut	0.63
Garden grass Seeds	0.59
Groundnut, roasted	0.39
Almonds	0.24
Spices or Condiments	
Chillies, dry	0.93
Cumin Seeds	0.55
Fenugreek Seeds	0.34
Nutmeg	0.33
Cardamom	0.22
Coriander	0.22
Fruits	
Apricot, dried	0.22
Melon, musk	0.11
Pineapple	0.20
Vegetables	
Chekkur Manis	0.48
Turnip, greens	0.31
Beat, greens	0.26
Knol knol, greens	0.25
Tamarind, Leaves	0.24
Colocasia, Leaves	0.22
(Green vareity)	
Agathi (Sesbania)	0.21
Pulses or Legumes	
Soyabean	0.73
Cow Peas	0.51
Bengal Gram dal	0.48

Table 6.13 (*contd.* on page 123)

Table 6.13 (*contd.* from page 122)

Green Gram dal	0.47
Green Gram whole	0.47
Peas dry	0.47
Peas roasted	0.47
Lentils	0.45
Moth Beans	0.45
Red Gram, dal	0.45
Horse Gram	0.42
Black Gram, dal	0.42
Cereals or Cereal Products	
Rice bran	2.70
Wheat Germ	1.40
Wheat bulger	0.74
Italian Millet	0.59
Barley	0.47
Wheat Whole	0.45
Maize dry	0.42
Ragi	0.42
Jowar	0.37
Bajra	0.33
Wheat Bread Brown	0.21
Rice Flakes	0.21
Rice Puffed	0.21

Source: Nutritive Value of Indian Foods, National Institute of Nutrition, Hyderabad.

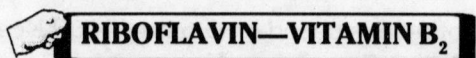

RIBOFLAVIN—VITAMIN B$_2$

Riboflavin derives its name from the Latin word for yellow. Since it also contains a sugar named ribose, hence the chemical name riboflavin was adopted. It is a yellow-green fluorescent pigment that forms yellowish brown needle-like crystals. It is water-soluble and relatively stable to heat. But light and radiation readily destroy riboflavin. It is stable in acid medium and is not easily oxidized.

Absorption and Storage

Absorption occurs readily in upper part of small intestines, assisted by phosphorus in the intestinal mucosa. In the body it is present as the co-enzyme or flavoproteins. Storage is limited, although small amounts are found in liver and kidneys. However, day-to-day needs must be supplied in the diet.

Regular use of bulk fibre laxatives like psyllium hinder the riboflavin and can contribute to its deficiency in body metabolism.

Function of Riboflavin

1. **Co-enzymes Protein Metabolism:** Major role of riboflavin is to act as a control agent in both energy production and tissue building. Herein, it plays the vital role of co-enzymes.

The cell enzymes of which riboflavin is an important constituent are called flavoproteins. The de-amination is the key reaction that removes the nitrogen containing amino groups from certain amino acids.

2. **Co-enzymes in Carbohydrate Metabolism:** The two co-enzymes herein are riboflavin monophosphate or flavin mononucleotide (FMN) and the more common flavin adenin dinucleotide (FAD). Some of these flavin enzymes contain metallic constituents like iron, copper or molybdenum. These flavins act as oxidizing agents within the cells. These flavoproteins show a wide range of redox potential and hence can play a wide variety of roles in oxidative metabolism.

Deficiency

1. **Ariboflavinosis:** This brings in a combination of symptoms such as tissue inflammation and breakdown and poor wound healing. Lips become swollen and crack easily. Cheilosis or cracking of corners of mouth develops, accompanied often by swollen and reddened tongue-glossitis, Skin become scaly and greasy. Eyes become sensitive to light *i.e.* photophobia and corneal vascularisation or proliferating capillaries result.

2. **Deficiency in New-borns:** Because riboflavin is light-sensitive, new-born infants treated with photo therapy show riboflavin deficiency.

Requirement

The RDA standard for riboflavin is based on 0.6 mg/1000 Kcal, *i.e.* for an average adult, it ranges from 1.2 to 1.7 mg/day. However, risk groups or vulnerable sections need extra dosage of riboflavin.

Food Sources

Milk, which contains lactoflavins, is the most important source of riboflavin. Other fairly good sources are organ meats like liver, kidney and eggs. Some fruits and vegetables contain riboflavin in very small amounts. If foods are cooked uncovered or with excess water, it results in a considerable loss of riboflavin.

TABLE 6.14: FOOD SOURCES OF RIBOFLAVIN (VITAMIN B_2) (mg/100 g Edilble Stuff)

Food	Vitamin B
Milk or Milk Products	
Skimmed Milk Powder (Cow's Milk)	1.64
Whole Milk Powder (Cow's Milk)	1.36
Khoa (Whole Cow's Milk)	0.41
Cow's Milk (Whole)	0.19

Table 6.14 (*contd.* on page 125)

Table 6.14 (*contd.* from page 124)

Meat or Poultry	
Liver, Sheep	1.70
Beef meal	0.44
Hen's Egg	0.44
Duck's Egg	0.26
Nuts or Oilseeds	
Niger Seeds	0.97
Garden Cess Seeds	0.61
Almonds	0.57
Coconut meal	0.57
Walnut	0.40
Chilgoza	0.30
Spices or Condiments	
Chillies, dry	0.43
Mace	0.42
Chillies, green	0.39
Cumin Seeds	0.36
Coriander	0.35
Fruits	
Papaya ripe	0.25
Raspberry	0.19
Raisins	0.19
Seethaphal	0.17
Currants black	0.14
Jack Fruit	0.13
Mulberry	0.13
Vegetables	
Manathakkali Leaves	0.59
Turnip, greens	0.57
Beet greens	0.56
Colocasia, Leaves (Black variety)	0.45
Soyabeans	0.39
Carrot Leaves	0.37
Red Grams, tender	0.33
Green Gram Whole	0.27
Curry Leaves	0.21
Lentils	0.20
Horse Gram	0.20
Cow Peas	0.20
Black Gram dal	0.20
Cereal or Cereal Products	
Wheat Germ	0.54
Rice Bran	0.48
Bajra	0.25
Barley	0.20
Ragi	0.19

Source: Nutritive Value of Indian Foods, National Institute of Nutrition, Hyderabad (India).

NIACIN—VITAMIN B$_3$

Nicotinic Acid (Niacin) and Nicotinamide (Niacinamide) are the isomeric compound having the same biological properties, known specially for 'Pellagra'. The P-P vitamin (Pellagra-preventing vitamin) is related to essential amino acid, tryptophan. Tryptophan, a precursor of niacin, can be converted by the body to niacin.

Niacin is water-soluble, fairly stable to acid alkali, heat, light and oxidation. Niacin is the most stable of all the vitamins. It forms a white powder when crystallized.

Absorption and Storage

Niacin is easily absorbed from the small intestine. Its precursor, trytophan is converted to vitamin in the presence of pyridoxine.

Functions

1. **Co-enzyme Role:** Two co-enzymes, nicotinamide adenine dinucleotide (NAD) and nicotinamide adenine dinucleotide phosphate (NADP), are present in the body.

   Niacin is partner with riboflavin in the cellular co-enzyme system that converts protein to glucose, which is then oxidized to release controlled energy.

2. **Drug Therapy:** Therapeutic doses of niacin are used in cardiovascular diseases to lower the elevated levels of cholesterol. High doses of nicotinic acid (not nicotinamide) act as vasodilators and cause gastro-intestinal distress, skin-flushing and itching. It helps lower serum cholesterol level.

Deficiency

Since both niacin and riboflavin are closely inter-related, as control agents in cell metabolism, their deficiencies are observed simultaneously.

Pellagra is the deficiency disease marked by rough skin. There is weakness, lassitude, loss of weight and appetite too, besides dermatitis. Prolonged deficiency affects the central nervous system, leading to confusion, disorientation and dementia.

Requirement

The RDA standard is 6.6 mg/1000 kcal, which equals 13 niacin equivalents (NE). The adult standard is 15-19 mg/day.

TABLE 6.15: NIACIN CONTENT OF COMMON WESTERN FOODS (mg/100 g)

Food	Niacin
Milk, Whole, pasteurised	0.08
Milk, semi-skimmed, pasteurised	0.09
Milk, skimmed, pasteurised	0.09
Milk, Whole sterilised	0.09
Soya Milk	0.11
Double Cream	0.04
Yoghurt, low fat	0.12-0.19
Cheese, cheddar	0.04-0.11
Cheese, cottage	0.14-0.26
Cheese, Brie, Camembert	0.48-1.57
Cheese, Roquefort	0.57-0.74
Egg, Whole	0.07
Beef, average	4.5
Pork, average	5.2
Lamb, average	5.0
Chicken, Meat only	7.8
Kidney, average	8.0
Liver, average	14.0
Cod	1.7
Herring	2.0-6.0
Wheat Bran	29.6
Bulgur Wheat	4.5
Oatmeal	1.0
Flour, Whole meal	5.7
Flour, White	0.7
Broad Beans	3.2
Butter Beans, Haricot Beans	2.5
Lentils, red, split	2.0
Soya Beans	2.2
Potato, average	0.4-5.0
Asparagus	1.0
Broccoli	0.9
Brussels Sprouts	0.2
Carrots	0.2
Lettuce	0.3-0.6
Mushrooms	3.2
Plantain	0.7
Seaweed, Irish Moss	0.6
Spinach	1.2
Sweet Potato	0.5
Sweetcorn	1.9
Tomato	1.0
Yam	0.2
Yeast Baker's, dried	36
Coffee, ground, roast	10-40

Source: *The Technology of Vitamins in Food*, Ed. Berry Ottaway.

TABLE 6.16: INDIAN FOOD SOURCES OF NIACIN (mg/100 g Edible Stuff)

Food	Vitamin B
Milk or Milk Products	
Very poor source of Niacin	
Meat or Poultry	
Liver, Sheep	17.6
Mutton	6.8
Beef, lean	6.4
Beef, meal	5.8
Nuts and Oilseeds	
Groundnut, roasted	22.1
Groundnut	19.9
Garden Cess Seeds	14.3
Niger seeds	8.4
Coconut, meal deoiled	6.0
Sunflower Seeds	4.5
Gingelly (Sesame Seeds)	4.4
Mustard Seed	4.0
Spices or Condiments	
Chillies, dry	9.0
Fruits or Vegetables	
Very poor source of Niacin	
Turnip Leaves	5.4
Tamarind Leaves	4.1
Beat, greens	3.3
Apricots, dry	2.3
Curry Leaves	2.3
Pulses or Legumes	
Peas roasted	3.5
Peas, dry	3.4
Soya Beans	3.2
Red Gram, tender	3.0
Kesari, dal	2.9
Lentils	2.6
Green Gram, dal	2.4
Green Gram, whole	2.1
Black Gram, dal	2.0
Cereals and Cereal Products	
Rice, Bran	29.8
Wheat, Whole	5.5
Barley	5.4
Wheat, bulger	4.8
Rice Parboiled, hand pounded	4.0
Rice flakes	4.0
Rice puffed	4.1
Rice milled	3.8
Wheat, flour	2.4

Source: Nutritive Value of Indian Foods, National Institute of Nutrition, Hyderabad (India).

Food Sources

Protein-rich like poultry, fish, meat, peas, beans and peanuts are good sources of niacin. Though corn and rice are poor, yet most of the grains are a fair source of niacin. Green leafy vegetables, potatoes, legumes, milk, eggs and cheese, though poor in niacin, are rich source of tryptophan. Table 6.15 gives the niacin content of some common foods.

Table 6.15 and 6.16 gives the Niacin contents of common Western and Indian foods.

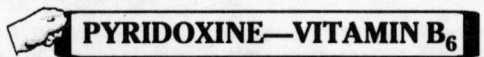 **PYRIDOXINE—VITAMIN B$_6$**

Vitamin B$_6$ derives its chemical name pyridoxine, because of a pyridin ring in its structure. The three basic forms, viz. Pyridoxol, pyridoximine and pyridoxine— all these are converted to the co-enzyme, pyridoxal phosphate (B$_6$-PO$_4$), which is the most potent form of this vitamin. Pyridoxine is water soluble, stable to heat and acids. But it is very sensitive to light and alkalies.

Absorption and Storage

Pyridoxine is easily absorbed in the upper portion of small intestine. The active form of pyridoxal phosphate can be formed from any of the three isomeric compounds. It is stored in all the tissue throughout the body.

Functions

1. *Co-enzymes in Protein Metabolism:* In its active form, pyridoxal phosphate (PLO) acts as a co-enzyme in many amino acid reactions, such as:

    1. Carboxylation converts glutamic acid to γ-aminobutyric acid (GABA) and tryptophan to serotonin, both vital regulatory substances in brain activities.
    2. Deamination: It transfers nitrogen from one amino acid to the other and releases carbon residues for energy.
    3. Trans-sulfuration: Moves sulfur from sulfur-containing methionine to form other sulfur compounds like cysteine.
    4. Niacin: It controls formation of nitrogen from tryptophan.
    5. Hemoglobin Synthesis: It incorporates amino acids into 'heme' - the essential non-protein core of hemoglobin.
    6. Amino Acid Transport: It actively transports amino acids from the intestine into circulation and across cell walls into the body cells.

2. *Co-enzyme in Carbohydrate and Fat Metabolism:* It provides metabolites for energy-producing fuel. It also converts the essential fatty acid, linoleic acid to arachidonic acid.

Deficiency

From the wider array of multiple functions, it is evident that pyridoxine holds a key to many clinical problems like:

1. Anemia, since heme is not formed.
2. Central Nervous System—hyper-irritability and convulsions.
3. Pregnancy: There are signs of pyridoxine deficiency during pregnancy.
4. Oral Contraceptives: These contraceptive measures call for additional dosage.
5. Drug Therapy: Isoniazid (INH) for TB is an antagonist to pyridoxine. It also inhibits the conversion of glutamic acid, the only amino acid the brain metabolizes and this causes neuritis.

Requirement

Since pyridoxine is involved in amino acid metabolism, so its demand varies with protein intake in the diet. For adults, a minimum 1 mg/day is essential. The RDA standard is 1.6-2.0 mg/day.

Food Sources

Pyridoxine is quite widespread in foods, though it is found only in small doses. Good sources of pyridoxine include grains, seeds, liver, kidneys and other meats. However, it is found in a very limited amount in milk, eggs and vegetables.

TABLE 6.17: VITAMIN B_6 (PYRIDOXINE) CONTENT OF COMMON FOODS (mg/100 g)

Food	Vitamin B
Milk, Whole, pasteurided	0.06
Milk, semi-skimmed, pasteurised	0.06
Milk, skimmed, pasteurised	0.06
Milk, sterilised	0.04
Soya Milk	0.07
Double Cream	0.03
Yoghurt, low fat	0.08
Cheese, chedder	0.06-0.13
Cheese, cottage	0.08
Cheese, Brie, Camembert	0.15-0.28
Cheese, Roquefort	0.1
Eggs	0.12
Beef, average	0.25
Lamb, average	0.2
Pork, average	0.4
Chicken, meat only	0.4
Kidney, average	0.3
Liver, average	0.5

Table 6.17 (*contd.* on page 131)

Table 6.17 (*contd.* from page 130)

Cod	0.3
Herring	0.5
Shrimps	0.1
Cod roe	0.32
Wheat Bran	1.38
Oatmeal	0.12
Flour, Whole meal	0.5
Flour, White	0.15
Rice, Brown	0.55
Rice, White	0.17-0.3
Broad Beans	0.06
Butter Beans, Haricot Beans	0.53
Chick Peas	0.53
Green Beans	0.05
Lentils, red, split	0.6
Red Kidney Beans	0.4
Soya Beans	0.38
Potato, average	0.4
Asparagus	0.09
Broccoli	0.14
Brussels Sprouts	0.37
Carrot	0.14
Lettuce	0.03-0.08
Mushrooms	0.18
Spinach	0.17
Sweetcorn	0.15
Yam	0.16
Apple	0.03
Banana	0.51
Melon	0.04-0.07
Orange	0.06
Raisins	0.3
Yeast, Baker's, dried	2.0

Source: The Technology of Vitamins in Food, Ed. Berry Ottaway.

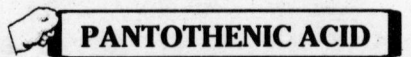 **PANTOTHENIC ACID**

Its name is derived from Greek word, Pantheon, meaning all over or everywhere. It shows that pantothenic acid is very widely present in nature and is also freely synthesised by the bacteria in the intestine. Hence, there is never any deficiency of pantothenic acid.

Pantothenic acid is a white crystalline compound, a free acid, unstable viscous yellow oil which is stable in water. It is sensitive to acids, alkalies and heat. Absorbed readily in the intestine, it combines with phosphorous to form the active co-enzyme, 'Co-enzyme A', which has widespread metabolic presence throughout the body.

TABLE 6.18: PANTOTHENIC ACID CONTENT OF COMMON FOODS (mg/100 g)

Food	Pantothenic Acid
Milk, Whole, pasteurised	0.35
Milk, semi-skimmed, pasteurised	0.32
Milk, skimmed, pasteurised	0.32
Double Cream	0.19
Low fat Youghurt	0.45
Cheese, cheddar	0.3-0.5
Cheese, cottage	0.2-0.4
Cheese, Brie, Camembert	0.36-1.4
Cheese, Roquefort	0.5-1.73
Egg, Whole	1.77
Egg, Yolk	4.6
Beef, Lamb, average	0.6
Pork, average	0.7-1.1
Chicken	1.2
Kidney, average	3.0-3.85
Liver, average	8
Heart, Lamb's	2.5
Brain, Calve's, Lamb's	2.0-2.6
Wheat Bran	2.4-2.9
Flour Whole meal	0.8
Flour, White	0.3
Rice, Brown	1.1
Rice, polished	0.4
Oatmeal	1.0
Wheat Germ	1.2-1.9
Broad Beans	4.9
Butter Beans	1.3
Soya Beans	0.8-1.7
Potato	0.4
Broccoli	1.2
Cabbage	0.2
Carrot	0.25
Mushroom	2.0
Sweetcorn	0.7
Yam	0.3
Avocado	1.1
Dates, dried	0.8
Watermelon	1.6
Almonds	0.5
Hazelnuts	1.2
Peanuts	2.7
Yeast, Baker's, dried	11.0

Source: The Technology of Vitamins in Food, Ed. Berry Ottaway.

Functions

Co-enzyme A, owing to its involvement in many vital reactions, has great significance in the body metabolism, as under:

1. By forming active acetate, it is very important in the process of energy production in the cells from both fats and carbohydrates.
2. The active form of acetate is also a precursor of cholesterol and other steroid hormones.
3. Activation of succinic acid and glycine is part of the primary step in the formation of heme in hemoglobin synthesis.
4. Combination with sulfonomide drugs facilities their excretion.

Requirement

Owing to its easy availability, its RDA has not been stated. The estimated safe range of panothenic acid for adults is 4-7 mg. In USA, the average intake is about 10-20 mg/day.

Food Sources

Yeast, liver and kidney are the rich sources of pantothenic acid. Other sources are egg yolk, milk, sweet potatoes, cheese, legumes and yellow corn.

Table 6.18 shows the pantothenic acid content of common foods.

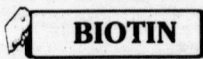

BIOTIN

Found in minute traces, Biotin is an essential sulfur-containing vitamin that performs multiple tasks. Biotin functions in partnership with acetyl-Co-enzyme A in reactions that transfer carbon dioxide from one compound to another. These may be

1. Initial steps in the synthesis of some fatty acids.
2. Conversion reactions in the synthesis of amino acids: Through its contributory role in the production of antibodies, it helps increase the effectiveness of the immune system.
3. Carbon dioxide fixation in the formation of purines.

Deficiency

Biotin deficiency is very rare. But in patients on parenteral nutrition, it does show Biotin deficiency. Long term alcohol abuse may also lead to biotin deficiency.

Requirement

The RDA for adult is stated between 30-100 mg/day.

Food Sources

In the nature, biotin is widely available. While in the corn and soyameals, it is completely available, that in wheat is virtually unavailable. Good food sources of biotin are egg yolk, liver, kidney, besides yeast and tomatoes.

TABLE 6.19: BIOTIN CONTENT OF COMMON FOODS (µg/100g)

Food	Biotin
Milk, Whole, pasteurised	2
Milk, semi-skimmed, pasteurised	2
Milk, skimmed, pasteurised	2
Milk, Whole, sterilised	1.8
Double Cream	1.1
Yoghurt, low fat	2.9
Cheese, cheddar	1.7-3.6
Cheese, cottage	3
Cheese, Brie, Camembert	2.8-7.6
Cheese, Roquefort	2.3
Egg, Whole	11-20
Beef, average	trace
Lamb, average	1-2
Pork, average	1-3
Chicken	2
Kidney, average	24-37
Liver, average	27-41
Liver, Chicken	210
Cod	3
Herring	10
Wheat Bran	14-45
Flour, Whole meal	7-9
Flour, White	1
Wheat Germ	25
Broad Beans	3
Soyabeans	65
Tempeh, fermented soya curd	53
Potato	trace
Green Beans	1
Cauliflower	2
Mushrooms	12
Quorn, myco-protein	9
Spinach	trace
Tomato	2
Apple	1
Currant, black	2
Orange	1-2
Almonds	18-23
Chestnuts	1-2
Walnuts	2-37
Yeast, Baker's dried	85-200

Source: *The Technology of Vitamins in Food*, Ed. Berry Ottaway.

FOLIC ACID

The name folic acid is derived from the latin word *'folium'*, meaning leaves, since folic acid is derived from dark green vegetables like spinach. Another form is folinic acid, which is a reduced form of folic acid is made of 3 linked compounds- a pteridine group, para-amino benzoic acid and glutamic acid. It is slightly water -soluble and is unstable in acid medium and is sensitive to light. Small amount of folic acid is synthesized by the intestinal microflora.

Absorption and Storage

About 25% of folacin in free form in foods is completely absorbed. But the polyglutamate form can only be absorbed after they are acted upon by the intestinal mucosal enzyme, Conjugase. By removing the extra glutamate group, conjugase releases the absorbable folic acid. In the body, the active form of folic acid is tetrahydrofolic acid.

Functions

Basic Co-enzyme role: Folic acid is an important agent in the task of attaching single carbon to compounds. Such key compounds are:

1. Purines: Nitrogen-containing compounds essential to all living cells and involved in the cells division and in the transmission of inherited traits.
2. Thymine: Essential compounds forming a key part of deoxyribonucleic acid (DNA), the important material in the cell nucleus that controls and transmits genetic characters.
3. Hemoglobin: Heme, the iron-containing non-protein portion of hemoglobin —folic acid, is one of the important haemopoietic agents necessary for the proper blood formation.

Deficiency

1. Megaloblastic anemia occurs in simple folic acid deficiency.
2. Spruce, a celiac disease, is a gastrointestinal problem characterized by intestinal lesions, malabsorption defects and general malnutrition.
3. Chemotherapy: Amethopterin, drug used in cancer chemotherapy, acts as a folic acid antagonist to reduce tumour growth.
4. Stress and Growth: All these call for increased folic acid dosage.

Requirement

The average American diet contains about 0.6 mg of total folic acid.

The RDA for adults ranges from 180 to 200 mg/day. But for pregnant women, the RDA is 400 mg/day.

TABLE 6.20: FOLATE CONTENT OF COMMON WESTERN FOODS (µg/100 g)

Food	Folates
Milk, Whole, pasteurised	6
Milk, semi-skimmed, pasteurised	6
Milk, skimmed, pasteurised	5
Milk, Whole, sterilised	0.2
Milk, Soya	17
Yoghurt, low fat	17
Soyabean oil	450-630
Cheese, cheddar	16-42
Cheese, cottage	12-27
Cheese, Brie, Camembert	56-100
Cheese, Roquefort	45-49
Egg, Whole	50
Egg, Yolk	130
Beef, average	trace
Lamb, average	1-2
Pork, average	1-3
Chicken	2-4
Kidney, average	24-37
Liver, average	27-210
Herring	10
Wheat Bran	80-260
Flour, Whole meal	57
Flour, White	22
Rice, Brown	49
Rice, polished	20
Oatmeal	60
Wheat germ	330-370
Broad Beans	145
Lentils, red, split	35
Miso, Fermented Soy bean paste	33
Potato	20-35
Green Beans	14-80
Peas	10-60
Asparagus	57-175
Broccoli	65-200
Brussels Sprouts	135
Carrots	10-20
Cassava	24
Lettuce	55
Spinach	130-330
Sweetcorn	41
Tomatoes	11-24
Watercress	120
Yeast, Baker's dried	4000

Source: The Technology of Vitamins in Food, Ed. Berry Ottaway.

Food Sources

Fresh green leafy vegetables like spinach, lettuce, liver, kidney, dry beans and pulses are good sources of folic acid. But fruits, milk, poultry and eggs are a poor source of this vitamin. Table 6.20 shows the folate content of common Western foods while Table 6.21 gives the folic acid content of Indian food.

TABLE 6.21: FOOD SOURCES OF FOLIC ACID (µg/100 g Edible Stuff)

Food	Folates
Milk or Milk Products	
Nil	
Meat or Poultry	
Liver, Sheep	188.0
Liver, Goat	176.2
Duck's Egg	80.0
Hen's Egg	78.3
Nuts	
Nil	
Condiments or Spices	
Fenugreek Seeds	84.0
Coriander	32.0
Chillies green	29.0
Turmeric	18.0
Fruits	
Nil	
Vegetables	
Amaranth tender	149.0
Spinach	123.0
Mint	114.0
Curry Leaves	93.9
Cabbage	23.0
Pulses or legumes	
Bengal Gram, Whole	186.0
Bengal Gram, dal	147.5
Green Gram, dal	140.0
Bengal Gram, roasted	139.0
Cow Peas	133.0
Black Gram dal	132.0
Red Gram dal	103.0
Soya beans	100.0
Cereals or Cereals Products	
Bajra	45.5
Wheat, Whole	36.6
Wheat, flour whole	35.8
Jowar	20.0
Maize	20.0
Italian Millet	15.0

Source: Nutritive Value of Indian Foods, National Institute of Nutrition, Hyderabad.

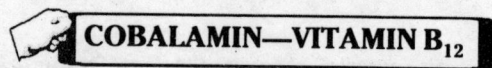 **COBALAMIN—VITAMIN B$_{12}$**

Vitamin B$_{12}$ is named cobalamin, because of its unique structure with a single red atom of the trace element cobalt at its centre.

Absorption and Storage

Being very large, its cobalamin is first split from its protein complex by the hydrochloric acid in the stomach. It is then bound to a specific glycoprotein, called 'Intrinsic Factor', secreted by gastric mucosal cells. This complex then moves into the intestines where it is absorbed by special receptors in the ileal mucosa.

Cobalamin is stored in active body tissues like liver, heart, pancreas, testes, brain, blood and bone marrow.

TABLE 6.22: VITAMIN B$_{12}$ (CYANOCOBALAMINE) CONTENT OF COMMON FOODS (µg/100 g)

Food	Vitamin B$_{12}$
Milk, Whole, pasteurised	0.4
Milk, semi skimmed, pasteurised	0.4
Milk, skimmed, pasteurised	0.4
Milk, Whole sterilised	0.1
Double Cream	0.2
Yoghurt, low fat	0.2
Cheese, cheddar	0.8-15
Cheese, cottage	0.7
Cheese, Brie, Camembert	1.1-3.1
Cheese, Roquefort	0.5
Egg, Whole	2.5
Egg, Yolk	6.9
Beef, average	1-2
Lamb, average	1-2
Pork, average	1-3
Chicken	trace
Kidney, average	30-50
Liver, average	50-100
Brain, Calves, Lambs	9
Cod	1-2
Herring	6
Mackerel	10
Sardines, canned in oil, fish only	28
Cod roe	10
Oysters	15
Seaweed, dried	2.5-47
Miso, fermented Soybean paste	0.2
Tempeh, fermented Soybean curd	0.1
Marmite, Yeast extract	0.5

Source: The Technology of Vitamins in Food, Ed. Berry Ottaway.

Food Sources

Cyanocobalamin is supplied by animal foods. The richest source are liver, kidneys, beef meat, eggs and cheese. Vegetables and fruits do not contain any vitamin B_{12}. Table 6.22 gives the vitamin B_{12} content of common foods.

Table 6.23 gives the comparative summary of all water-soluble vitamins.

TABLE 6.23: SUMMARY OF WATER-SOLUBLE VITAMINS

	Physiological Functions	Clinical Applications	Requirement	Food Sources
Vitamin C Ascorbic Acid	Antioxidation Collagen biosynthesis General metabolism: Makes iron available for Hb synthesis. Influences conversion of folic acid to folinic acid. Oxidation-reduction of amino acids—Phenylalanine and Tyrosine	Scurvy (deficiency) Wound healing, tissue formation; Fevers and infections; Stress reactions Growth	60 mg	Fresh fruits, especially citrus; Vegetables, such as tomato, cabbage, potatoes, chillies, Peppers, and broccoli
B Complex Vitamins				
Thiamine Vitamin B_1	Carbohyd. metabolism: Thiamine pyrophosphate (TPP): oxidative decarboxylation	Beri-beri (deficiency), Neuropathy Wernicke-Korsakoff Syndrome (alcoholism) Depressed muscular and secretory symptoms	1.1-1.5 mg	Pork, beef, liver whole or enriched grains, legumes
Riboflavin Vitamin B_2	General Metabolism: Flavin adenine Flavin mono-nucleotide (FMN)	Dinucleotide (FAD), Cheilosis, glossitis, seborrheic dermatitis	1.2-1.7 mg	Milk, liver, Enriched cereals
Niacin - Nicot.acid, Nicotinamide	General metabolism: Nicotinamide adenine Dinucleotide (NAD) Nicotinamide adenine Dinucleotide phosphate (NADP)	Pellagra (deficiency) Weakness, anorexia Scaly dermatitis Neuritis	15-19 mg NE	Meat, peanuts, enri-ched,grains (protein foods containing tryptophan)
Vitamin B_6 (Pyridoxine,) Pyridoxal, Pyridoxamin)	General metabolism: Pyridoxal phosphate (PLP) transamination and decarboxylation	Reduced serum levels associated with pregnancy and use of oral contraceptives. Antagonized by ixoniazid, pencillamine and other drugs	1.6–2.0 mg	Wheat, corn meat, liver
Pantothenic acid	General metabolism CoA (Coenzyme A) acetylation	Many roles through acyl transfer reactions (e.g. lipogenesis, amino acid activation and formation of cholesterol, steroid hormones, heme)	4-7 mg	Liver, egg, milk

Table 6.23 (*contd.* on page 140)

Table 6.23 (*contd.* from page 139)

Biotin	General metabolism: N-carboxybiotiny1 Lysine :CO_2 transfer reactions	Deficiency induced by Avidin and by antibiotics. Synthesis of some fatty acids and amino acids.	30-100 mg	Egg yolk, liver Synthesized by intestinal microorganisms.
Cobalamin Vitamin (B_{12})	General metabolism: Methylcobalamin: Methylation reactions (e.g. Synthesis of amino acids, heme)	Pernicious anemia, Megaloblastic anemia, Methylmalonic acidura, Homocystinuria, Peripheral neuropathy (strict vegetarian diet)	2.0 mg	Liver, meat, milk, egg, cheese.
Folic acid (Folacin)	General metabolism: Single carbon transfer reactions (e.g., purine nucleotide, thymine, heme synthesis)	Megaloblastic anemia	Infants: 25-35 mg Children: 50-180 mg Adults: 150-180 mg	Liver, green leafy vegetables

Source: *Essentials of Nutrition and Diet Therapy*. Pub. Mosby

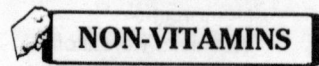

NON-VITAMINS

Some other compounds are inappropriately called B Vitamins, because of the fact that they serve as co-enzymes in metabolism. Among these non-B vitamins are the trio of co-enzymes inositol, choline and carnatine. However, only chorine has been assigned an Adequate-Intake' (AI) value.

Other substances have also been mistaken for essential nutrients. These include

(1) Para-amino benzoic acid (PABA).
(2) Bioflavonoids (Vitamin P or Hespiridin)
(3) Ubiquinone

Other names one occasionally comes, without any degree of veracity, are

(1) Vitamin B_{15}
(2) Vitamin B_{17} (Laetrile, a fake cancer drug)

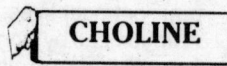

CHOLINE

Choline is a component of lecithin, which participates in lipid metabolism. It can reduce cholesterol level in the blood. It is reported to improve memory.

Deficiency

Its deficiency is associated with kidney damage, increased cholesterol and higher blood pressure and atherosclerosis.

Food Sources

Food sources of Choline are brain offals, wheat bran, brewers' yeast and egg yolk. It also found in lecithin, vegetables and milk.

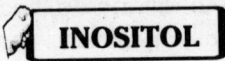 **INOSITOL**

Inositol is a structural component of lecithin. It is absorbed from intestine. Some proportion becomes sugar and some of it is led to heart muscles, brain and other organs.

Deficiency

For mice, it is considered as a dietary essential. Its deficiency shows up as loss of hair, reduced growth and milk secretion, constipation and congenital eye defects.

Food Sources

Inositol occurs naturally in liver, brewer's yeast, wheat bran, whole grains, nuts, oats, and milk. It is also found in small quantities in cabbage, peanuts, raisins and grapefruits.

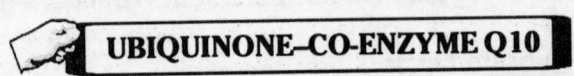 **UBIQUINONE–CO-ENZYME Q10**

Occurring everywhere in nature, this biologically active co-enzyme is called Ubiquinone. It participates in a variety of energy producing processes in the cells. It is an important anti-oxidant, which is effective in preventing heart patients from reperfusion injury.

Ubiquinone is registered as a medicine in Japan and heart patients take it as a daily supplement.

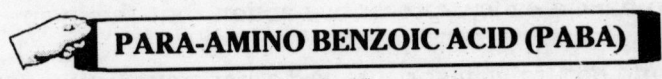 **PARA-AMINO BENZOIC ACID (PABA)**

PABA participates in the synthesis of folates. In the experimental animals, it prevents the hair from turning gray and can even restore normal hair colour.

PABA is non-toxic. For its sun-protective properties, it is used in sun-tan lotions.

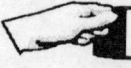 ## BIOFLAVONOIDS—VITAMIN P, RUTIN, HESPERIDIN

Rutin functions as an antioxidant. In the erstwhile Soviet Union, it was viewed as a promising antioxidant supplement, an effective daily dose of one gram is prescribed. Athletes are given bioflavonoids, because these are believed to speed up the healing of pulled muscles, sprained, joints and chafed skin.

Some studies have suggested a dose of 100 mg bioflavonoids per 500 mg vitamin C, because it helps improve the absorption of vitamin in the intestine and reinforces the beneficial effect of vitamin C on the connective tissues.

Bioflavonoids occur naturally in the plants.

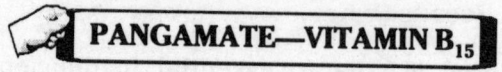 ## PANGAMATE—VITAMIN B_{15}

Pangamate is considered to be an antidote to toxins and can cure cancer, hepatitis, diabetes and other diseases. But its claims have yet to be scientifically vouchsafed.

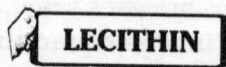 ## LECITHIN

Lecithin has become a popular food supplement. It occurs in soyabeans and vegetable oils and is one of the phospholipids produced in the liver. It is found in large quantities in brain tissue.

Phospholipids are required in food metabolism for the transport of lipids and production of energy. Lecithin is also reputed to improve memory and the mental well-being of the old people. It also has a potential beneficial effect on certain neurological diseases and myasthenia gravis.

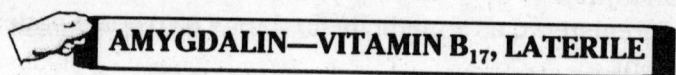 ## AMYGDALIN—VITAMIN B_{17}, LATERILE

It is reported to have a cancer-preventive action, but this point has yet to be fully vindicated.

Laetrile is found naturally in apricots and other stone fruits.

VITAMINS AND FREE RADICAL DAMAGE

Free Radicals are highly reactive oxygen-containing molecules which develop in the body as a result of both normal and abnormal metabolic processes.

Free Radicals are formed within the tissue as a result of normal metabolic activity of body. The main oxygen radicals which have pathological ramification are:

O_2'	Superoxide anions
H_2O	Hydrogen perioxide
HO'	Hydroxyl radical
HO_2'	Perhydroxy radical
RO'	Alkoxy radical
ROO'	Peroxy radical
O_2'	Singlet oxygen

Since many vitamins play a very important role as antioxidants, the Table 6.24 gives the list of such vitamins which provide protection against free radicals.

There is no denying the fact many of these vitamin antioxidants only influence the situation adequately in presence of various non-dietary defences and mineral constituents of the diet. Because whatsoever the case, one of the most important general function of vitamins lies in the field of antioxidant protection.

TABLE 6.24: VITAMINS AND ANTIOXIDANT ACTION

Vitamin A	Fat-soluble, weak free radical scavenger
β-Carotene	Lipid-soluble antioxidant and very powerful singlet oxygen quencher
Taurine	Hypochlorus acid scavenger
Vitamin C	Water-soluble extracellular antioxidant which reacts directly with hydroxyl, super oxide radical and singlet oxygen Mutually regenerates with Vitamin E.
Vitamin E	An important lipid membrane antioxidant. Reacts directly with peroxy, hydroxyl, superoxide radical and singlet oxygen. Mutually regenerates with Vitamin C. Also mutually spares with selenium.

Source: J Mark, Biological Functions of Vitamin In: *The Technology of Vitamins in Food*, Pub. Blackie Academic and Professional, 1973.

SUMMATION

In summation, one may mention the key points about all the vitamins - both fat-soluble water-soluble, as under:

1. Vitamins are essential, non-caloric organic nutrients needed in very minute doses in the diet.
2. Vitamins A, D, E and K are fat-soluble vitamins, while Vitamin C and Vitamin B group are water-soluble vitamins.
3. Vitamins can cure only those disease that are caused by the deficiency of that particular vitamin.
4. Vitamins do not yield energy when broken down, but they facilitate the release of energy from carbohydrates, fats and proteins.
5. It is not the supplement but the nutritious foods that are the best source of vitamins.

HYPERVITAMINOSIS

Many a time, some of the leading medicos consciously or otherwise recommend very high doses of vitamins in routine. This could lead to 'Hypervitaminosis', which could further aggravate the worsening conditions of the geriatrics. These complications due to excessive usage of vitamins have been categorically spelt out in Appendix Table 6.1.

APPENDIX TABLE 6.1: COMPLICATIONS OF HYPERVITAMINOSIS IN THE AGED

1.	**Vitamin A**	Gastrointestinal symptoms, Liver dysfunction, Headache, Desquamation and Xerosis.
2.	**Vitamin C**	Decreased absorption of vitamin B_{12}, Rebound Scurvy and Renal Stones.
3.	**Vitamin D**	Hypercalcemia, Hyperphosphatemia, Ectopic Calcification, Confusion and Lethargy.
4.	**Vitamin E**	Potentiates the effect of Coumadin by inhibiting vitamin K.
5.	**Vitamin B_6**	Ataxia, Loss of Vibrations and Position sense and Perioral Numbness.

Source: Duthie and Katz: *Practice of Geriatrics*. Pub. W B Saunders.

FACTORS INFLUENCING VITAMINS

The natural tendency of the compulsive 'Pill Pushers' can, to some extent, be reigned in by the family doctor or the nutritionist taking into consideration the 'Attenuating Factors', which directly influence the stability of vitamins and their retention in foods.

Appendix Figure 1 lists the eleven such factors that affect their stability.

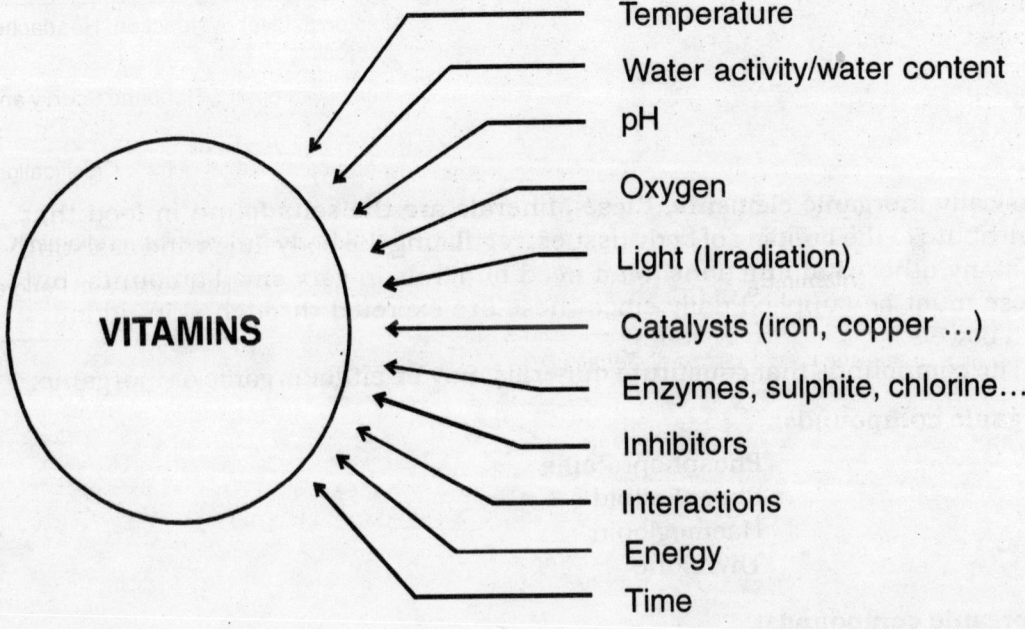

Appendix Figure 1: Factors influencing the stability of vitamins and their retention in foods (Killeit, 1988)

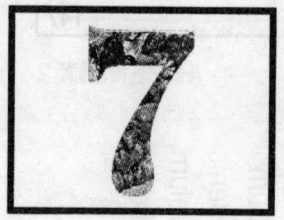

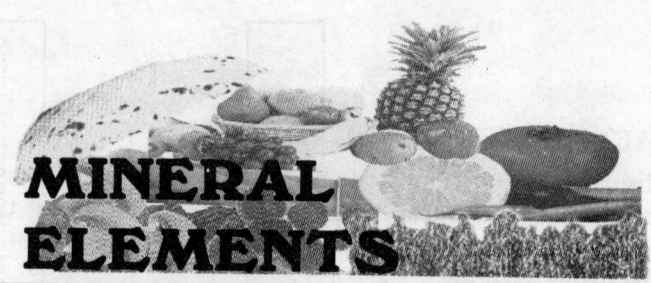

MINERAL ELEMENTS

Basically inorganic elements, these Minerals are the salts found in food that contribute to the building of body tissues, regulating the body fluids and assisting in many other vital functions. Man need minerals in very small amounts, but these must be supplied daily since these are excreted through skin, kidneys and bowels.

The compounds that constitute minerals may be either organic or inorganic:

Organic compounds:

> Phosphoproteins
> Phospholipid
> Haemoglobin
> Thyroxine

Inorganic compounds:

> Sodium chloride
> Calcium phosphate
> Free ions

Composition wise, mineral elements may be divided into three groups, viz.

(1) Major Minerals or Macro-minerals

These salts are required in relatively larger doses, more than 100 mg/day. There are five major minerals, viz., calcium, phosphorus, sodium, potassium and chlorine.

(2) Micro Minerals

This group includes salts that are required in less than a few mg/day. These examples are iron, sulfur and magnesium.

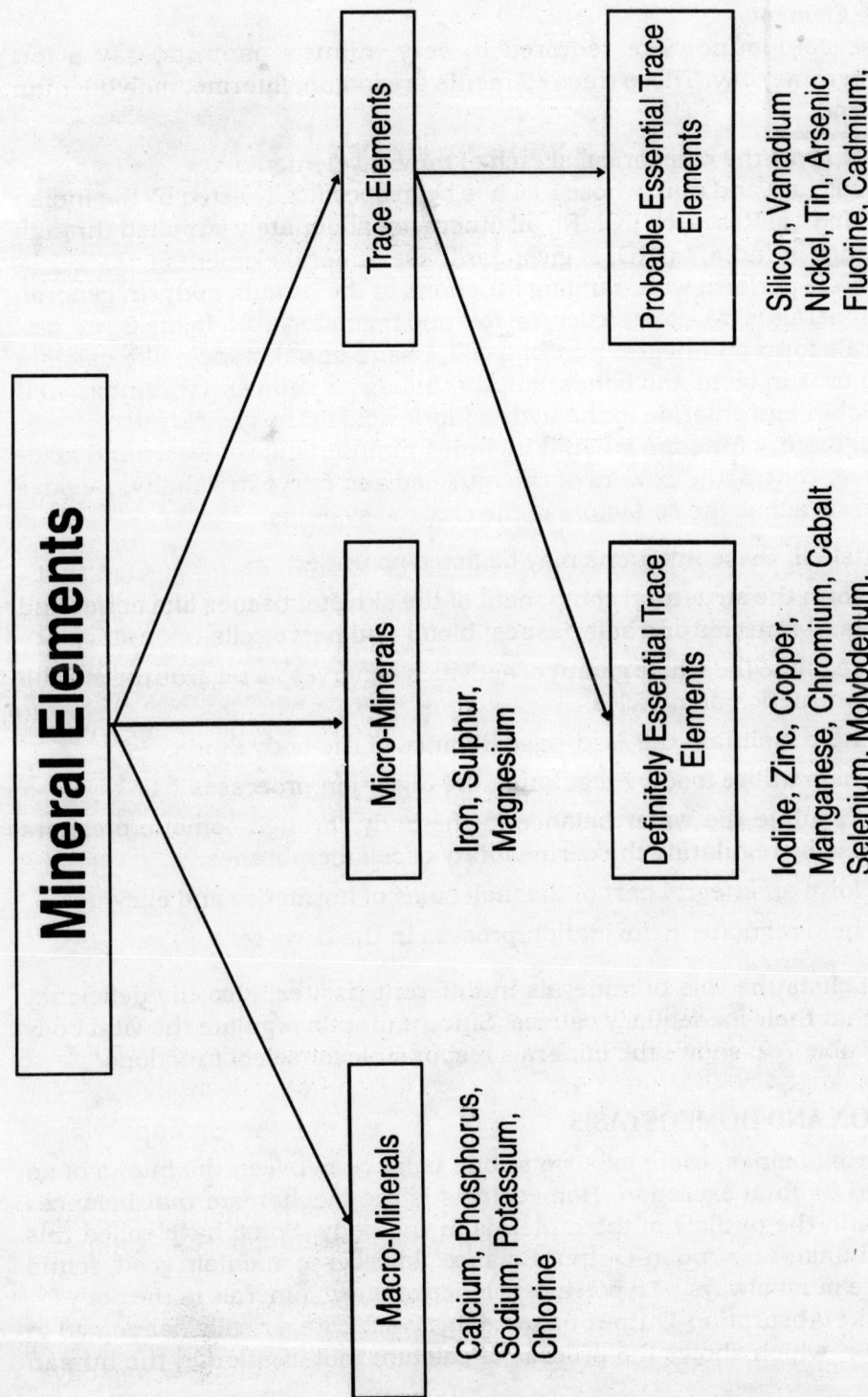

Fig. 7.1: Categorization of Mineral Elements

Mineral Elements

Trace Elements

Micro-Minerals

Macro-Minerals

Probable Essential Trace Elements

Silicon, Vanadium Nickel, Tin, Arsenic Fluorine, Cadmium, Aluminum, Boron

Definitely Essential Trace Elements

Iodine, Zinc, Copper, Manganese, Chromium, Cabalt Selenium, Molybdenum,

Iron, Sulphur, Magnesium

Calcium, Phosphorus, Sodium, Potassium, Chlorine

(3) Trace Elements

These compounds are required in very minute amounts, say a few micrograms/day. These trace elements are iodine, fluorine, molybdenum and zinc.

Figure 7.1 gives the categorical sketch of mineral elements.

Save for calcium and iron, whose RDI has been specifically listed by the Indian Council of Medical Research (ICMR), all others are adequately supplied through the diet, hence in India, no RDI is given for these mineral elements.

The minerals perform wide-ranging functions in the human body. In general, the role of minerals is two-fold: structural role and regulatory role. In the Structural role, minerals form an integral part of a cell, tissue or substance, like calcium and phosphorus in teeth and bones, sulphur in hair, insulin and thrombin, iron in haemoglobin and chloride in the hydrochloric acid of the gastric juice.

It is a Regulatory function when it includes maintenance of water and acid-base balance, contractile powers of the muscles and nerve irritability. Besides these minerals act as the co-factors of the enzyme systems.

In nutshell, these functions may be listed as under:

1. They form the structural component of the skeletal tissues like bones and teeth and muscles and soft tissues, blood and nerve cells.
2. They regulate the whole gamut of activities of nerves as regards the stimuli and contraction of muscles.
3. They help maintain the Acid-base Balance of the body fluids.
4. They help utilize food by regulating the digestion processes.
5. They regulate the water balance in the body through osmotic pressure and also by regulating the permeability of cell membranes.
6. They form an integral part of the molecules of hormones and enzymes.
7. They help regulate the oxidation process in the body cells.

Table 7.1. lists the role of minerals in different tissues, also the deficiency syndrome that their inadequacy causes. Since minerals regulate the vital body functions. Table 7.2. shows the minerals responsible for select functions.

ABSORPTION AND HOMEOSTASIS

In all the living beings, there exists a subtle balance between the intake of an element and its final excretion. Homeostasis is the mechanism that balances the inflow and the outflow of the minerals in the body. Some have called this process as 'Intake-Absorption-Output Balance'. In order to maintain good, sound health, there must always be a positive balance of these minerals in the body.

This Intake-Absorption-Output balance has been categorically delineated in Fig. 7.2 later, which shows the process of calcium mobilization in the human body.

TABLE 7.1: MINERAL REQUIREMENTS OF BODY TISSUES

Tissues	Minerals Needed	Deficiency Syndrome
Bones and Teeth	Calcium and Phosphorus	Stunted growth, soft bones, malformed or decaying teeth and rickets
Hair, Nails, Skin and Soft Tissues	Potassium, Phosphorus, Sulphur and Chlorine	—
Nervous Tissues	Phosphorus	—
Blood	Iron, Calcium, Sodium, Phosphorus and Copper	Lack of Fe or Cu results in low hemoglobin in blood —nutritional anaemia
Glandular Secretions		
Gastric	Chlorine	
Intestinal	Sodium	
Thyroid	Iodine	Inadequate iodine results in enlargement of thyroid gland—simple goitre
Pancreas (Insulin)	Zinc	

TABLE 7.2: BODY REGULATION OF MINERALS

1.	To maintain the normal exchange of body fluids (osmosis)	Sodium, potassium, chlorine, magnesium
2.	Maintaining muscle contractility	Ca, Na and K balance
3.	Nerve irritability	Potassium
4.	Clotting of blood	Calcium
5.	Oxidation processes	Fe, I, Se and Mn
6.	Maintaining pH of body	Balance between basic elements and acid fluids

Normally, the diet in countries like India is deficient in calcium, iron and iodine. If by judicious planning, these three most crucial elements are taken care of, then all the other elements will be automatically taken care of.

Table 7.3 at the end presents a comprehensive summary of these Macro minerals, and their sources of origin.

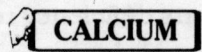 **CALCIUM**

Of all the minerals present in the body, Calcium is found in by far the largest amount. It constitutes about 1.5 to 2% of the total body weight, approximating about 1200 grams in an average adult. Almost 99% of the total calcium is found in the teeth and bones, the remainder 1% of calcium in the circulatory system helps in the blood clotting process, as under:

$$\text{Blood Platelets} \xrightarrow{\text{Ca}^{++}} \text{Thromboplastin}$$

Thromboplastin + Prothrombin $\rightarrow$ Thrombin

Thrombin + Fibrinogen $\xrightarrow{\text{Ca}^{++}}$ Fibrin (Clot)

The bulk of the skeletal calcium in the body is deposited in the form of Hydroxyapatite $[Ca_{10}(PO_4)_6(OH_2)]$. The bone tissue is constantly being reshaped according to various body needs and stresses, with as much as 700 mg of calcium entering and leaving bones each day.

Absorption

On an average, between 10% to 30% of all the dietary calcium is absorbed. Most of the food calcium occurs in complexes with other dietary components. These complexes have to be broken down and calcium released in a soluble form, before it can be absorbed in the small intestines, mainly duodenum.

Factors Favouring Ca Absorption

1. **Vitamin D Hormone:** This hormone controls the synthesis of a calcium-binding protein carrier in the duodenum that transports calcium into the mucosal cells and blood circulation.

2. **Body Need:** More Ca is absorbed during the stress period. Hence conditions like growth, pregnancy, lactation and aging have strong influence on absorption. In the post-menstrual period and old age, the ability to absorb Ca is very much diminished.

3. **Dietary Proteins and Carbohydrates:** High protein levels mean still greater absorption. But this increased absorption leads to enhanced renal excretion, which ultimately results in a negative Ca balance. Lactose also enhances Ca absorption through the action of lactobacilli.

4. **Acidity:** Lower pH favours solubility of Ca and hence contributes to its ready absorption.

Factors Hindering Ca Absorption

1. **Vitamin D deficiency:** Vitamin D, along with parathyroid hormone, is essential for Ca absorption; its deficiency retards absorption.

2. **Dietary Fat:** Excess fat in food or poor absorption of fat results in increased fat in the intestines. This fat combines with Ca to form insoluble soaps, which are excreted, thus causing loss of Ca.

3. **Binding Agents:** An excess of dietary fibre binds Ca and hinders its absorption. Other binding agents meeting the same fate are calcium oxalates and phytic acid.

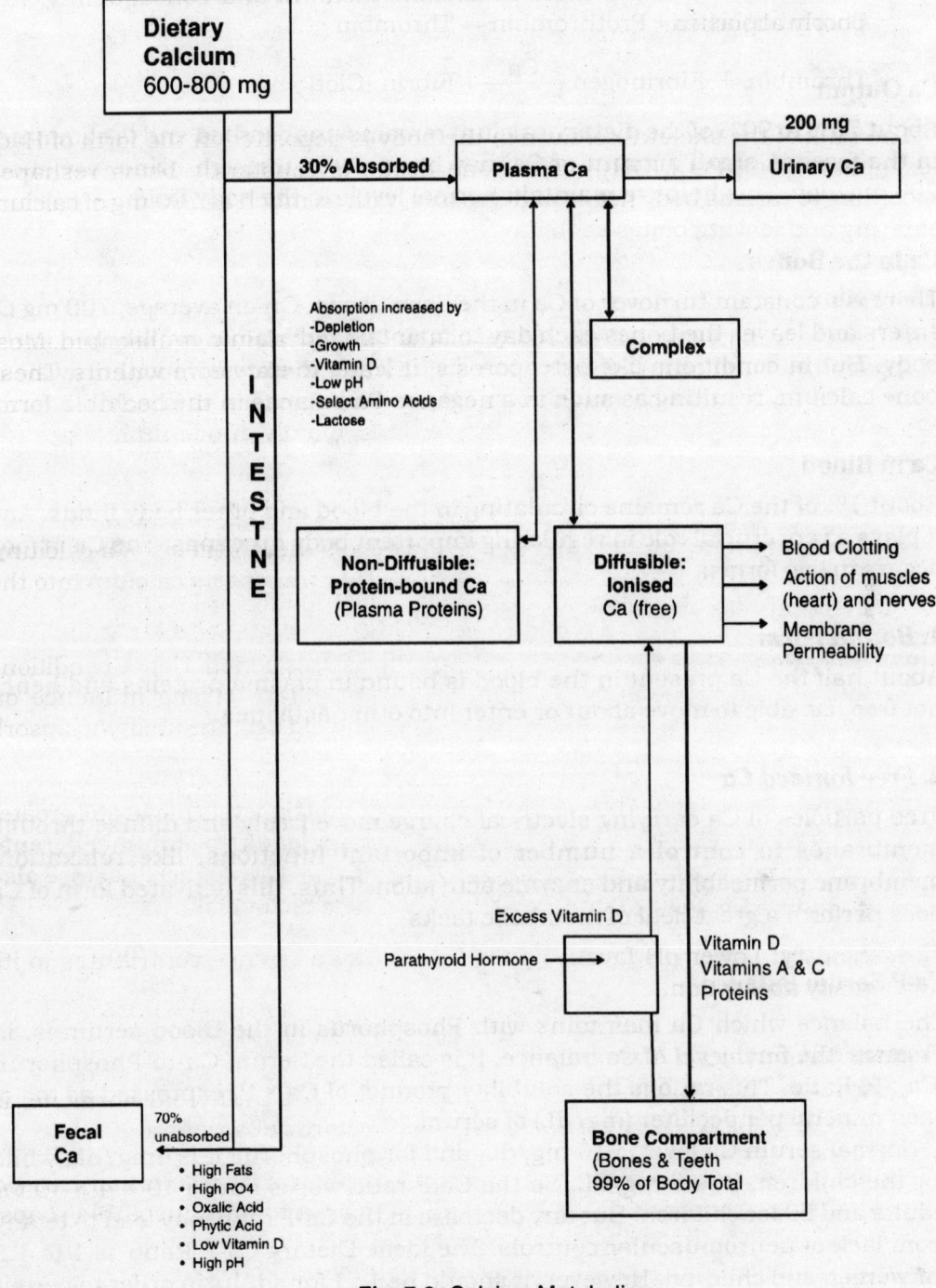

Fig. 7.2: Calcium Metabolism

(Source: Essentials of Nutrition and Diet Therapy by Sue Rodwell Williams, Mosby Pub., 1993)

4. **Alkalinity:** Ca is insoluble in alkaline medium and consequently, it is poorly absorbed.

Ca Output

About 70% to 90% of the dietary calcium remains unabsorbed and is eliminated in the feces. A small amount of Ca may be excreted through urine, say about 200 mg/day. This helps to maintain normal levels in the body fluid.

Ca in the Bones

There is a constant turnover of Ca in the bone tissue. On an average, 700 mg Ca enters and leaves the bones each day to maintain a dynamic equilibrium in the body. But in conditions like osteoporosis, it leads to excessive withdrawals of bone calcium, resulting as such in a negative Ca balance in the body.

Ca in Blood

About 1% of the Ca remains circulating in the blood and other body fluids. And it plays a very crucial role in regulating important body functions. The Ca in food occurs in two forms:

1. *Bound Form*

About half the Ca present in the blood is bound in plasma proteins and hence not free, *i.e.* able to move about or enter into other activities.

2. *Free Ionized Ca*

Free particles of Ca carrying electrical charge move freely and diffuse through membranes to control a number of important functions, like relaxation, membrane permeability and enzyme activation. Thus, this activated form of Ca does perform a great deal of metabolic tasks.

Ca-P Serum Balance

The balance which Ca maintains with Phosphorus in the Blood serum is, in essence, the final level of Ca balance. It is called the Serum Ca-to-Phosphorus (Ca : P) Ratio. This ratio is the solubility product of Ca × P, expressed as mg of each mineral per deciliter (mg/dL) of serum.

Normal serum Ca level is 10 mg/dL, and for phosphorus it is 4mg/dL, while for the children, it is 5 mg/dL. So the Ca:P ratio works out to 10 × 4 = 40 for adults and 50 for children. But any decrease in the Ca-P ratio may lead to tetany from lack of neuromuscular controls. The ideal 'Dietary Ca-P Ratio' is 1 to 1.5 for women and children. However, it should be 1 : 1 for adults in order to permit ideal absorption and utilization of calcium.

Deposition-Mobilization Balance

The second largest homeostatic balance control involves bones as a major site of Ca storage. Bone is a dynamic tissue, characterized by constant turn-over of Ca. The circulating ionized Ca is being constantly deposited in bone, while Ca stored in the bone is being perpetually cannabalized and withdrawn.

Three inter-related hormones regulate this exchange and maintain the Ca balance.

1. *Vitamin D (Calcitrol)*

Vitamin D plays a major role in the intestinal absorption of Ca and later its deposition in bone matrix. That way, it directly affects the calcification of bone tissue.

2. *Parathyroid Hormone*

Parathyroid hormone acts in concert with vitamin D hormone to control plasma changes of free ionized Ca. When the plasma level drops, parathyroid glands react by producing parathyroid hormone, which acts at three levels to restore calcium level. These phases are:

1. It stimulates intestinal mucosa to increase the absorption of Ca,
2. It mobilizes Ca rapidly from the bone compartment by activating osteoclasts to demineralise the bone,
3. To increase resorption of Ca from glomerular filtrate and decrease resorption of phosphates, thus conserving Ca and increasing renal excretion of phosphates.

   These combined activities restore Ca and P to their correctly-balanced ratio in the blood. Tetany results from a decrease in the free ionized serum Ca. This action of parathyroid hormone prevents tetany.

3. *Calcitonin*

Calcitonin, a hormone involved intimately in Ca metabolism, is produced by the special C cells in the thyroid gland. Calcitonin prevents abnormal rise in serum Ca by decreasing the release of Ca from bones. Thus, its action counterbalances the action of parathyroid hormone to regulate the serum Ca at normal levels in balance with bone calcium.

Figure 7.2 illustrates the overall balance relationship of various factors in Calcium metabolism.

Physiological Functions

The metabolic function of 99% of the Ca in the body is to build and maintain skeletal tissues, developing cartilage into bone. This delicate task is carried out by two types of cells, viz. osteoblasts and osteoclasts. The osteoblasts continually form new bone matrix in which calcium phosphate is deposited and bone crystals develop. Osteoclasts continually balance this activity by absorbing bone tissue. They engulf (phagostise) and digest minute bone crystals.

Tooth Formation: Special tooth-forming organs in the gums deposit Ca to form teeth. This exchange in dental tissue occurs mainly in the dentin and cementum.

General Metabolic Functions

The remaining 1% of the body Ca performs a number of vital metabolic functions like:

1. **Blood Clotting:** Serum Ca ions are required in blood clotting for cross-linking fibrin, as shown earlier.

2. **Nerve Impulse Transmission:** A current of Ca ion triggers the flow of signals from one nerve cell to another and then onward to the target muscles.

3. **Muscle Contraction/Relaxation:** Ionized serum Ca initiates contraction of muscle fibres. This factor is very important in the contraction-relaxation cycle of the heart muscles.

4. **Cell Membrane Permeability:** It controls the passage of fluids through cell membranes. It also influences the integrity of the intercellular cement substance.

5. **Enzyme Activation:** Ca ions are important activators of specific enzymes, particularly the one that provides energy for muscle contraction.

Clinical Problems (Deficiency)

Tetany

Low ionized serum Ca results in Tetany, which is marked by severe intermittent spastic contraction of muscles and also by muscle pains.

Rickets

Deficiency of Vitamin D causes Rickets. Inadequate exposure to sunlight or deficient dietary intake of vitamin precursors impedes the formation of bones.

Osteoporosis

Osteoporosis is characterized by bone-mineral loss, which usually occurs in older persons, all the more so in the postmenstrual women. Repeated pregnancy and low intake of vitamin D and calcium are the predisposing causes of osteoporosis. There is a negative Ca balance of about 40 to 120mg/day during the first five years after the menopause. Afterwards, this bone loss amounts to about 1% a year. It is also seen in case of interference with fat absorption and the consequent vitamin D mal-absorption and in the patients with renal diseases. There is a softening of leg bones, spine, thorax and pelvis, which get bent or deformed. Hormonal therapy with both vitamin D and estrogens proves beneficial in osteoporosis.

Hypercalcemia

The excessive rise in blood Ca level is caused by the greater intake of Ca. This results in increased Ca deposition in soft tissues and increased excretion of Ca in the urine. This is usually observed in peptic ulcer cases. The symptoms herein are vomiting, gastrointestinal bleeding and an increased blood pressure.

Toxicity

No adverse effects have been found with the ingestion of Ca supplements up to 2400 mg Ca/day, except for constipation in some cases. However, dietary intake of more than 2400 mg Ca may impair renal function. There is a risk of stone formation in patients with renal hypercalciuria, primary hyperthyroidism and sarcoidosis.

Ca Requirement

The RDA standard for Ca for adults is 800 mg/day, which goes up to 1200 mg/day in the case of pregnant and lactating women. Children need relatively more Ca. A generous intake of milk and green leafy vegetables are recommended during lactation, as also quick-growing infancy periods.

A majority of studies have shown that Ca supplementation for the post-menopausal women helps delay or even treat osteoporosis condition.

Dietary calcium intake of most individuals in the United States is less than recommended (Table 7.3). Median intake of males is above the RDA until about 40 years of age while the mean intake exceeds the RDA until age 80. Median intake of females drops below the RDA in the 12- to 15-year range while the mean intake does not fall below the RDA until age 30-39 years. Therefore, in more than 50% of women the calcium intake is below the recommended intake for the critical ages of bone deposition.

Food Sources

Dairy products like skim milk, butter milk and cheese provide the bulk of dietary calcium. A glass of milk (8 oz) contains about 300 mg Ca. Other non-dairy sources of Ca (in moderate amounts) are eggs, green leafy vegetables, broccoli, legumes, nuts and the whole grains. Amongst cereals, Ragi (Finger Millets) is a very rich source of Ca; so also grain Amaranth. Table 7.4 shows the composition of Ca-rich foods.

TABLE 7.3: RECOMMENDED DIETARY ALLOWANCES FOR CALCIUM

Age (years)	RDA (mg)
Infants	
0.0-0.5	400
0.5-1.0	600
Children	
1-3	800
4-6	800
7-10	800
Males	
11-14	1200
15-18	1200
19-24	1200
25-50	800
51+	800
Females	
11-14	1200
15-18	1200
19-24	1200
25-50	800
51+	800
Pregnant	1200
Lactating	
1st 6 month	1200
2nd 6 month	1200

RDA = Recommended dietary allowance.

Source: Kathleen Mahan and Escott Stump in *Food, Nutrition and Diet Therapy*. Pub. W.B. Saunders.

PHOSPHORUS

Phosphorus is one of the most important mineral which forms the very matrix of the genetic substances—DNA and RNA—that are the real core of heredity. Phosphorus is found in all cells and is the sixth most abundant element in the body. Phosphorus accounts for about 1% of the total body weight. Phosphorus is deeply involved in the process of metabolism in each and every cell.

Phosphorus is associated very closely with Ca, hence it is also called 'Metabolic Twin'. Both phosphorus and Ca are involved in bone formation and are related to vitamin D and parathyroid hormone in absorption and excretion processes. They both exist in the blood serum in a certain ratio. The adult serum phosphate level normally ranges from 2.5 mg/dL to 5 mg/dL.

Chemically, Phosphorus can exist in a variety of oxidation states—from PH_3 to P_2O_5. From Nutritional Biochemistry angle, PO_4, rather than phosphorus per se, becomes the main center of attention.

TABLE 7.4: DIETARY SOURCES OF CALCIUM

Excellent Sources (over 200 mg per serving)		Good Sources (100-200 mg per serving)		Fair Sources (50-100 mg per serving)	
Source	Quantity	Source	Quantity	Source	Quantity
Milk	290 mg/cup	Cottage		Sandwich	
Cheddar		Cheese	100 mg/½ cup	Bread	50 mg/2 slices
Cheese	200 mg/oz	Broccoli	100 mg/cup,	Bran	
Yogurt	271 mg/cup		cooked	Muffin	57 mg/muffin
Sardines	375 mg/3-oz can	Okra	147 mg/cup, cooked	Lobuster	94 mg/cup of meat
Canned salmon	550 mg/7-oz can	Mustard greens	193 mg/cup, cooked	Potato Salad	80 mg/cup
Turnip greens	267 mg/cup, cooked	Blackstrap Molasses	137 mg/tbsp	Lima Beans	80 mg/cup, cooked
Collard greens	357 mg/cup, cooked	Cornbread	133 mg/2-in square	Onions	50 mg/cup, boiled
Spinach	232 mg/cup, cooked	Pancakes Ice cream	150 mg/3 pan- 194 mg/cup	Lentils	50 mg/cup, cooked
Macaroni and Cheese	362 mg/cup	Tofu	154 mg/2-in square (1 in thick)	Oranges Raisins	70 mg/orange 54 mg/3 oz

Source: Alice A. Chenault in *Nutrition and Health*, Pub., Hott, Rinehart and Winston.

Phosphorus in extracellular fluid accounts for only 1% of the total phosphorus in the body. The majority, say about 70% of the total phosphorus in human plasma is found as a constituent of organic phospholipids, though the clinically useful fraction in plasma is the total inorganic phosphorus concentration.

Absorption-Excretion Balance

Free phosphate is absorbed in the jejunum in small intestines and is regulated by calcitrol, the active form of vitamin D. When the serum phosphate level is low, the kidney is stimulated to provide vitamin D hormone, which, in turn, enhances phosphorus absorption from the intestines. This is called the 'Feedback Mechanism' of hormone action. Excess of Ca or other binding materials like aluminium and iron inhibit the absorption of phosphorus.

The primary tissue sites of phosphorus storage are in bone hydroxapatite (85%) and skeletal muscle (14%). Kidneys provide the main excretion route for regulation of serum phosphate level. The amount of phosphorus excreted in urine in a person on an average diet varies from 0.6 to 1.8 g/day.

Physiologic Functions
1. *Glucose and Glycerol Absorption*

Phosphorus combines with glucose and glycerol to assist in their absorption in the intestines. Phosphorus also promotes renal tubular reabsorption of glucose to release the sugar into blood.

2. Transport

Phospholipids provide a mode of fat transport.

3. Energy Metabolism

The phosphorus-containing compound, Adenosine triphosphate (ATP) is the key cell substance in energy metabolism.

4. Buffer System

The phosphate buffer system of phosphoric acid and phosphate helps control acid-base balance in the blood.

4. As Activators in Vitamins

The active form of many vitamins are their phosphorus-derivatives like B_1, B_2, B_6 and pantothenic acid.

6. As Storage Compound

High energy storage compounds are phosphate esters of organic compounds, like ATP, creatine phosphate, etc.

Deficiency and Imbalance

Since our diet contains adequate proteins and calcium, so the incidence of Phosphorus deficiency are very rare. The conditions which involve physiologic and clinical changes in serum Phosphorus level include stunted growth, poor teeth and bone formation. Rickets, weakness, pain and anorexia are the symptoms of phosphorus deficiency. Most of the deficiency syndrome resembles that of calcium. Phosphorus deficiency is accompanied by a reduction in the urinary phosphorus excretion and an increase in urinary calcium, magnesium and potassium excretion.

Hyperphosphatemia and Hypophosphatemia may result when the serum-Phosphorus levels deviate from the normal, either they go up or come down due to the impaired phosphorus metabolism. Excessive amount of phosphorus can be lost in the urine of uncontrolled diabetic patients who have polyuria and acidosis.

Hyperphosphatemia is usually seen in chronic renal failure, wherein reduced renal function results in increased sensitivity to large dietary loads of phosphorus. It is also seen with severe hemolysis, tumour lysis syndrome and various endocrine dysfunction like hyoperthyroidism.

Phosphorus Requirements

During growth, pregnancy and lactation, the ratio of dietary P to Ca should preferably be 1 : 1.5. Since both Ca and phosphorus are found in the same foods, hence if Ca needs are met, then adequate P will be automatically ensured for the body metabolism.

The RDA standard for phosphorus is the same as that of Ca ranging between 800-1200 mg/day. But for the infants, it is 300-500 mg/day.

The average adult intake of phosphorus in the United States is approximately 1500 mg/day for males and 1000 mg/day for females. Most phosphorus (about 60%) comes from milk, meat, poultry, fish and eggs. Another 20% comes from cereals and legumes, and approximately 10% comes from fruits and their juices. Soft drinks, tea and coffee supply about 3%.

Phosphorus is well absorbed from meat. Phosphorus bound to milk casein, which is approximately 20% of total amount, is much less available.

Table 7.5 shows the RDA for phosphorus for different age groups and sex.

TABLE 7.5: RECOMMENDED DIETARY ALLOWANCES FOR PHOSPHORUS

Age (years)	RDA (mg)
Infants	
0.0-0.5	300
0.5-1.0	500
Children	
1-3	800
4-6	800
7-10	800
Males	
11-14	1200
15-18	1200
19-24	1200
25-50	800
51+	800
Females	
11-14	1200
15-18	1200
19-24	1200
25-50	800
51+	800
Pregnant	1200
Lactating	
1st 6 month	1200
2nd 6 month	1200

RDA = Recommended dietary allowance.

Source: Kathleen Mahan and Escott Stump in *Food, Nutrition and Diet Therapy*. Pub. W.B. Saunders.

Food Sources

Milk and meat are the most important sources of phosphorus in the food, accounting for almost 50% of the dietary phosphorus supplied. Cereals, particularly whole grains, flours, legumes and nuts are the other fairly good sources for obtaining phosphorus. Table 7.6 shows the phosphorus content of selected foods.

TABLE 7.6: PHOSPHORUS CONTENT OF SELECT FOODS

Food	Quantity (mg)
Grilled Cheese Sandwich, 1	531
Macaroni and Cheese, 1 cup	322
Milkshake, vanilla, 10 oz	289
Sole, baked, 3 oz	248
Tostada with Beans and Beef, 1	247
Tofu, firm, ½ cup	239
Milk, 2% fat, 1 cup	232
Pizza, 1/8 of 15" diameter	216
Cheese, Swiss, processed, 1 oz	216
Split Pea Soup, 1 cup	213
Cheese, American, 1 oz	211
Ham, 3 oz	210
Ice milk, soft serve, 1 cup	202
Almonds, ¼ cup	184
Oatmeal, 1 cup	178
Lentils, cooked, ½ cup	178
Cheese, cottage, 2% fat, ½ cup	170
Cheese, cheddar, 1 oz	146
Yeast, Brewer's, 1 tsp	140
Cashews, ¼ cup	138
Shrimp, boiled, 2 large	137
Baked Beans (white), ½ cup	137
Ground Beef, 3 oz	135
Tofu, regular, ½ cup	120
Potato, baked, ith skin, 1	115
Cheese Sauce, ¼ cup	109
Garbanzo Beans, canned, ½ cup	108
Egg, 1	86
Milk, dry, nonfat, instant, 2 tsp	84
Bread, Whole Wheat, 1 slice	74
Peas, frozen, cooed, ½ cup	72
Cola Beverage, 1 can (12 oz)	46
Baking Powder, 1 tsp	45
Potato Chips, 14	43
Chocolate, dark, 1 oz	41
Cocoa Powder, 1 tsp	38
Bread, White, 1 slice	30
Lettuce, Romaine, 1 cup	25
Cauliflower, fresh, ½ cup	23
Orange, 1	18

Source: USDA: Composition of Foods. USDA Handbook, 1976-1986.

SODIUM

Sodium is the one mineral salt that is available most abundantly in the human body. Sodium chloride is the basic element of food—something which lends special taste to the diet.

An adult body has got 120 mg (4 oz) of sodium. Of this, about one-third present in the skeleton is an inorganic-bound material. The remaining two-thirds is the free ionized sodium in the extracellular fluids, which forms the main electrolyte in the body fluids outside the cells. The latter is largely distributed in plasma and in nerve and muscle tissues. Normal serum values range from 310 mg to 340 mg/dL (136 to 145 mEq/L).

Absorption-Excretion Balance

Sodium is readily absorbed from the intestines; only 5% is left behind to be eliminated through feces. However, in conditions like diarrhea, there is too much loss of sodium salt. The sodium-conserving hormone, Aldosterone from the adrenal glands, regulates the excretion of sodium through the kidneys. The aldostrone mechanism for conservation is one of the major homeostatic controls of body sodium, and hence of the body water too.

Physiologic Functions

1. *Water Balance*

Ionized sodium is the major regulator of water-balance, outside the cells.

2. *Acid-Base Balance*

Along with chloride and bicarbonate ions, ionized sodium helps regulate the acid-base balance of the body.

3. *Cell Permeability*

The sodium pump in all cell membranes helps exchange sodium and potassium and other cellular materials. Glucose is the one major element carried by this active transport system.

4. *Muscle Irritability*

Sodium ions play a major role in transmitting electro-chemical impulses along the nerve and muscle membranes and thus, help maintain the normal muscle irritability or excitability.

Deficiency

The abundance of sodium chloride in the food does not permit any sort of deficiency to occur in the system. However, in the case of athletes and others engaged in hard manual labour, there can be sodium depletion. This is due to excessive sweating. Herein, the symptoms are giddiness, nausea, weakness and muscle cramps. In very advanced case, it could lead to circulatory failure even. This deficiency syndrome could be easily overcome by the greater intake of common salt as also more fluids being taken with the diet.

In case of cardiac and renal failure, the sodium excretion is reduced, which results in swelling of the extremities and edema.

Requirements

The RDA standards for sodium are estimated at 500 mg/day. However, sodium in the average American diet comprising mainly of processed foods far exceeds this amount. A judicious intake of about 2 g sodium, equal to about 5 g table salt (one teaspoon) is advisable, looking to the association of hypertension with high salt intake. Indians are accustomed to a very high intake of salt, averaging 15-20 g/day. For them, it is advisable to bring down the level of salt consumption to 8-10 g/day. This would also compensate for excessive sweating or hard manual labour.

Food Sources

Common salt is the main source of sodium. One teaspoonful salt contains 2000 -2400 mg sodium. Other sources of sodium are milk, egg-white, meat, poultry, fish and some vegetables and fruits, besides cereals and legumes. For more categorical details, one may refer to sodium levels in different food stuffs in Chapter 19.

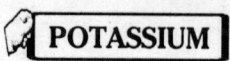 **POTASSIUM**

The mineral, Potassium is abundantly present in the body—being twice as plentiful as sodium. An average adult body contains 270 mg potassium (9 ounces or 4000 mEq/L). By far the largest amount is found inside the cells, since potassium is reckoned as the major regulator of body water inside the cells. And the smaller moiety found in the extracellular fluid plays a very significant role in muscle activity, especially for the heart muscles. The normal serum value for potassium range from 14 mg to 20 mg/dL.

Absorption-Excretion Balance

The dietary potassium is readily absorbed in the small intestines. But it also circulates in gastro-intestinal secretions, having earlier been absorbed in the digestive process. Renal excretion is the principal route for potassium loss. Since maintenance of serum potassium within a certain range is vital to the heart muscle action, as also the electrolyte balance, the kidney carefully guards potassium, although it may not be as effective as that of sodium. In the renal aldosterone mechanism for sodium conservation, it is the potassium which is lost in exchange for sodium. Normally, this potassium loss is estimated at about 160 mg per day.

Physiologic Functions

1. *Water and Acid-Base Balance*

Potassium balances with sodium outside the cells to maintain normal osmotic pressures and water balance to protect the cellular fluid. Along with ionized sodium and ionized hydrogen, potassium also works to maintain the acid-base balance.

2. *Muscle Activity*

Potassium plays a significant role in the activity of skeletal and cardiac muscle. Supported by Na and Ca, it regulates neuromuscular stimulation, transmission of electrochemical impulses and contraction of muscle fibres. This action is particularly notable in the action of the heart muscles, which show up any inadequacy in the ECG. In acute cases, the heart may develop a 'Gallop Rhythm', that could even lead to cardiac arrest. Low serum potassium and hypertension causes muscle irritability and paralysis.

3. *Carbohydrate Metabolism*

For each gram of glycogen converted from blood sugars for storage, potassium to the tune of 0.36 mmol is stored. When a diabetic patient is treated with insulin and glucose, rapid glycogen production draws potassium from the serum. Serious Hypokalemia results if adequate potassium replacement does not accompany the treatment.

4. *Protein Synthesis*

Potassium is vitally needed for the storage in muscle protein and general cell protein. When a tissue breaks down, potassium is lost together with nitrogen. To ensure N retention, amino acid replacement must include potassium.

Deficiency Syndrome

Hypokalemia

Potassium deficiency is noticed only in the case of prolonged malnutrition, as also in chronic alcoholism, anorexia nervosa and low carbohydrate diets. It also occurs in weight reduction when the diet is very much restricted. In case of accidents, burns and after surgery, potassium loss may exceed replacement, thus leading to deficiency. The symptoms herein are low plasma level of potassium, *i.e.* Hypokalemia accompanied by nausea, vomiting, muscle weakness, increased heart beat (tachycardia), besides arrhythmia and an altered electrocardiogram. In severe cases of potassium deficiency, it could even led to cardiac arrest.

Hypertension

Recent studies show that inadequate intake of potassium contributes to the development of hypertension. Reports also indicate that a high potassium intake lowers blood pressure.

Toxicity: Hyperkalemia

The excess of potassium shows up in cases of severe dehydration, renal failure, adrenalin insufficiency and after very rapid administration of potassium. The main symptoms are paresthesias (sensation of numbness, pricking or tingling) of scalp, face and tongue; muscle weakness, breathing troubles, cardiac arrhythmia and changes in the ECG.

Potassium Requirement

The RDA standards estimate a minimum daily intake of 2000 mg potassium per day for an average adult. This is normally met by most of the diet which contain potassium from 2000 to 4000 mg/day. The increased intake of fruits and vegetables helps raise potassium level to 3500 mg/day.

Food Sources

Fruits and many vegetables are considered to be the richest sources of potassium. Other good sources are meat, poultry, fish, milk and curds. Other foods rich in potassium are whole grain cereals and legumes, fruits and vegetables like bananas, potatoes, tomatoes, carrots, celery, broccoli, orange, grapes, chikus and custard apple. For more categorical details, one may refer to Potassium level of different food stuffs in Chapter 19.

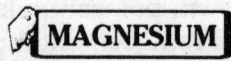 **MAGNESIUM**

Magnesium is found in all the body cells. An average adult body contains about 25 grams of magnesium. Three-fourths of this amount is combined with calcium and phosphorus in the bone. The remaining 30% is distributed in various tissues and body fluids.

Absorption-Excretion Balance

Magnesium is absorbed throughout small intestines. On a high magnesium diet, only about one-fourth of the limited intake is absorbed, but this level goes up to three-fourths in case of low magnesium diets. High levels of dietary calcium, phosphorus and proteins diminish magnesium absorption from intestines. Aldosterone increases the renal clearance of magnesium.

Physiologic Functions

1. *Catalyst*

Magnesium plays the role of a catalyst in many a metabolic function for energy production and building the body tissues.

2. *Muscle Action*

Magnesium aids in normal muscle action. It is very essential for the functioning of heart beat and maintenance of blood pressure. Any change in intracellular fluid concentration of magnesium ions produces neuromuscular irritability.

3. *Enzyme Activation*

It is required to activate the enzyme involved in the oxidative phosphorylation of ADP to ATP and for the return of ATP to cyclic AMP, which then regulates parathormone secretions.

Deficiency Syndrome

Magnesium deficiency is not found under normal conditions. But prolonged malnutrition and increased excretion may lead to lowering of the plasma magnesium. This shows up like the hypocalcemic tetany, convulsions and delerium. Magnesium deficiency is often seen in cases of chronic alcoholism, cirrhosis of liver, kwashiorkor, diabetes and diuretic therapy.

Requirement

The 1989 RDA for adults was accepted at 4.5 mg/kg body weight. The RDA standards for an adult male is 350 mg/day and 280 mg for women. This level can be increased to 320 mg/day during pregnancy, to further go upto 355 mg/day for lactating women. Table 7.7 shows the RDA for magnesium for different age groups and sex.

Food Sources

Magnesium is relatively widespread in nature. Green vegetables are a good source of magnesium complex found in the chlorophyll. Its main sources are soyabeans, nuts, cocoa, sea-foods, whole grains and dried peas and beans, besides fresh green vegetables and legumes. Table 7.8 shows the magnesium content of different food stuffs and Table 7.9 shows the hierarchy of different food stuffs as regards magnesium.

TABLE 7.7: RECOMMENDED DIETARY ALLOWANCES FOR MAGNESIUM

Age (years)	RDA (mg)
Infants	
0.0-0.5	40
0.5-1.0	60
Children	
1-3	80
4-6	120
7-10	170
Males	
11-14	270
15-18	400
19-24	350
25-50	350
51+	350
Females	
11-14	280
15-18	300
19-24	280
25-50	280
51+	280
Pregnant	300
Lactating	
1st 6 month	355
2nd 6 month	340

RDA = Recommended dietary allowance.
Source: Kathleen Mahan and Escott Stump in *Food, Nutrition and Diet Therapy*. Pub. W.B. Saunders.

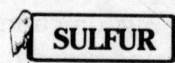

SULFUR

Sulfur is an essential element that contributes to a wide range of metabolic functions. As a constituent of cell proteins, it is found in all the cells of body. Sulfur is also a constituent with many other protein compounds like:

(1) Sulfur-containing amino acids like methionine, cystine and cysteine,
(2) Glycoprotein in cartilage, tendons and bone matrix,
(3) Detoxification products formed by bacterial activity in the intestines, e.g. cresol sulphuric acid and indoxyl sulphate.
(4) Other organic compounds like heparin, insulin, Co-enzymes A, lipoic acid, and water soluble vitamins, thiamine and biotin.
(5) Keratin, the protein of hair and nails.

The plasma sulfate levels range from 50 mmol to 150 mmol/L.

TABLE 7.8: MAGNESIUM CONTENT OF SELECTED FOODS

Food	Quantity (mg)
Tofu, firm, ½ cup	118
Chili with Beans, 1 cup	115
Wheat Germ, toasted, ¼ cup	90
Cashews, roasted, ¼ cup	89
Halibut, baked, 3 oz	78
Swiss Chard, cooked, ½ cup	75
Peanuts, roasted, ¼ cup	67
Chocolate Chips, semisweet, ¼ cup	58
Baked Potato with skin, 1	55
Cocoa Powder, 2 tsp	52
Molasses, blackstrap, 1 tsp	52
Cereal, Raisin Bran, 1 oz	48
Spinach, fresh, 1 cup	44
Cheerios, 1 oz	39
Milk, 2% fat, 1 cup	33
Bread, Whole Wheat, 1 slice	26
Chicken, Breast, 3 oz	25
Green Peas, frozen, cooked, ½ cup	23
Ground Beef, lean, 3 oz	16
bread, White, 1 slice	13
Fruits	10-25
Egg, 1	5

Source: As in Table 7.7.

TABLE 7.9: SOURCES OF MAGNESIUM

(mg/100 gm of Food)

Rich Sources (> 150)	Good Sources (150-100)	Fair Sources (25-50)	Poor Sources (<25)
Cocoa	Clams	Oysters	Lobster
Nuts	Cornmeal	Crab	Pork
Soybeans	Spinach	Fresh peas	Lamb
Whole grains		Liver	Milk
Molasses		Beef	Eggs
Spices			Veal
			Most Fruits and Vegetables
			Fowl

Source: Alice A. Chenault in *Nutrition and Health*, Pub., Hott, Rinehart and Winston.

Absorption-Excretion Balance

Elemental sulfur is absorbed in the intestines as such and goes directly into the portal blood circulation. The sulfur containing amino acids, methionine and cysteine are split off from protein during digestion and are also absorbed into the portal circulation.

Sulfur is excreted in urine. Excess serum-sulphate, Hypersulfatemia has been observed in infants fed on TPN formulas containing increased amounts of sulfur-containing amino acids.

Physiologic Functions

The organic sulfur performs important functions like:

1. A structural component of mucopolysachharides like chondroitin sulphate found in cartilage, tendons, bone, skin and the heart valves.

2. In the enzymes, sulfur is present as SH group.

3. Sulpholipids are found in liver, kidney, salivary glands and the white matter of brain in large amounts.

4. Sulfur compounds required in oxidation-reduction reactions are coenzymes of thiamine, biotin, Co-enzyme A, lipoic acid and glutathione.

Deficiency Syndrome

Sulfur deficiency is not known to exist anywhere. The clinical problems associated with sulfur are renal calculi and cystinuria.

Food Sources

All protein foods rich in methionine, cystine and cysteine supply large doses of sulfur. Meat, milk, eggs, fish poultry, cheese and nuts are good sources of sulfur.

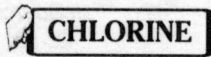 **CHLORINE**

Chlorine is found in all the body cells as chloride ion. It accounts for 3% of the body's total mineral content and is thus the major anion of the fluid outside the cells.

Large amounts are found in the extra-cellular fluid. It is also found in the red blood cells. Gastrointestinal secretions, specially HCl contain very large amounts of chlorine. A healthy adult body contains about 50 mEq of chloride per kg of body weight. The normal serum levels range from 340 mg to 370 mg/L.

Absorption-Excretion Balance

Chlorine is almost completely absorbed in the small intestines with only a small amount lost through feces. Excretion occurs through kidneys. Like sodium, chloride is a renal threshold substance, largely conserved under the hormonal influence of aldosterone, reabsorved in the renal tubules and returned to the circulating plasma.

Physiologic Functions

1. *Water and Acid-base Balance*

Chloride is necessary in the extra-cellular fluid for regulating the osmotic pressure, water balance and acid-base balance.

2. *Gastric Acidity*

In the gastric juice, it is the chief anion along with H ion and provides the acid medium for activating digestive enzymes. It also helps initiate digestion process in the stomach.

3. *Enzyme Activator*

Chlorides also help activate other enzymes like the amylases.

Deficiency

Severe deficiency occurs in case of vomiting and diarrhoea, when very large amounts of chloride are lost. This may lead to alkalosis, wherein the chlorides have been replaced with bicarbonates.

Requirement

The abundance of chlorides do not call for any specifications for men. In general, an adult needs about 750 mg chlorine per day and the growing children 350 - 750 mg. Prolonged intake of sodium chloride has been associated with elevated blood plasma in the case of very sensitive persons.

Food Sources

In the average diet, table salt provides the most abundant source of chloride. The amount of chloride consumed is as much as the sodium. Table 7.9 shows a very comprehensive picture of the major minerals.

TABLE 7.9: SUMMARY OF MINERAL ELEMENTS

Element	Food Source	Functions	RDA	Elimination
Calcium	Milk, cheese, some green vegetables	Bone and tooth formation, blood coagulation; regulates muscle contraction,	0.8 g daily, Pregnancy and Lact.—1.2 g	Urine and feces
Phosphorus	Milk, poultry, fish, meat, cheese, nuts, cereals, legumes	Muscle and cell activity; part of DNA and RNA, phospholipids and buffer system	0.8 g daily, Pregnancy and Lact., 1.2 g	Urine and feces
Magnesium	Nuts, cereals, milk, meat, legumes, green vegetables	Regulates muscles and nerves, part of bones	Women, 300 mg Men, 350 mg	Urine and feces
Sodium	Table salt, animal products	Regulate electrolyte and water balance in extracellular fluids and cell metabolism	Approx. 0.5 g	Urine and sweat
Potassium	Meat, cereals, legumes, fruits and vegetables	Regulates electrolyte/water in intracellular fluid	0.8 – 1.3 g	Urine and sweat
Chlorine	Table salt, animal products	In gastric juice, regulates elect. and water balance	About 0.5 g	Urine and sweat
Sulfur	Protein foods	In body tissues, especially hair and nails	Adequate if proteins right amount	Urine and in feaces

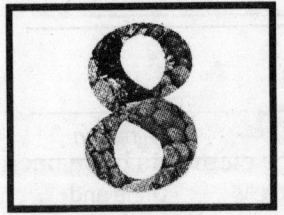

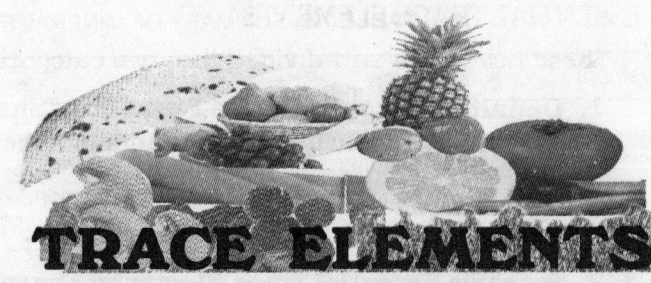

8 TRACE ELEMENTS

Of the 54 known chemical elements in the Periodic Table, 27 elements have been reckoned as essential for man's diverse biological functions. Since most of these are found in fairly large amounts, hence their physiologic presence is easily determined. But a still large number of elements exist, albeit in very minute or infinitesimally small amounts. These are called Trace Elements. In general, trace elements are the chemicals which have the required intake of less than 100 mg/day. Yet some of these elements exist in our diet or the environment in fairly large amounts.

ESSENTIAL FUNCTIONS

Notwithstanding the technical difficulty in assessing and evaluating these small amounts in our body, their essential nature can be determined on the basis of their physiological functions, else by the severity of their deficiency syndrome.

An element is reckoned as essential when its inadequacy in diet leads to impairment of some body functions. And their administration helps prevent the aforementioned malfunctioning. Field investigations have shown two basic functions in terms of catalysts and structural component of the larger molecules.

REQUIREMENT

Owing to very minute amount of trace elements that occasion difficulty in categorical measurement, specific needs and RDA have been stated only for

(1) Iron, because of its long history
(2) Zinc, because of its high concentration,
(3) Iodine, because of its one known specific function.

For most other trace elements, the RDA are given merely as guestimates or empirical projections.

ESSENTIAL TRACE ELEMENTS

These have been sub-divided into two categories:

1. **Definitely Essential Trace Elements:** Ten such trace elements have been identified from their definite functions. These are:

    | Iron | Iodine | Zinc | Copper | Manganese |
    | Chromium | Cobalt | Selenium | Molybdenum | Fluorine |

2. **Probable Essential Trace Elements:** The remaining eight have been called Probable elements, because notwithstanding some essentiality, they still need greater research and validation. This group includes:

    | Silicon | Vanadium | Nickel | Tin |
    | Cadmium | Arsenic | Aluminium | Boron |

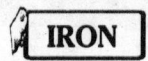

IRON

Iron is an essential nutrient responsible for the formation of haemoglobin of the red blood cells and plays an important role in the transport of oxygen.

In most of the developing countries, including India, the diet is very much deficient in iron. And anaemia is the most widely prevalent of all the deficiency diseases reported in human nutrition. An average Indian diet contains about 20-30 mg of iron, sufficient to meet the body needs of an adult.

The human body contains about 45 mg iron/kg body weight. This iron is distributed in four forms that relate to its basic metabolic function.

1. *Transport Iron*

A minute trace of iron (0.05 to 0.18mg/dL) is found in the plasma bound to its transport carrier protein, transferrin.

2. *Haemoglobin*

About three-fourths of the body iron is to be found in the red blood cells as a vital constituent of the 'heme' portion of Hb. Another smaller moiety (5%) is a part of the muscle haemoglobin, 'myoglobin'.

3. *Storage Iron*

Nearly 20% of all the body iron is stored as the protein-iron compound, 'Ferritin', which is found in liver, spleen, and bone marrow.

4. *Cellular Tissue Iron*

About 5% of the body iron is distributed throughout all the cells of the body as a major component of oxidative enzyme systems for producing energy.

Absorption–Storage–Excretion Balance

Dietary iron enters the body in two forms, Heme and Non-heme, as shown in the tabulation below. Non-Heme, the largest part is absorbed very slowly, since it is tightly bound in its food source to organic molecules in the form of ferric iron (Fe^{+++}). In the acid medium of stomach, it must be delinked and reduced to more soluble ferrous (Fe^{++}). A protein receptor in the intestinal mucosal cells, 'apoferritin' then receives iron to form ferritin. Only 10% to 30% of the total ingested iron is absorbed, mostly in duodenum. The remaining 70% to 90% of the iron is eliminated from the body.

Heme iron is absorbed more readily than non-heme iron and it is independent of vitamin C and iron-binding chelates. The absorption of non-heme iron can be enhanced by vitamin C.

Factors Favouring Fe Absorption

1. Body Need

In deficiency or stress situations like pregnancy or growth, the mucosal ferritin stored in the liver and other tissues is lower and hence, more iron is absorbed. But when the tissue reserves are saturated, any extra iron is rejected and excreted.

DIETARY IRON

	Heme (Smallest Part)	Non-Heme (Largest Part)
Food Sources	None in plants; 40% in animal sources	All iron in plants; 60% iron in animal sources
Absorption Rate	Rapid; transported and absorbed intact	Slow, tightly bound in organic molecules

2. Acidity and Reduction Agents

Vitamin C aids iron absorption by its reducing action that affects acidity. So also gastric hydrochloric acid which offers acid medium for iron utilization.

3. Calcium

Ca helps bind and remove agents like phosphates and phytates which would otherwise combine with iron and prevent its absorption.

Factors Hindering Fe Absorption

1. Binding Agents

Agents like phosphates, phytates and oxalates bind iron and hinder absorption. Tea and Coffee inhibit non-heme iron absorption.

2. *Reduced Gastric Acid*

Gastrectomy (stomach removal) reduces hydrochloric acid secretion, thus reducing absorption of iron.

3. *Infection*

Any sort of severe infection affects the rate of iron absorption.

4. *Gastrointestinal Diseases*

Malabsorption or any other condition that cause diarrhoea hinders the absorption of iron.

Transport and Storage

Haemoglobin in the red blood cells and myoglobin in the tissue cells are vital for the transport of oxygen to the cells and storage within the cells, whereas the iron-containing enzymes within the cells are associated with metabolic oxidation.

Iron is oxidized and bound with plasma ferritin in duodenum and jejunum. It is transported by blood as 'Transferrin' to the storage sites in bone marrow for haemoglobin synthesis. Iron is stored in the liver as ferritin, to be drawn upon whenever needed for haemoglobin in RBCs and also for general body metabolism. In the liver, it is stored in a less soluble form, 'Hemosiderin'. Iron is mobilized for haemoglobin synthesis as needed, from 20-25 mg/day in an adult. Fig. 8.1 vividly illustrates this process.

Absorbed iron is lost by desquamation from alimentary tract, respiratory tract and by skin and hair. Iron released from the breakdown of haemoglobin is reutilized. In adults, the total iron loss that needs replacement is 1 mg/day. But in women, there is an additional loss of 5-32 mg per month owing to menstrual losses.

Only small amounts of iron are lost by renal excretion. But any surgery or heavy menstrual flow, parasitic infestations or gastrointestinal diseases could lead to severe losses of iron from body.

Physiologic Functions

1. *Oxygen Transport*

Hb acts as a carrier of oxygen from lungs to the tissues and thus indirectly helps CO_2 return to lungs. After the RBCs have completed their 120 days life cycle, the iron is removed and sent to the bone marrow for synthesis of new RBCs, i.e. 'Haemopoiesis'.

Myoglobin is the iron-protein complex in the muscles that stores oxygen for immediate use by the cells. Transferrin is the circulating form of iron, while ferritin or hemosiderin is the storage form of iron. As such, iron functions as a major transport medium of vital oxygen to the cells for both respiration and metabolism.

2. *Cellular Oxidation*

Many an oxidase enzyme like catalase, cytochrome oxidase and xanthine oxidase contain iron as an integral part of their molecular structure.

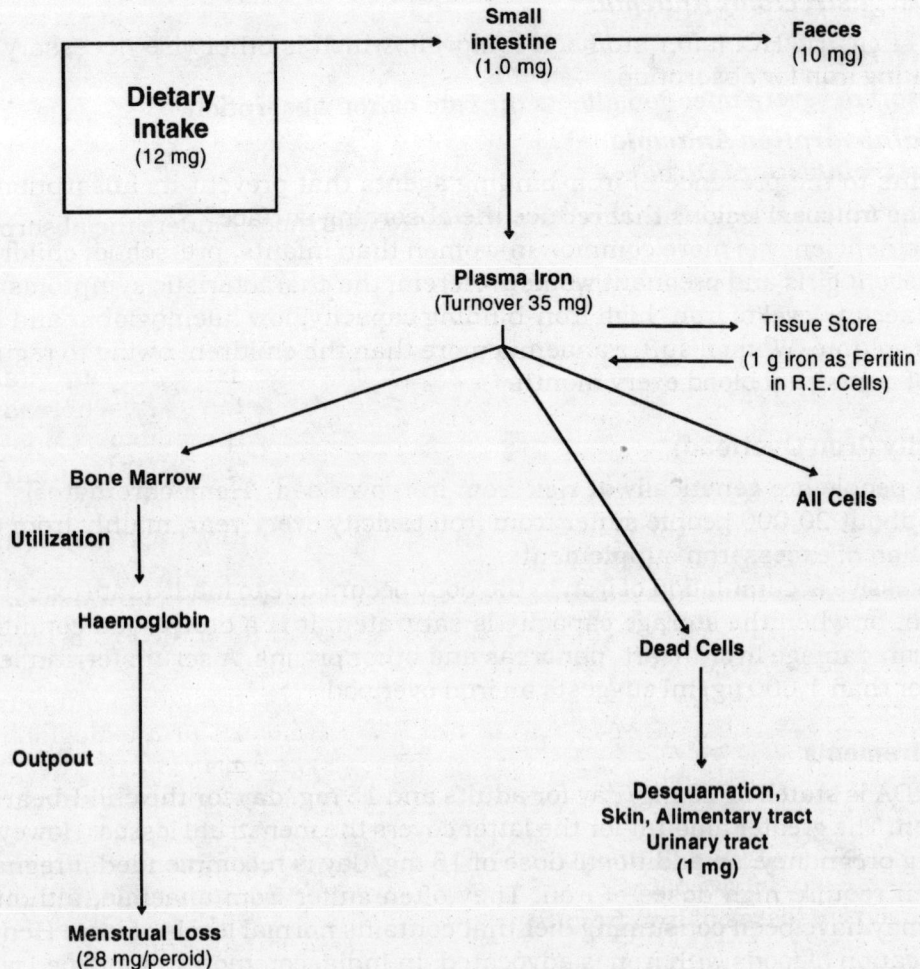

Fig. 8.1: Summary of Iron Metabolism
(Adapted from Moore, 1961)

Deficiency Syndrome

The well known and most common iron deficiency syndrome is anaemia. Four types of iron deficiency manifesting as anaemia is reported from the field.

(a) *Nutritional Anaemia*

It is due to inadequate dietary supply of iron and other nutrients for haemoglobin and red blood cell production.

(b) Hemorrhagic Anaemia

It means excessive loss of blood iron.

(c) Post-gastrectomy Anaemia

Lack of gastric HCl (after stomach removal), which is otherwise necessary for liberating iron for absorption.

(d) Malabsorption Anaemia

It is due to the presence of iron-binding agents that prevent its absorption or else the mucosal lesions that reduce the absorbing surface.

Iron deficiency is more common in women than infants, pre-school children, adolescent girls and pregnant women. Herein, the characteristic symptoms are a low serum level of iron, high iron-binding capacity, low haemoglobin and low RBCs volume. Women suffer anaemia more than the children, owing to regular loss of menstrual blood every month.

Toxicity (Iron Overload)

Some people are genetically at risk from iron overload, 'Hemochromatosis'. In USA, about 20,000 people suffer from iron toxicity every year, mainly from the ingestion of excess iron supplements.

Excessive accumulation of iron in the body occurs due to inadequate excretion of iron, or when the storage capacity is saturated. It is a dangerous condition that can damage liver, heart, pancreas and other organs. A serum ferritin level greater than 1,000 µg/ml suggests an iron overload.

Requirements

The RDA is stated at 10 mg/day for adults and 15 mg/day for the child-bearing women. The greater amount for the latter covers the menstrual losses. However, during pregnancy, an additional dose of 15 mg/day is recommended. Pregnant women require high doses of iron. They often suffer from anaemia, although they may have been consuming diet that contains normal levels of iron. Hence, fortification of foods with iron is advocated. In India, common salt fortified with iron has been successfully developed, so also the fortified wheat flour.

Table 8.1 shows the RDA for Iron for different age groups and sex.

Food Sources

Good sources of iron (heme) are lean meat, liver, fish and poultry. Cereal grains and millets are rich source of iron. Herein, Bajra (Pearl Millets) and Ragi (Finger millets) are unusually rich sources. Other sources of iron are legumes, whole grains and hand-pounded cereals, as well as green leafy vegetables and dried fruits. The inorganic form of iron is to be found in jaggery and rice flakes, since these are made in iron pans in the villages. However, from the absorption angle, heme iron is considered much better than the non-heme iron variety.

TABLE 8.1: RECOMMENDED DIETARY ALLOWANCES FOR IRON

Age (years)	RDA (mg)
Infants	
0.0-0.5	6
0.5-1.0	10
Children	
1-3	10
4-6	10
7-10	10
Males	
11-14	12
15-18	12
19-24	10
25-50	10
51+	10
Females	
11-14	15
15-18	15
19-24	15
25-50	15
51+	10
Pregnant	30
Lactating	
1st 6 months	15
2nd 6 months	15

RDA = Recommended dietary allowance.
Source: Kathleen Mahan and Escott Stump in *Food, Nutrition and Diet Therapy*. Pub. W.B. Saunders.

The inclusion of 50 g of green leafy vegetables in the diet helps provide a fair amount of iron, besides providing Ca, β carotenes and vitamin C.

Table 8.2 shows the relative hierarchy of iron-rich foods.

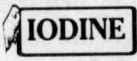 **IODINE**

Though required in very minute amounts, yet this trace element, iodine very significantly affects the growth and metabolism of man. Its deficiency leads to Goitre. In an average adult body iodine ranges from 20 to 50 mg. Its distribution in the body tissues is as under:

Muscles	Approx. 50%
Thyroid Gland	20%
Skin	10%
Skeleton	6%

TABLE 8.2: FOOD SOURCES OF IRON

Excellent Sources (> 2.0 mg/serving)		Good Sources (1.0-2.0 mg/srving)	
Food	Quantity (mg)	Food	Quantity (mg)
Liver, 3 oz		Egg, 1 Whole	1.3
Pork	24.7	Vegetables	
Lamb	15.2	Greens, 1 cup cooked:	
Calf	12.1	Collards	1.5
Chicken	7.2	Kale	1.8
Beef	7.5	Dandelion	1.8
Legumes, cooked, 1 cup		Potato, baked, one	1.1
Navy Beans	5.0	Broccoli, cooked, 1 cup	1.3
Lima Beans	4.9	Acorn squash, cooked, 1 cup	1.8
Blackeyed Peas	4.8	Meats, Poultry, Fish	
Green Peas	2.9	Flounder Fillet, one	1.4
Spinach, cooked, 1 cup	4.3	Lamb Leg, 3 oz	1.9
Meats		Chicken Breast, one	1.3
Roast Beef, 3 oz	3.1	Grains	
Beef Stew, 1 cup	2.9	Rice, 1 cup cooked (brown or	
½ cup Beef Heart	4.2	enriched white)	1.0
Pork roast, lean	3.2	Bread, 2 slices (whole wheat or	
Prunes		enriched white)	1.5
Cooked, 1 cup	4.2	Macaroni, enriched, cooked, 1 cup	1.3
Prune Juice, 1 cup	10.5	Oatmeal, cooked, 1 cup	1.4
Blackstrap Molasses		Shredded Wheat,	
1 tbsp	3.2	spoon-size, 1 cup	1.8
Shellfish		Wheat germ, 3 tbsp	1.5
Oysters, 4	3.6		
Cherrystone Clams, 4	4.0		
Grains			
40% Bran Flakes, 1 cup	12.0		
Wheat Flakes, 1 cup	1.1-3.5		

Source: US Department of Agriculture.

The balance 14% iodine is shared by other endocrine tissues, central nervous system and plasma. However, the greatest concentration of iodine is found in the thyroid glands, wherein it participates in the synthesis of thyroid hormone, thyroxine.

Absorption–Excretion Balance

Dietary iodine is absorbed in the small intestine in the form of iodides. Bound loosely with proteins, it is carried by the blood to thyroid gland. Nearly one-third of the iodide is absorbed by the thyroid cells and is thus removed from circulation. The remaining two-thirds is usually excreted through the urine route within three days of its ingestion.

The Thyroid Stimulating Hormone (TSH), secreted by the pituitary glands, stimulates the iodine uptake by the thyroid cells. This normal physiologic 'feedback mechanism' helps maintain a healthy balance between the supply and demand of iodine.

Physiologic Functions of Iodine

1. *Thyroid Hormone Secretion*

The main function of Iodine is the synthesis of thyroid hormone in body metabolism. The hormone, Thyroxine, in turn, stimulates cell oxidation and helps regulate the basic metabolic rate (BMR). Thus, iodine exerts important influence on our body metabolism.

2. *Plasma Thyroxine*

The free thyroxine is secreted into the blood stream and then bound down to plasma proteins for being transported to body cells, as and when needed. After it has been used to stimulate oxidation in the cells, the hormone is degraded in the liver and the iodine is excreted through bile in the form of inorganic iodine.

Deficiency Syndrome

The world over, about 150 million people suffer from Iodine deficiency. During the early fetal stages, this deficiency could lead to mental retardation and stunted growth. The daily requirement of iodine is reported to be 100-150 µg. In the endemic goiter areas, there is a built-in iodine deficiency in the soil, water and the locally-grown foods. Administration of iodized salts containing 15 µg iodine per gram cold easily meet the daily iodine requirements. To meet any losses during transport, iodisation up to 30 ppm is recommended.

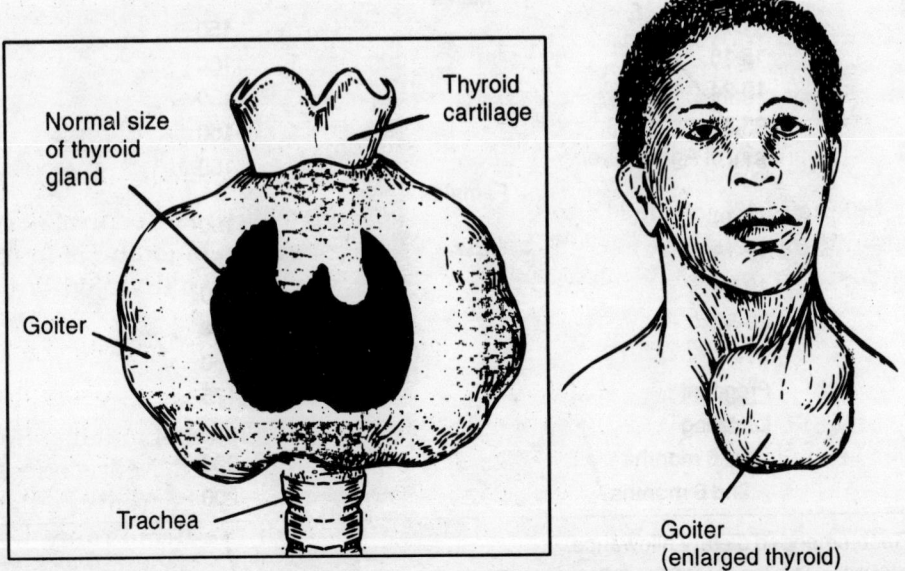

Fig. 8.2: Goiter. The extreme enlargement shown here is a result of extended duration of iodine deficiency

Goitre is the principal deficiency disease, since the size (hypertrophy) and the number (hyperplasia) of epithelial cells in the gland increases. Women are more affected than men. Cretinism is characterized by low basal metabolic rates, muscular flabbiness and weakness, besides dry skin, rough hair, enlarged tongue, thick lips, skeletal retardation and also mental retardation.

Goitrogens: These are the substances that interfere with thyroxine activity to produce goiter. Goitrogens are to be found in vegetables like cabbages, cauliflower, brussel sprouts, peanuts and mustard. However, these goitrogens are inactivated during the high temperature cooking process.

Requirements

The RDA for iodine is 150 µg /day for an average adult. But this amount goes up during the period of growth or pregnancy. On the other hand, this requirement goes down in the older people. Table 8.3 shows the RDA for iodine for different age groups and sex.

TABLE 8.3: RECOMMENDED DIETARY ALLOWANCES FOR IODINE

Age (years)	RDA (µg)
Infants	
0.0-0.5	40
0.5-1.0	50
Children	
1-3	70
4-6	70
7-10	120
Males	
11-14	150
15-18	150
19-24	150
25-50	150
51+	150
Females	
11-14	150
15-18	150
19-24	150
25-50	150
51+	150
Pregnant	175
Lactating	
1st 6 months	200
2nd 6 months	200

RDA = Recommended dietary allowance.
Source: Kathleen Mahan and Escott Stump in Food, Nutrition and Diet Therapy. Pub. W.B. Saunders.

Food Sources

Seafoods, particularly saltwater fish and seaweeds are rich source of iodine. In case of animal sources, their iodine content depends upon the iodine level of the feeds consumed by the animals. Similarly, vegetables and fruits grown in the lands inherently rich in iodine have plentiful iodine to offer.

Normally, fortification of common salt with potassium iodate is the ideal practice to supply the much-needed iodine. Many countries have made it mandatory to supply the iodized salt for public consumption. Table 8.4 shows the iodine content of some important foods.

TABLE 8.4: IODINE CONTENT OF SELECTED FOODS

Food	μg
Salt, Iodized, 1 tsp	400
Bread, made with Iodate dough conditioner and continuous mix process, 1 slice	142
Haddock, 3 oz	104-145
Bread, made with regular process, 1 slice	35
Cheese, cottage, 2% fat, ½ cup	26-71
Shrimp, 3 oz	21-37
Egg, 1	18-26
Cheese, cheddar, 1 oz	5-23
Ground beef, 3 oz	8

Source: USDA: Composition of Foods. USDA Handbook, Washingtan DC, 1976-1986.

OTHER ESSENTIAL TRACE ELEMENTS

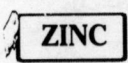 ZINC

Zinc is an important element performing a range of functions in body as a co-factor for a number of enzymes. Of late, zinc has gained considerable nutritional prominence. Its wider tissue distribution reflects its broad metabolic activity as a component of key cell enzymes.

In the body, it is found in pancreas, liver, kidneys, lungs, muscle, bones and eyes, endocrine glands, prostrate secretions and sperms. An adult body contain 1.3 to 2.3 g of zinc. The plasma zinc levels range from 75 to 120 μg/dL.

Absorption–Excretion Balance

Zinc is absorbed mostly in the upper jejunum in small intestines. A Zinc-Binding Ligand (ZBL) from pancreas serves as a transparent carrier into the mucosal cells. There it is picked up by albumin molecules on the serosal membranes and transported to liver for storage or redistribution.

Zinc is excreted mainly through feces; only a small amount is excluded through pancreas.

Physiologic Functions

Zinc mainly functions as an essential component of cell enzyme system, particularly metalloenzymes. These enzymes include:

Carboxypeptidase   Carbonic anhydrase
Lactate dehydrogenase   Superoxide dismutase
Glutamate dehydrogenase   Thymidine kinase
Alkaline phosphatase

As such, any deficiency of zinc brings multiple problems in the dysfunction of many body systems.

Zinc supplementation helps effect clinical improvement in

(a) Hypogeusia—impairment of the sense of taste
(b) Hyposmia—impairment of the sense of smell

Further, chronic or debilitating diseases in aging also respond to the supplementation with zinc.

Deficiency Syndrome

Deficiency of Zinc leads to failure of growth and poor development of gonadal functions. It has been reported as dwarfism and hypogonadism in Iran and Egypt.

Zinc deficiency affects the speedy healing of wounds. In the aged, the deficiency leads to reduced immune response.

In India, no definitive deficiency syndrome has been observed. However, sub-clinical Zn deficiency does exist in many parts of the country, although not much clinical abnormality has been witnessed.

Requirement

The RDA for zinc is estimated as 15 mg/day for men and 12 mg/day for women. Table 8.5 shows the RDA for zinc for different age groups and sex.

Food Sources

Meat products like liver, kidneys, eggs and sea-foods are rich sources of zinc. Plant products like grains and legumes also provide fair amount of dietary zinc.

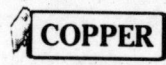

COPPER

Copper has often been labeled as the 'Iron Twin'. Both these elements exhibit the same functions as cell enzyme components. Both are related to energy production and also haemoglobin synthesis.

A typical Indian diet provides about 2 mg copper per day.

TABLE 8.5: RECOMMENDED DIETARY ALLOWANCES FOR ZINC

Age (years)	RDA (µg)
Infants	
0.0-0.5	5
0.5-1.0	5
Children	
1-3	10
4-6	10
7-10	10
Males	
11-14	15
15-18	15
19-24	15
25-50	15
51+	15
Females	
11-14	12
15-18	12
19-24	12
25-50	12
51+	12
Pregnant	15
Lactating	
1st 6 months	19
2nd 6 months	16

RDA = Recommended dietary allowance.

Source: Kathleen Mahan and Escott Stump in *Food, Nutrition and Diet Therapy*. Pub. W.B. Saunders.

Physiologic Functions

Copper is an essential element and plays an important role in iron absorption. Copper is also involved in cross linkages of connective tissues, neurotransmission and lipid metabolism. Part of the body copper circulates in plasma as Ceruloplasmin. Copper is also present in oxidative enzymes like cytochrome.

As a co-enzyme, copper is involved in:

(1) The release of energy in cytochrome system,
(2) Melanin production in skin,
(3) Absorption and transport of iron,
(4) Formation of calicholamine in brain and adrenal glands,
(5) Formation of haemoglobin and transferrin,
(6) Metabolism of glucose, cholestrol and phospholipids,
(7) Synthesis of collagen and elastin,
(8) Detoxification of superoxide radicals.

Copper metabolism in the body is under homeostatic regulation; in case of low intake, copper excretion is reduced. There is little storage in excess, except in conditions like Wilson's disease. Copper toxicity is often seen in renal dialysis.

Deficiency

The dietary deficiency of copper is rare. Deficiency syndrome shows up in organs rich in connective tissue, central nervous system disorders, with impaired myelination and catecholamine metabolism.

Symptoms of acute poisoning are vomiting, dizziness and diarrhoea and in severe cases circulatory collapse, severe hemolysis and liver and kidney failure.

Food Sources

Copper is widely distributed in natural foods. The main food sources are meat, shell-fish, nuts, seeds, legumes and whole grains.

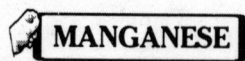 **MANGANESE**

Manganese is an essential element, since it participates in a number of reactions as metal-enzyme or Co-factor. Manganese is directly associated with the defence mechanism of the body. It helps in the proper utilization of vitamins B and E groups. It supports digestion, removes fatigue, helps in blood clotting and in adequate production of milk in the lactating mothers. Manganese increases glucose tolerance, hence it is considered beneficial for the diabetics.

Manganese is a component of two metallo-enzymes and is a catalyst for a number of enzymes involved in glucose and fatty acid metabolism and urea formation. It is also needed for bone formation, skin integrity and utilization of thiamine.

An average adult body contains about 20 mg manganese, found mainly in liver, bones, pancreas and pituitary glands.

Physiologic Functions

Manganese functions like other trace elements as an essential part of cell enzymes that catalyze many important metabolic reactions. Its function in glycosyl transferase is well recognised and its deficiency leads abnormality in skeleton bone mineralisation. Manganese also participates in carbohydrate and lipid metabolism.

Deficiency

Normally, manganese deficiency is not seen in the Indian conditions. Manganese deficiency, as evidenced by low serum levels, has been reported in diabetes and pancreas insufficiency, as well as in protein-energy malnutrition in the form of Kwashiorkor.

Cases of sub-optimal manganese status have been reported in children born with metabolic disorders and in men with rheumatic arthritis.

Toxicity

Manganese toxicity shows up as an industrial disease syndrome, 'Inhalation Toxicity' in miners and others exposed to manganese dust for long time. Herein, excess manganese accumulates in the liver and central nervous system. Toxicity results in dementia and psychiatric disorders resembling schizophrenia, followed by a crippling neurologic disorder that is similar to Parkinson's disease.

Requirement (ESADDI)

The RDA standard for an adult is 2 to 5 mg manganese per day. And for the children, it is 1 to 5 mg. In 1989 an ESADDI for manganese for adults and children 11 years and older in the range of 2 to 5 mg/day was established. For children, 1 to 3 mg/day is suggested depending on age (Table 8.6).

TABLE 8.6: ESTIMATED SAFE AND ADEQUATE DAILY DIETARY INTAKES FOR MANGANESE

Category	Age (years)	ESADDI (mg)
Infants	0-0.5	0.3-0.6
	0.5-1	0.6-1.0
Children and adolescents	1-3	1.0-1.5
	4-6	1.5-2.0
	7-10	2.0-3.0
	11+	2.0-5.0
Adults		2.0-5.0

Source: Kathleen Mahan and Escott Stump in *Food, Nutrition and Diet Therapy.* Pub. W.B. Saunders.

Food Sources

The manganese content of foods varies greatly. The richest sources are whole grains, legumes, nuts and tea. Fruits and vegetables are moderate sources. Animal tissues, seafood, and dairy products are poor sources. Relatively high amounts occur in instant coffee and tea. Human milk is relatively low in manganese.

An average Indian diet contains 4-10 mg manganese per day. The absorption rate of manganese from the diet ranges from 5% to 20%.

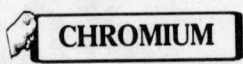

CHROMIUM

Chromium is an essential element necessary for life. The total chromium content of the body is very low, less than 6 mg. Highest concentrations have been found in skin, adrenal glands, brain muscle and fat. The serum levels are normally less than 10 mg/ml.

Absorption-Excretion Balance

Only a small amount of dietary chromium is absorbed in the intestines. While only 0.5% of the inorganic chromium is absorbed, it now appears that 25% of the organic chromium can be assimilated in the body. Chromium absorption is inhibited by iron, manganese, copper, zinc and titanium.

In the blood, chromium is bound to protein, transferrin. Chromium is later released from blood and is then stored in liver, spleen and bone marrow.

Physiologic Functions

Chromium functions as an essential component of the organic complex, Glucose Tolerance Factor (GTF). The GTF stimulates the action of insulin in the body. Insulin resistance manifested by impaired glucose tolerance, has responded positively to chromium supplementation by restoring normal blood sugar. Significant reduction of elevated serum cholesterol has also been reported.

A Korean report has shown that 83 out of 100 diabetics experienced reduced dependence on insulin and an overall improvement in general condition after supplementation with chromium.

Deficiency Syndrome

Deficiency of chromium leads to impaired glucose tolerance. It is reported in persons who have been long on total parenteral nutrition (TPN). However, no deficiency syndrome has been noticed in India.

Requirement

The RDA standard for chromium is estimated as ranging from 50 to 200 mg per day. An average diet contains just enough chromium (about 70-150 mg) to satisfy the basic requirement of a man. Table 8.7 shows the estimated safe and adequate daily dietary intakes for chromium for different categories and age groups.

TABLE 8.7: ESTIMATED SAFE AND ADEQUATE DAILY DIETARY INTAKES FOR CHROMIUM

Category	Age (years)	ESADDI (mg)
Infants	0-0.5	10-40
	0.5-1	20-60
Children and adolescents	1-3	20-80
	4-6	30-120
	7-10	50-200
	11+	50-200
Adults		50-200

Source: Kathleen Mahan and Escott Stump in *Food, Nutrition and Diet Therapy*. Pub. W.B. Saunders.

Food Sources

Precise assessment of chromium in foods is difficult; biologically available chromium and inorganic chromium cannot be distinguished from each other. Analyses done before 1980 must be viewed with caution because determinations were flawed by contamination and analytical problems.

Brewer's yeast, oysters, liver and potatoes have high chromium concentrations; seafoods, whole grains, cheeses, chicken, meats, and bran, are intermediate in content. Refining of wheat removes chromium along with the germ and the bran; refining sugar fractionates the chromium into the molasses portion. Dairy products, fruits and vegetables are low in chromium.

A study of usual chromium intake showed an average of 33 μg/day in self-selected diets containing 2300 kcal and 25 μg/day in 1600-kcal diets.

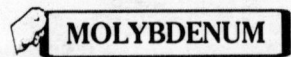 **MOLYBDENUM**

Molybdenum functions as a catalyst component in several cell enzyme systems. As such, it is essential for a number of metabolic reactions. The body tissue amount of molybdenum is exceedingly small about 0.1 to 1 mg/g of wet tissue.

Molybdenum is an essential constituent of Xanthin and aldehyde oxidases and is instrumental in uric acid metabolism. The occurrence of molybdenum in human tissue is still under investigation—body tissues contain a minimal of molybdenum approximately 0.1 to 1.0 mg/g of wet tissue. However, it is reported to be present in small amounts in the animal tissues.

In the human body, it is found deposited in the liver, kidneys, bone and skin.

Physiologic Functions

Molybdenum is required as a catalytic component of the metalloenzyme, Xanthin oxidase, aldehyde oxidase and sulfite oxidase. As such, it is essential for many metabolic functions.

Toxicity

High molybdenum and low calcium intake can lead to endemic 'Genu vulgam' and bone disorders, which occur in the endemic fluorosis cases.

Requirement (ESADDI)

The daily requirement of molybdenum is not known; however, the ESADDI standards for molybdenum for an adults is stated as 75 to 250 μg/day. Depending on the age of the child, the estimated safe intake is 25 to 150 μg/day (Table 8.8).

An excessive intake of 10 to 15 mg/day is associated with incidence of a goutlike syndrome.

Food Sources

Molybdenum is distributed widely in commonly used foods, such as legumes, whole grain, cereals, milk and milk products and dark green leafy vegetables. Intakes range from 50 µg/day in infants to peaks of 80 and 126 µg/day for 1 to 16-years-old females and males, respectively. Intakes decrease slowly to 74 and 101 µg/day for 60 to 65 year old females and males respectively.

TABLE 8.8: ESTIMATED SAFE AND ADEQUATE DAILY DIETARY INTAKES FOR MOLYBDENUM

Category	Age (years)	ESADDI (mg)
Infants	0-0.5	15-30
	0.5-1	20-40
Children and adolescents	1-3	25-50
	4-6	30-75
	7-10	50-150
	11+	75-250
Adults		75-250

Source: Kathleen Mahan and Escott Stump in *Food, Nutrition and Diet Therapy.* Pub. W.B. Saunders.

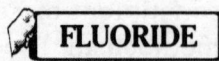 **FLUORIDE**

Fluoride is an important element for human health and plays a very important role in the prevention of dental caries. The trace element fluorine accumulates in all body tissues, showing calcification mostly in bones and teeth. Whole blood fluoride levels in USA have been reported in the range of 0.04 to 0.4 mg/g.

Absorption-Excretion Balance

Absorption of fluorides takes place in small intestines, though very little is known about its bio-availability. Their absorption is affected by other dietary minerals and fats. Absorption of fluorides is reduced by aluminium, calcium, and sodium chloride. Fats, on the other hand, increase the rate of absorption. Up to 80% of fluorides are excreted through urine.

Physiologic Functions

In human nutrition, fluorides are mainly responsible for inhibiting dental caries. Fluoride therapy enhances the ability of tooth structure to withstand the erosive effect of the bacterial acids.

Fluorides also play an important role in helping control the development of osteoporosis. It may thus provide protection from the mineralisation of bone that characterizes this condition. It has been established that fluorides, together with vitamin D and calcium help increase the bone mass in cases of osteoporosis.

Fluorides have also been associated with both increased and decreased incidence of cardiovascular diseases.

Toxicity

High doses of fluorides, 2-3 ppm in water lead to fluorosis. In the endemic areas of Andhra Pradesh in India, another clinical manifestation of fluoride toxicity, Genu valgam has been reported.

Requirement

The RDA for adults for fluorine ranges between 1.5 mg to 4 mg/day.

Public fluoridation at the rate of I part per million parts of water supply is adequate to supply the essential body needs for fluorides.

The estimated safe and adequate intake of fluoride for adults is 1.5 to 4 mg/day. Depending on the age, it is 0.5 to 2.5 mg/day for children and adolescents and 0.1 to 1 mg/day for infants (Table 8.9). An 8 oz glass of fluoridated water (1 part per million or 1 mg/day) provides about 0.2 mg of fluoride.

TABLE 8.9: ESTIMATED SAFE AND ADEQUATE DAILY DIETARY INTAKES FOR FLUORIDE

Category	Age (years)	ESADDI (mg)
Infants	0-0.5	0.1-0.5
	0.5-1	0.2-1.0
Children and adolescents	1-3	0.5-1.5
	4-6	1.0-2.5
	7-10	1.5-2.5
	11+	1.5-2.5
Adults		1.5-4.0

Source: Kathleen Mahan and Escott Stump in *Food, Nutrition and Diet Therapy*. Pub. W.B. Saunders.

Food Sources

The major dietary sources of fluoride are drinking water and processed foods that have been prepared or reconstituted with fluoridated water. The reported difference in intake is 0.9 mg/day in an area with unfluoridated water to 1.7 mg/day in a fluoridated area (Singer *et al.*, 1980). Although fluorides are widespread in fruits and vegetables, the amounts are not significant. However, the amount in tea leaves can be important, depending on the brewing strength and the extent of tea consumption. One cup of tea can contain as much as 1.0 mg of fluoride (Sweeney and Shaw, 1988). Soups and stews made with fish and meat bones also provide fluoride in societies that depend extensively on such foods. Mechanically deboned meat and fowl, as well as seafood and beef liver are high in fluoride. Cooking foods in Teflon pans (a fluoride-containing polymer) increases its fluoride content.

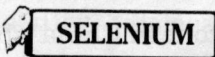 SELENIUM

The increasing evidence that excessive activity of free radicals is associated with the occurrence of some chronic diseases, particularly those relating to the heart and some forms of cancer, has led to growing interest in the use of selenium as a supplement, because of its sparing action on vitamin E and its direct involvement in the enzyme glutathione peroxidase.

Occurrence in the Body

The highest concentrations of selenium in the body are found in the liver, kidneys, heart and spleen; and the lowest, in the lungs and brain.

Absorption–Excretion Balance

Absorption depends on the solubility of the selenium compound ingested and on the dietary ratio of selenium to sulfur. Intestinal absorption of selenium compounds generally is about 80% or more of the total intake.

Metabolic Functions

1. *Enzyme Component*

Selenium is an integral component of antioxidant enzyme glutathione peroxidase, a catalyst transferring reducing agents from reduced glutathione to hydrogen peroxide or to lipid peroxides, which protects cells and membranes against oxidative damage. In this role, selenium balances with vitamin E, each sparing the other. The protective function of selenium is widespread, for the enzyme is found in most body tissues.

2. *Structural Component*

Selenium is also incorporated into the protein matrix of the teeth.

Deficiency

The selenium deficiency disease is named Keshan disease in China. It is a congestive heart disease first observed in Chinese children and young women of child-bearing age and then successfully prevented and treated with selenium supplements. In the United States, selenium deficiency has been observed in persons on TPN feeding, and their symptoms of muscular pain and weakness completely reversed with selenium supplementation in their TPN formulas.

Toxicity

Toxicity from excess selenium in soil and plants has long been a problem in livestock management. More recently it has become a problem in humans, with reports from one high-selenium zone in China where intakes were about 5 mg/day from local foods. The symptoms included nail and hair changes, nerve damage, irritability, fatigue, nausea, abdominal pain, and diarrhea.

Requirement

The new RDA standard for adults has been established at 70 µg/day for men and 55 µg/day for women. The average increase for pregnancy is 10 µg/day and for lactation, 20 µg/day. The Table 8.10 shows the RDA for selenium.

TABLE 8.10: RECOMMENDED DIETARY ALLOWANCES FOR SELENIUM

Age (years)	RDA (µg)
Infants	
0.0-0.5	10
0.5-1.0	15
Children	
1-3	20
4-6	20
7-10	30
Males	
11-14	40
15-18	50
19-24	70
25-50	70
51+	70
Females	
11-14	45
15-18	50
19-24	55
25-50	55
51+	55
Pregnant	65
Lactating	
1st 6 months	75
2nd 6 months	75

RDA = Recommended dietary allowance.
Source: Kathleen Mahan and Escott Stump in *Food, Nutrition and Diet Therapy*. Pub. W.B. Saunders.

Food Sources

Food sources vary with the selenium soil content. Thus grains and other seeds are more variable in selenium. Consistently good sources are seafoods, kidney and liver with lesser amounts in other meats. Fruits and vegetables generally contain little selenium.

ULTRA-TRACE ELEMENTS WITH PROBABLE ESSENTIALITY

Ultra-trace elements are those elements with estimated dietary requirements usually less than 1 mg/g and often less than 50 ng/g of diet for lab animals. They are considered essential for humans, although their essentiality has not been firmly established, as these are required in infinitesimally small amounts. This group includes 13 elements:

Arsenic	Bromine	Boron	Cadmium
Fluorine	Lead	Lithium	Manganese
Molybdenum	Nickel	Silicon	Tin
Vanadium			

Since early 1970s, it has been speculated that the lack of any one of these trace-elements does contribute to the occurrence of some human disease, such as atherosclerosis, osteoporosis, osteoarthritis and hypertension, albeit with incomplete understanding of their cause.

When animals or human beings are exposed to some form of stress, viz., nutritional, metabolic, hormonal or physiological stress, some of these trace-elements may be of great nutritional significance. However, with the increasing dependence upon long-term 'Total Parenteral Nutrition (TPN)', as in critical or terminally ill cases, these ultra-trace elements are bound to acquire greater practical relevance.

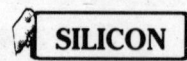 **SILICON**

Silicon-deficient diets, when fed to the animals, have shown up in the form of bone deformities, specially that of skull. Animals given silicon supplements showed growth stimulation, besides maintaining normal bone structure. Apparently, silicon provides a general cross-linking in collagen in the early development of bone tissue. Others have postulated a protective role of silicon against cardiovascular diseases. Silicon is reported to preserve the structural integrity of aorta.

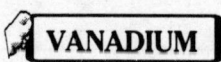 **VANADIUM**

Vanadium is involved in lipid metabolism. Its deficiency leads to elevated cholesterol levels. It accumulates in the dentin of teeth, where it promotes mineralization. Bone releases vanadium slowly and acts as a storage tissue.

An average American diet provides about 20 µg/day. An intake of 0.0320 µg of diet provides signs of deficiency in test animals.

Sea foods, whole grains, root vegetables, nuts and seeds are considered to be good sources of vanadium.

NICKEL

Nickel is an essential ultra trace element for mammals. In lab animals, nickel activates a number of enzymes, such as arginase and deoxyribonuclease, besides helping maintain the structure of nucleic acids and membranes. It also participates in lipid metabolism.

A dietary requirement of 50-80 ng/g of diet or about 30 µg/day has been projected for the human beings. The normal American diet usually has got about 100 - 200 µg/day, thus supplying the human needs. Nickel is mainly found in plant foods, especially grains and vegetables.

TIN

Tin is reported to contribute to the tertiary structure of proteins and other large molecules. Its concentration is the highest in bones and teeth, but it is also found in many other tissues like gastrointestinal tract, lungs, liver, kidneys, heart, spleen and muscles. High tin levels in the diet are not fully absorbed, hence its accumulation in tissues interferes with calcium balance and increases its excretion.

American diets normally provide 4-17 mg/day of tin, enough to meet all the body requirements. Organ meats and cereals are good food sources. However, storing left-over or half-used canned acid food in the refrigerators or in the open extracts more tin from the unlaquered cans that lends unpleasant odor and could add to some liabilities.

CADMIUM

This heavy metal cadmium is an integral component of proteins, 'Metal-thionein' indicating that it is a normal constituent of biologic matter. It has potential toxic effects on human health. Higher doses can lead to foetal retardation and interference with zinc metabolism as also cardiovascular system in the mammals.

Cadmium is absorbed poorly in the intestines and excreted slowly in the urine. It accumulates in the renal cortex and liver, but is also found in other tissues.

ARSENIC

Though an acknowledged poison, arsenic is reckoned as a beneficial ultra-trace element in very minute doses. Our diet usually contains 0.2 to 1 mg/day of arsenic. It is readily absorbed and excreted in urine. Blood levels in humans are about 0.2 to 0.4 µg/g.

In animal husbandry, arsenic supplements are used as growth promoters in piggery and poultry. Arsenic deficient lab animals have low hematocrit levels and increased red blood cell fragility.

Arsenic is widely distributed in foods like fish, shellfish and cereals.

ALUMINIUM

Aluminium is the third most abundant naturally occurring element, comprising about 8.8% of the earth's crust. In the normal course, adults consume about 3 to 5 mg/day in diet, apart from drinking it in water.

Aluminium is reported to participate in non-enzymatic cross-linking that occurs in brain with aging. In the normal aging process, there is a slow but steady increase in the aluminium level in the brain and this process accelerates sharply in the age group 70 to 100.

BORON

The real potentiality of boron has only recently been discovered. It apparently functions with major minerals in human metabolism. It is also considered essential for plant growth. Boron has a role to play in relation to human estrogen and metabolism of calcium, phosphorus and magnesium.

The human requirement for boron is projected between 0.5 and 1 mg/day.

Plant foods, especially fruits, leafy vegetables, legumes and nuts are very rich sources of boron. While animal products are poor source, wines and beers are fairly high in boron.

These eight ultra trace elements listed above are now considered essential in human nutrition, both as co-factors for cell enzymes in key metabolism reactions (i.e. activating these enzymes) and as structural components in special tissues, like the role of boron with calcium in bone formation.

Trace Elements in Food Stuffs

mg/100 g

Food Name	Iron	Zinc	Copper	Selenium	Manganese
Dairy Products					
Egg, whole, raw, large	1.440	1.100	0.014	0.044	0.024
Cheese, cottage, uncreamed	0.228	0.469	0.028	0.023	0.003
Cream, sour, cultured	0.061	0.270	0.019	—	0.003
Milk, buttermilk, fluid	0.049	0.420	0.011	0.001	0.002
Milk, whole, 3.3% fat, fluid	0.049	0.381	0.010	0.001	0.004
Milk, nonfat/skim, fluid	0.041	0.400	0.011	0.003	0.002
Fats					
Butter, regular, tablespoon	0.157	0.050	0.014	0.000	0.007
Vegetable oil, corn	0.000	0.000	0.000	—	0.000
Vegetable oil, olive	0.384	0.060	0.074	—	—
Margarine, reg, hard, unsalted	0.000	0.000	—	0.000	—
Cereals					
Bran flakes, Kellogg's	63.590	13.205	0.741	0.010	4.333
Corn flakes, Kellogg's	6.300	0.282	0.066	0.004	0.084
Oatmeal, cooked	0.679	0.491	0.055	0.009	0.585
Wheat, puffed, plain	4.733	2.358	0.408	—	1.758
Wheat, shredded, buiscuit	3.136	2.500	0.500	—	3.072
Rice Krispies	6.303	1.690	0.250	0.014	0.989
Breads, Cookies, Crackers					
Bread, white, soft	2.840	0.620	0.140	0.028	0.280
Bread, whole-wheat, soft	3.373	1.655	0.338	0.046	—
Muffin, English, plain	2.821	0.720	0.311	0.027	—
Roll, hamburger/hotdog	2.975	0.620	0.165	0.030	—
Meat, Fish					
Beef, cooked	3.790	8.660	0.164	0.006	0.019
Hamburger patty, beef/lean	2.106	5.365	0.066	0.024	0.014
Steak, lean, broiled	3.357	6.518	0.146	0.034	0.018
Chicken, leg, no skin, roasted	1.305	2.853	0.080	0.014	0.021
Chicken, breast, roasted	1.061	1.020	0.050	0.027	0.018
Lamb, all cuts, lean/fat, cooked	1.871	4.459	0.119	—	0.022
Turkey, dark meat, no skin	2.336	4.464	0.160	0.025	0.023

Table (*contd.* on page 196)

Table (contd. from page 195)

Food Name	Iron	Zinc	Copper	Selenium	Manganese
Veal, all cuts, lean, cooked	1.165	5.094	0.120	—	0.038
Bluefish	0.480	0.807	0.053	—	0.021
Flatfish, raw	0.353	0.459	0.032	—	0.016
Shrimp, raw, mixed species	2.400	1.114	0.271	—	0.057
Tuna, can/oil, drained	1.388	0.900	0.071	0.072	0.015
Tuna, diet, low sodium	1.201	0.500	0.060	0.116	0.039
Sweets					
Honey, strained/extracted	0.476	0.095	0.038	0.005	0.029
Jams/preserves, regular	1.000	—	0.310	0.000	—
Sugar, brown	0.409	—	0.350	0.001	—
Sugar, white, granulated	0.00	0.050	0.017	0.000	—
Juices					
Apple juice, can and bottle	0.371	0.028	0.022	0.001	0.113
Apricot nectar, can	0.382	0.092	0.073	—	0.032
Cranberry juice, bottle	0.150	0.070	0.018	0.000	0.193
Grape juice, can	0.096	—	—	—	—
Grapefruit juice, can, unsweetened	0.200	0.090	0.038	0.000	0.020
Lemon juice, can and bottle	0.130	0.060	0.037	0.000	0.020
Orange juice, can	0.442	0.070	0.067	0.000	0.030
Pear Nectar, can	0.260	0.070	0.067	0.000	0.030
Pineapple juice, can	0.260	0.110	0.090	0.001	0.992
Prune juice, can and bottle	1.180	0.210	0.068	0.000	0.151
Tomato juice, can	0.582	0.140	0.101	0.000	0.077
Tomato juice, low sodium	0.582	0.140	0.101	0.000	0.077
Vegetables					
Asparagus, can, spears	1.831	0.400	0.096	0.004	0.170
Beans, snap, green, can, cuts	0.904	0.290	0.038	0.001	0.200
Beets, can, whole	0.671	0.230	0.097	0.000	0.241
Beets, can, diet, low-sodium	0.671	0.230	0.097	0.001	0.241
Broccoli, raw, boiled, drained	0.839	0.380	0.043	0.002	0.218
Cabbage, common, boiled, drained	0.390	0.160	0.028	0.002	0.129
Carrots, can, sliced, drained	0.640	0.260	0.104	0.001	0.450
Carrots, can, low sodium	0.610	0.290	0.103	0.001	0.451
Carrot, raw, whole, scraped	0.500	0.200	0.047	0.003	0.142
Cauliflower, raw, boiled, drained	0.419	0.242	0.090	0.001	0.177
Celery, raw, stalk	0.400	0.130	0.035	0.000	0.035

Table (contd. on page 197)

Table (*contd.* from page 196)

Food Name	Iron	Zinc	Copper	Selenium	Manganese
Corn, sweet, can, drained	0.861	0.390	0.058	0.001	0.173
Corn, sweat, can, low sodium	0.350	0.359	0.056	0.000	0.033
Cucumber, raw, sliced	0.280	0.230	0.040	0.001	0.061
Peas, green, can, drained	0.953	0.712	0.082	0.001	0.303
Peas, green, can, low sodium	0.953	0.712	0.082	0.001	0.303
Tomato, raw, red, ripe	0.450	0.089	0.074	0.001	0.105
Tomato, red, can, stewed	0.729	0.170	0.112	0.001	0.059
Tomato, can, low sodium, diet	0.608	0.160	0.110	0.001	—
Potato, boiled, peeled before cooked	0.310	0.270	0.167	0.001	0.140
Noodles, Egg, enriched, cooked	0.875	—	0.169	0.059	—
Rice, white, parboiled, cooked	1.126	0.310	0.094	0.020	0.260
Fruits					
Apples, raw, unpeeled	0.181	0.036	0.041	0.001	0.045
Apple, raw, peeled	0.070	0.039	0.031	0.001	0.023
Apricots, can, light syrup	0.391	0.107	0.079	0.000	0.052
Bananas, raw, peeled	0.307	0.160	0.104	0.001	0.152
Blueberries, raw	0.170	0.110	0.061	0.001	0.282
Cherries, sweet, can/juice	0.580	0.100	0.073	0.000	0.061
Grapefruit, red/pnk/wht, raw	0.087	0.070	0.047	—	0.012
Oranges, raw, all varieties	0.100	0.069	0.045	0.002	0.025
Peaches, raw, whole	0.110	0.140	0.068	0.001	0.047
Peaches, can, light syrup	0.359	0.088	0.052	—	0.046
Pears, raw, unpeeled	0.250	0.120	0.113	0.001	0.076
Pineapple, can/juice	0.280	0.100	0.086	0.001	1.120
Strawberries, raw, whole	0.380	0.130	0.049	0.001	0.290

Source: *Modern Nutrition in Health and Disease*, Vol. 2.

Summary of Trace Elements (Required intake less than 100 mg/day)

Element	Physiologic Functions	Clinical Applications	Requirements	Food Sources
Iron (Fe)	Hemoglobin synthesis, oxygen transport Cell oxidation, heme enzymes	Anemia (hypochromic, microcytic) Excess: hemosiderosis, hemochromatosis Growth and pregnancy needs	Adults: men—10 mg, women—15 mg Pregnancy and Lactation: 30 and 15 mg, respect. Infants: 6-10 mg Children: 10-12 mg	Liver, Meats, Eggs Whole Grains Enriched breads and Cereals Dark Green Vegetables Legumes, Nuts (Iron cookware)
Iodine (I)	Synthesis of thyroxin, which regulates cell metabolism, basal metabolic rate (BMR)	Endemic colloid goiter, cretinism Hypothyroidism and hyperthyroidism	Adults: 150 µg Infants: 40-50 µg Children: 70-150 µg	Iodised Salt Seafood
Zinc (Zn)	Essential coenzyme constituent: carbonic anhydrase, lactic dehydrogenase	Growth: hypogonadism Sensory impairment: taste and smell Wound healing Malabsorption disease	Adults: 12-15 mg Infants: 5 mg Children: 10-15 mg	Widely distributed Seafood, Oysters Liver, Meat Milk, Cheese, Eggs Whoe Grains
Copper (Cu)	Associated with iron in enzyme systems, hemoglobin synthesis Metalloprotein enzyme constituent	Hypocupremia: nephrosis and malabsorption Wilson's disease, excess copper storage	Adults: 1.5-3 mg Infants: 0.4-0.7 mg Children: 0.7-2.5 mg	Widely distributed Liver, Meat Seafood Whole Grains Legumes, Nuts (Copper cookware)
Manganese (Mn)	Enzyme component in general metabolis	Low serum levels in diabetes, protein-energy malnutrition Inhalation toxicity	Adults: 2-5 mg Infants: 0.3-1.0 mg Children: 1-5 mg	Cereals, Whole Grains Legumes, Soybeans Leafy Vegetables

Table (contd. on page 199)

Table (*contd.* from page 198)

Element	Physiologic Functions	Clinical Applications	Requirements	Food Sources
Chromium (Cr)	Associated with glucose metabolism; improves faulty glucose uptake by tissues; glucose tolerance factor	Potentiates action of insulin in persons with diabetes Lowers serum cholesterol, LDL-cholesterol Increases HDL	Adults: 50-200 µg Infants: 10-60 µg Children: 20-200 µg	Cereals Whole Grains Brewer's Yeast Animal Protein
Cobalt (Co)	Constituent of vitamin B_{12}, functions with vitamins	Deficiency associated only with deficiency of vitamin B_{12}	Unknown; evidently minute	Vitamin B_{12} source
Selenium (Se)	Constituent of enzyme glutathione peroxidase Synergistic antioxidant with vitamin E Structural component of teeth	Marginal deficiency when soil content is low Deficiency secondary to parental nutrition (TPN), malnutrition Toxicity observed in livestock	Adults: 55-70 µg Infants: 10-15 µg Children: 20-50 µg	Varies with soil content Seafood Legumes Whole Grains Low-fat Meats and Dairy products Vegetables
Molybdenum (Mo)	Constituent of oxidase enzyme, xanthine oxidase	Deficiency unknown in humans	Adults: 75-250 µg Infants: 15-30 µg Children: 25-250 µg	Legumes Whole grains Milk Organ Meats Leafy Vegetables
Fluoride (F)	Accumulates in bones and teeth, increasing hardness	Dental caries inhibited Osteoporosis: may help control Excess: dental fluorosis	Adults: 1.5-4 mg Infants: 0.1-0.5 mg Children: 0.5-2.5 mg	Fish Fish products Tea Foods cooked in fluoridated water Drinking water

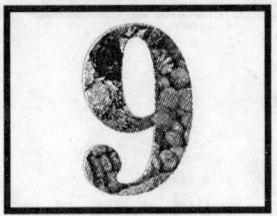

9

WATER AND ELECTROLYTES

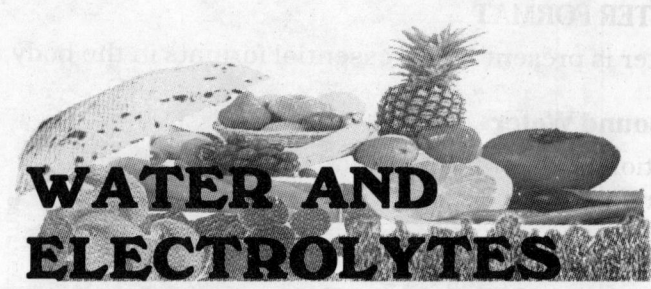

Water is Life !

We live on a planet of water. All the living forms, plants, animals or human beings, need regular uninterrupted supply of water. It is our moving cycle of surging, nourishing water that sustains life. Water is only second to oxygen in maintaining life. The body can survive without food for several weeks, but dies within 5-10 days, if deprived of water. Technically, a loss of 20% of body water results in death. Such is the great contribution of water.

Indeed, our body, without adequate water, would soon be poisoned to death under the weight of its internal waste products. Toxic elements like urea and uric acid, need water to be flushed out of the body, as does skin. Our lungs need to be kept in a moistened state in order that they can absorb oxygen and excrete carbon dioxide. Water is the best *'Cleansing and Scavenging Agent'*, since all the chemical reaction of the body processes take place in the presence of water. Blood is 90% water and urine is 97% water. An incidence of acute diarrhoea, all the more so in the case of infants can lead to dehydration, which may eventually result in death. Even a momentary shortage of water can severely disrupt the body chemistry. Such is the *quintessential role* that water plays in a man's life.

A large number of minerals, described in the earlier chapters, have been functioning as 'Electrolytes' in controlling the body's vital water balance. This collective function is fundamental to the human health and often plays a vital part of patient's care. Thus, one has to look into the three basic inter-dependent factors that control this balance.

(1) Water itself is the solvent base for solutions.
(2) Various particles or 'solute' in solution in water.
(3) The separating membranes that control the flow.

WATER FORMAT

Water is present in five essential formats in the body, as under:

1. Bound Water

Portion of water in food and body tissues that is attached to the colloids and is therefore more difficult to release than free water.

2. Exogenous Water

Water in the body coming from dietary sources, either as liquid or as a food component.

3. Endogenous Water

Water derived from the metabolism of food in the body. Its also called 'Metabolic Water'.

4. Free Water

That portion of water in the body or food that is not closely bound by attachment to the colloids.

5. Metabolic Water

Also called 'Water of Combustion', *i.e.* provided by the combustion of foodstuffs.

Oxidation of all the foodstuffs yields water, as under:

$$C_6H_{12}O_6 \xrightarrow{\text{Oxidation}} CO_2 + H_2O \ (\text{Water} + \text{Energy})$$

Glucose (Sugar)

Thus, one hundred grams of foodstuffs would yield:

Carbohydrates	→	55 g water
Proteins	→	41 g water
Fats	→	107 g water

On an average, water produced by the body's metabolic activity aggregates to about 200-300 ml per day.

BODY WATER DISTRIBUTION

A man's body is about 55%-65% water, while in the women, this share comes to about 50%-55%. The higher water proportion is accounted by the greater muscular mass. Striated muscles contain more water than any other body tissue, except blood. The remaining 40% of a man's weight comprises of:

Proteins	-	About 18 %
Fats	-	15 %
Minerals	-	7 %

A woman's remaining body content is about the same, except for the smaller muscle mass, but it has larger fat deposits.

WATER DEFICIT

It is an established fact that abnormal loss of water may occur in diarrhoea, excessive vomiting and severe burns. The following formula is used to calculate the water status:

$$(100 \text{ TBW} \times \text{BW}) \times \left\{ 1 - \frac{(\text{Sodium predicted})}{(\text{Sodium measured})} \right\}$$

TBW is the percent total body water (about 60% for an average adult, 42% for lean female, 30% for obese male and 70% for lean male). BW is the actual body weight in kgs.

Sodium predicted is the constant average serum sodium level—140 mEq/L

Sodium measured is the actual measurement of serum sodium .

WATER FUNCTIONS

Water in the body performs three essential functions:

1. Turgor

The cell water and its contents in solution provide a normal turgor or fullness to the tissue, a degree of rigidity that results from liquid pressure of cell contents on the cell membranes. Just as a balloon requires air pressure for its form and functions, so also the human body requires water.

2. Solvent

Water provides the necessary chemical solvent on which the tremendous variety of body tissue solutions are based. This water environment provides the base of tissue fluid circulation that supply nutrients to the cells and also accounts for the large multitude of cell chemical reactions that fulfil the body's needs.

3. Body Temperature

Water is the indispensable medium that maintains body temperature. The loss of water through skin helps maintain a steady body temperature. When the weather is hot or in case of increased body exercise, more water is eliminated by the skin as perspiration, the evaporation of which helps remove excess body heat to a comfortable level.

WATER COMPARTMENTS

The body water may be divided into 2 compartments:

(1) The Extracellular Fluid Compartment (ECF) that contains water outside the cells.

(2) The Intracellular Fluid Compartment (ICF) is the total water inside the cells.

(A) Extracellular Fluid (ECF): Water present outside the cells accounts for about 20% of the body weight. The ECF comprises of four parts, viz.

1. Blood Plasma which forms about 25% of the ECF, but only 5% of the body weight.
2. Interstitial Fluid is the water that surrounds the cells.
3. Secretory Fluid which is the water circulating in transit.
4. Dense Tissue Fluid is the water found in dense connective tissue, cartilages and bones.

(B) Intracellular Fluid (ICF): Total water present inside the cells makes up for about 40%-45% of the total body weight. Since the body cells perform a wide range of metabolic activity, hence the total water inside the cells is almost twice the amount present outside.

Overall Water Balance (Intake and Output)

An average adult metabolizes about 2.5-3 litres (10-13 cups) of water every day in a constant turnover balance between intake and output. Table 9.1 gives the detailed Water balance of the human body.

Normally, this water enters and leaves the body by various routes, controlled by the basic mechanisms like thirst and hormonal activity. Thirst and drinking mechanism are complex interactions involving control centres located in the brain and related hormonal activity that regulates water intake. Special pressure sensitive cells called 'Osmoreceptors' located in the brains' thirst centre in hypothalamus relay messages through nerve fibres that stimulate the conscious act of drinking.

TABLE 9.1: WATER BALANCE: WATER INTAKE AND LOSS FROM BODY

	Temperate climate (ml)	Tropical climate (ml)
Water Intake:		
Drinking water	1500	2000-5000
In Food	1000	1000-2000
By oxidation of Carbohydrates, Fats and Proteins in Tissues	300	300
Total	**2800**	**3300-7300**
Water Loss:		
In Urine	1500	1000-1500
Via Skin	800	1800-5200
Via Lungs	400	400
In Feces	100	100-200
Total	**2800**	**3300-7300**

The hormonal regulation of renal water excretion for maintaining water balance is under the control of 'Vasopressin', the anti-diuretic hormone (ADH) secreted by the pituitary gland.

Intake

Water enters the body in three principle forms:

(1) Preformed water as such and in other beverages and drinks.
(2) Preformed water in food that is eaten.
(3) Metabolic water which is a product of cell oxidation.

Output

Water is flushed out of body through kidneys, skin, lungs and feces. This intake-output must be maintained in a constant balance, as shown in Table 9.2. The infant's body contains greater percentage of total body water and more water is outside the cells and easily available for loss, hence, their greater vulnerability to dehydration.

TABLE 9.2: DAILY INTAKE AND OUTPUT OF AN ADULT

		Intake (ml/day) (Replacement)		Output (loss) ml/day	
				Obligatory (Insensible)	Additional (According to the needs)
A.	Preformed:				
	Liquids	1200-1500	Lungs	350	
	In foods	700-1000			
			Skin		
			- Diffusion	350	
			- Sweat	100	± 250
			Kidneys	900	± 250
			Feces	150	
B.	Metabolism: (Oxidation of Foods)	200-300			
	Total	2100-2800	Total	1850	750
				(Approximately 2600 ml/day)	

FORCES CONTROLLING WATER DISTRIBUTION

Two factors influence and control the distribution of body water. These are 'Solutes'—the particles in solution in body water, and 'Separating Membranes' between water compartments.

Solutes

There are three main types of particles with varying concentration in the body. These are electrolyte, plasma proteins and organic compounds.

1. *Electrolytes*

Several inorganic minerals provide electrolytes for the body. They move freely in solution, but carry an electrical charge. These free charged ions or atoms carry either a positive charge, when they acre called 'Cations'. For example, Sodium (Na^+) is the major cation outside the cells. And Potassium (K^+) the cation inside the cells, besides Calcium (Ca^{++}) and Magnesium (Mg^{++}).

Conversely, an ion with a negative charge is called 'Anions', e.g. chloride (Cl^-), carbonate (CO_3^-), phosphate (HPO_4^-) and sulphate (SO_4^-). Being of small size, these ions can diffuse freely across body membranes. These electrolytes are the major force controlling movement of water within the body.

2. *Plasma Proteins*

Plasma proteins are organic substances of larger molecular size, mainly albumin and globulin. They influence the shift of water in and out of the capillaries in balance with the surrounding water. The plasma proteins are called 'Colloids' (Greek: *Kolla* means glue) and form colloidal solutions. Because of their large size, these particles or molecules do not pass readily through separating capillary membranes. Thus, they normally remain in blood vessels, exerting colloidal osmotic pressure (COP) to maintain the integrity of blood volume.

3. *Organic Compounds*

Other organic compounds of small size, such as glucose, urea and amino acids diffuse freely but do not influence shifts of water, unless present in very large concentration. For example, large amount of glucose in urine in diabetes mellitus patients causes an abnormal osmotic diuresis or excess water output.

Separating Membranes

Two basic types of membranes are involved in the movement of water and solutes within the body: capillary membranes and cell membranes. The capillary membrane is relatively free and allows rapid change of substances. On the other hand, cell membrane is more complex semi-permeable structure. It is composed essentially of lipid material embedded within the protein molecule The metabolic processes within the cell usually govern the passage of electrolytes and therefore, water across this barrier. Water and solutes move freely across the body's separating membranes through physiologic mechanisms like osmosis, diffusion, filtration, active transport and pinocytosis.

Influence of Electrolyte on Water Balance

Measurement of Electrolyte

The number of particles in a solution, i.e. concentration determines the chemical activity of that solution. Electrolytes are measured according to the total number of particles, each one of which contributes its chemical combining power according to its valence. And the unit of measurement is called an 'Equivalent', rather milliequivalents owing to the very small amounts. It is usually expressed as milliequivalents per litre (mEq/L). This figure represents the number of ions—cations and anions in the solution.

Electrolyte Balance

The distribution of electrolytes in the body water compartments in a definitive pattern helps maintain stable 'Electrochemical Neutrality' in body fluid solutions. As per biochemical and electrochemical laws, a stable solution must have equal number of positive and negative particles. That means, it has got to be electrically neutral. Our system has got an automatic compensating mechanism to adjust and stabilise the essential electroneutrality.

Controlling Body Hydration

Ionized sodium is the chief cation of extracellular fluid (ECF) and ionized potassium is the chief cation of the intracellular fluid (ICF). These two electrolytes control the amount of water retained in any given compartment. The term hypertonic and hypotonic dehydration refers to the electrolyte concentration outside the cells, which, in turn, causes a shift of water into or out of the cell to maintain the balance.

Influence of Plasma Proteins

Capillary Fluid Shift Mechanism

Water circulating in the blood vessels has got to get out of these vessels in order to service various tissues and later on, it must be drawn back into circulation to maintain normal transporting flow. Two opposing pressures, viz. Colloid Osmotic Pressure (COP) from the plasma proteins (mainly albumin) and Hydrostatic Pressure (blood pressure) of the capillary blood flow, provide balanced control of water and solute movement across capillary membranes. It is indeed a filtration process operating according to the differences in osmotic pressure on either side of the capillary membrane.

When blood first enters the capillary system, the greater blood pressure forces water and small solutes out into the tissue to bathe and nourish the cells. But the plasma protein particles are too large to go through the pores of capillary membranes. The proteins remain in the vessels and exert greater colloidal osmotic pressure that draws the returning fluid and its materials back into circulation from the cells. This is called Capillary Fluid Shift Mechanism and provides the important homostatic mechanism in the body to maintain water balance, without which cells would die.

Cell Fluid Control

The cell proteins help provide the osmotic pressure that maintains integrity of fluid inside the cells. Ionized potassium within the cells guards cell water in balance with ionized sodium guarding water outside the cell. This balance supports the flow of water, nutrients and metabolites in and out of cells to sustain life.

Hormones and Water Balance

The antidiuretic hormone (ADH), also called Vasopressin, causes reabsorption of water by the kidney. This is a water-conserving mechanism. In any stress situation, this hormone is triggered to hold onto the precious body water.

Aldosterone Mechanism

Aldosterone is primarily a sodium-conserving mechanism related to renin-angiotension system. Besides, it also exerts secondary control over water loss. But aldosterone and ADH are activated by stress situations, such as injury or surgery.

Water Toxicity

Water intoxication is a condition that results from excessive intake of fluids, without an equivalent amount of salt, as in glucose drip in person with inadequate renal function. Since the kidney cannot excrete this extra load, the accumulated water enters all the fluid compartments, including cells and tissues which become water-logged. In case of severe water toxicity, there are symptoms of confusion, convulsions, coma and even death.

Water Requirements

Two vital conditions viz. removal of body heat and excretion of urea and other metabolic wastes need a constant supply of water. There is an obligatory daily loss of about 1500 ml water, as under:

Loss through Skin	600 ml
Loss through Expired Air	400 ml
Loss through Urine	500 ml.

But hot weather and any exertion demand more water. Water needs increase by 100 ml-150 ml per day for each one degree rise of body temperature (98.6°F). Based on body weight, the estimated daily requirement of water comes to:

New-born	140 - 150 ml/kg
2 years (12 kg)	115 - 125 ml/kg
6 years (20 kg)	90 - 100 ml/kg
25 years	40 ml/kg
60 years	30 ml/kg

Similarly, pregnancy and lactation also demand extra water.

PART 2

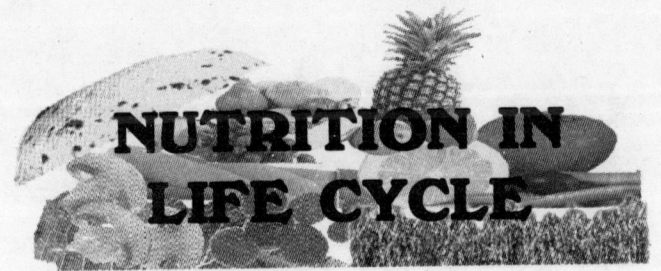

NUTRITION IN LIFE CYCLE

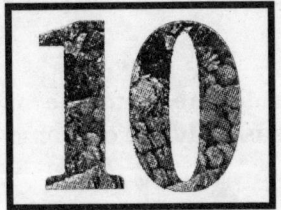

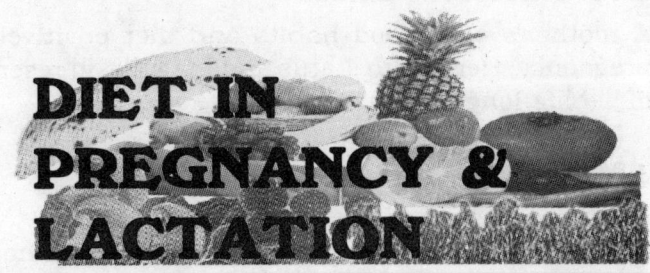

10

DIET IN PREGNANCY & LACTATION

It is a truism that healthy body tissues depend directly on certain essential nutrients in the food. Equally so is the infant's development related to the diet of the mother. Earlier, certain erroneous beliefs and fallacies persisted in regard to pregnancy. The old practices of semi-starvation of the pregnant women rested on the theory that it would produce a lighter baby, easy to deliver. This parasite theory was based on the belief that whatever the fetus needs will be drawn from the 'Reserve' store of the mother. And the maternal instinct theory believed that whatsoever the needs, the mother will instinctively crave and consume. However, positive nutritional support of pregnancy contradicts all the old fallacies and accounts for better health and vigor of both the infant and the mother.

FACTORS INFLUENCING NUTRITION NEEDS

Nutrition is the fundamental support system for successful pregnancy that manifests in the form of a healthy child and an equally healthy and happy mother. Three major factors that determine the nutrition need during pregnancy are:

1. Age and Parity
2. Pre-conception Nutrition
3. Complex Metabolic Interactions

1. Age and Parity

In the case of teen age pregnancies, the half-mature body and growth needs of this early-age mother further adds to the demands made by pregnancy. On the other hand, the late-age pregnancies involve some hazards. Also the number of pregnancies, parity and the interval between them severely impinge upon the mother's reserves.

2. Pre-conception Nutrition

A mother's early food habits and diet positively influence the outcome of pregnancy. Her health status and the built-in reserves are basically the outcome of her life-long dietary habits.

3. Metabolic Interactions of Gestation

The three distinct entities involved in pregnancy, viz. the mother, the fetus and the placenta form a unique biologic complex, whose interactions directly affect the course and the outcome of pregnancy.

BASIC CONCEPTS INVOLVED

1. Perinatal Concepts

This refers to the duration of pregnancy. The mother's food habits and nutritional status developed over the years are the important factors that significantly contribute to the outcome of pregnancy. Equally so are the social and cultural influences that bear upon pregnancy.

2. Synergism Concept

Synergism denotes the biologic systems wherein the cooperative action of two entities is far greater than their respective individual impact. Herein, maternal organism, fetus and placenta interact to produce a 'New Whole'. Many changes take place. Blood volume increases, so too the cardiac output and the breath rate, and the BMR too increases. Then, there is the generalised edema of pregnancy, which is a protective response, reflecting the normal increase in total body water required to support the extra-metabolic work of pregnancy.

3. Life Continuum Concept

Throughout her life, a mother is intuitively providing for this continuum of life through whatever food she consumes. This nutritional heritage passes from one generation to the other.

NUTRITIONAL DEMANDS OF PREGNANCY

The period of nine months gestation is a time of hectic growth. Starting from a single fertilized egg cell 'Ovum', the life grows to a full-fledged infant baby weighing about 3 kg. During this phase, the mother has to willy nilly meet all the demands of a growing fetus. Besides, there are the physiologic demands of her own changing body during this critical period of human growth. This increased need of nutrients further depends upon variations like size, activity and multiple pregnancy. Table 10.1 depicts a well articulated picture of the nutrition demands during pregnancy.

TABLE 10.1: NUTRIENT NEEDS DURING PREGNANCY

Nutrient	Amount (NRC)		Reasons for Increased Nutrient Need in Pregnancy	Food Sources
	Non-pregnant Adult Need	Pregnant Need		
Protein	46 gm	76-100 gm	Rapid fetal tissue growth Amniotic fluid Placenta growth and development Maternal tissue growth; uterus, breasts Increased maternal circulating blood volume: a. Hemoglobin increase b. Plasma protein increase Maternal storage reserves for labor, delivery and lactation	Milk Cheese Egg Meat Grains Legumes Nuts
Calories	2100	2400	Increased BMR, energy needs protein sparing	Carbohydrates Fats Proteins
Minerals				
Calcium	800 mg	1200 mg	Fetal skeleton formation Fetal tooth bud formation Increased maternal calcium metabolism	Milk Cheese Whole grains Leafy vegetables Some canned fish Egg yolk
Phosphorus	800 mg	1200 mg	Fetal skeletal formation Fetal tooth bud formation Increased maternal phosphorus metabolism	Milk Cheese Lean meats
Iron	18 mg	18+ mg (+30-60 mg increased hemoglobin supplement)	Increased maternal circulating blood volume, Increased hemoglobin Fetal liver iron storage High iron cost of pregnancy	Liver Meats Egg Whole or enriched grains Leafy vegetables Nuts Legumes Dried fruits

Source: Alice A. Chenault in *Nutrition and Health*, Pub., Hott, Rinehart and Winston.

The recommended daily dietary allowance (RDA), stipulated by the National Research Council, USA (1989 revision) is given in Table 10.2.

However, as the situation and also the genetic heritage varies considerably in the developing countries, the Indian Council of Medical Research (ICMR) has given the following stipulations for the RDA for the Indians (adapted from The Nutritive Values of Indian Foods), as shown in Table 10.3.

TABLE 10.2: RDA FOR PREGNANCY AND LACTATION (NRC-1989 REVISED)

Nutrients	Non-pregnant			Pregnancy				Lactation			
	Girls		Women	Added	Girls		Women	Added	Girls		Women
	12-14 yrs	14-18 yrs	25 yrs	Needs	12-14 yrs	14-18 yrs	25 yrs	Needs	12-14 yrs	14-18 yrs	25 yrs
Kilocalories	2200	2200	2200	300	2500	2500	2500	500	2700	2700	2700
Proteins(g)	46	46	50	10-15	60	60	60	15	65	68	65
Calcium(g)	1.2	1.2	0.8	0.4	1.6	1.6	1.2	0.4	1.6	1.6	1.2
Iron (mg)	15	15	15	15	30	30	30	0	15	15	15
Vitamin A (RE)	800	800	800	0	800	800	800	500	1300	1300	1300
Thiamine (mg)	1.1	1.1	1.1	0.4	1.5	1.5	1.5	0.5	1.6	1.6	1.6
Riboflavin (mg)	1.3	1.3	1.3	0.3	1.6	1.6	1.6	0.5	1.8	1.8	1.8
Niacin (NE)	15	15	15	2	17	17	17	5	20	20	20
Ascorbic Acid (mg)	50	60	60	10	60	70	70	35	95	95	95
Vitamin D (µg)	10	10	5	5	15	15	10	5	15	15	10

TABLE 10.3: ENERGY AND NUTRITIONAL REQUIREMENTS OF PREGNANCY (ICMR)

Nutrients	Non-Pregnant Girls		Non-Preg. Women	Pregnant Women	Lactating Mothers	
	13-15 yrs (47 kg)	6-18 yrs (50 kg)			0-6 mths	7-12 mths
Net Energy (kcal/day)	2060	2060	2225	2525	3210	2625
Proteins (g/d)	65	63	50	65	75	68
Fat (g)	22	22	20	30	45	45
Calcium(mg/d)	600	500	400	1000	1000	1000
Iron (mg/d)	28	30	30	38	30	30
Vitamin A (µg)						
Retinol +	600+	600+	600+	600+	950+	950+
β-Carotene	2400	2400	2400	2400	3800	3800
Thiamine (mg)	1.0	1.0	1.1	1.3	1.4	1.3
Riboflavin (mg)	1.2	1.2	1.3	1.5	1.6	1.5
NicotinicAcid (NE)	14	14	14	16	18	17
Ascorbic Acid (mg)	40	40	40	40	80	150
Folic Acid (mg)	100	100	100	100	80	150
Pyridoxine (Vitamin) B_6 (mg)	—	—	—	2.5	2.5	2.5
Vitamin B_{12} (mg)	0.2-1.0	0.2-1.0	1.0	1.0	1.5	1.5

Energy Needs

The kilocalories in energy must be sufficient to provide for

(a) Increased Metabolic workload.
(b) Extra Proteins needed for tissue building.

Normally, 36 kcal/kg is required for efficient use of proteins during pregnancy. The RDA stipulates an additional amount of energy—300 kcal, *i.e.* 10-15% increase or a total of about 2500 kcal. But this amount must go up for large sized women or those who are nutritionally deficit. Appropriate weight gains during pregnancy will show whether adequate kilocalories are being consumed.

Protein Needs

Proteins needed during pregnancy go up to 60 g/day, *i.e.* an increase of 20% over the normal RDA. This increased requirement provides for:

1. Rapid growth of fetus.
2. Enlargement of uterus, mammary glands and placenta.
3. Increased maternal blood volume.
4. Formation of amniotic fluid and storage reserve.

Milk, eggs, cheese and meat are the complete protein foods of high biologic value that would suffice for the state of pregnancy. Four cups of milk per day provide more than the additional 10 to 16 g of high-quality protein needed, increase the calcium intake to 1.2 g, and provide an additional 320 kcal from skim milk or 640 kcal from whole milk. A number of choices are available: whole milk low-fat milk, skim milk, non-fat powdered milk, buttermilk, acidophilus milk, evaporated milk, yogurt and cheese. Nonfat milk powder can be added in the preparation of meat loaf, soups, scrambled eggs, mashed and scalloped potatoes, sandwich spreads, cooked cereals, home-made breads, cookies, or pastries. Aproximately one-third cup of dried skim milk is equivalent to 1 cup of fluid milk. Milk can be made richer in calcium, protein and calories by adding 2 tablespoons of dried nonfat milk to a glass of fluid milk.

Mineral Needs

Amongst the minerals needed for proper maternal health, calcium and iron play an important role in pregnancy.

Calcium

As against the normal requirement of 800 mg/day calcium, the pregnant women need 1200 mg calcium, i.e. an increase of 50%. Calcium is needed for the formation of bones and teeth. It is also an important element in blood clotting and is also required for muscle action and other metabolic activities. Furthermore, the rapid fetal mineralisation of skeletal tissues during the final stages of rapid growth demands more calcium.

Milk and milk products, cheese and ice cream, are the main source of dietary calcium. Besides, green leafy vegetables and whole grains also contain calcium.

The NRC recommends an additional 150 mg of magnesium per day during pregnancy.

Iron

The 'Iron Cost' of pregnancy being very high, a woman must maintain a regular daily intake of 15 mg iron throughout her child-bearing age. This helps replenish the menstrual losses and store tissue and liver reserves after each pregnancy.

The women suffering from anemia need a large therapeutic dose of 120-200 mg of iron, which means 1-2 tablets of 300 mg ferrous sulfate every day.

During pregnancy, maternal circulating blood volume increases by 45-50%. Maternal iron is also needed to supply iron stores for the developing fetal liver. Adequate levels of iron also helps fortify the mother against serum iron losses at the time of delivery.

Liver is, by far, the richest source of iron. Iron is also present in meat, legumes, dried fruits, green vegetables, eggs and carrots.

The specification in regards to other vital minerals, as mentioned in Krause's book: *Food, Nutrition and Diet Therapy,* are given in Table 10.4.

TABLE 10.4: RDA FOR MINERALS

Mineral	15-18 yr.	19.24 yr.	25-50 yr.	Pregnant	Lactating 1st 6 months	2nd 6 months
Zinc (mg)	12	12	12	15	19	16
Iodine (mg)	150	150	150	175	200	200
Selenium (µg)	50	55	55	65	75	75

Vitamin Needs

A pregnant women needs extra amount of vitamins A, B complex, C and D. Their adequate supplies will also take care of vitamins E and K.

Vitamin A

A normal healthy woman does not need vitamin A during pregnancy. But malnourished mothers need extra vitamin A, since it is required for cell development, teeth formation and bone growth, besides the need for the epithelial tissue maintenance.

Liver, egg yolk, butter and fortified margarine, dark green and yellow vegetables and fruits are the main dietary source of vitamin A.

In particular, there is a great demand for folic acid during pregnancy. Its deficiency in malnourished women make it a high-risk case. Folic acid deficiency leads to megaloblastic anemia. The RDA standard is 400 mg of folic acid per day.

Group B Vitamins

The Group B vitamins are co-enzyme factors in many metabolic activities related to energy production, tissue protection, synthesis and functioning of muscle and nerve tissues.

In particular, there is a great demand for folic acid during pregnancy. Its deficiency in malnourished women make it a high-risk case. Folic acid deficiency leads to megaloblastic anemia. The RDA standard is 400 µg of folic acid per day.

Vitamin C

Ascorbic acid is specially needed for the formation of inter-cellular cement substance in developing connective tissue and vascular system. Vitamin C also helps increase the absorption of iron needed for the synthesis of increased volume of hemoglobin. An additional dose of 10 mg, over the normal 60 mg/day vitamin C, is recommended during the pregnancy.

Fruits like citrus and green vegetables are a good source of vitamin C in the mother's diet.

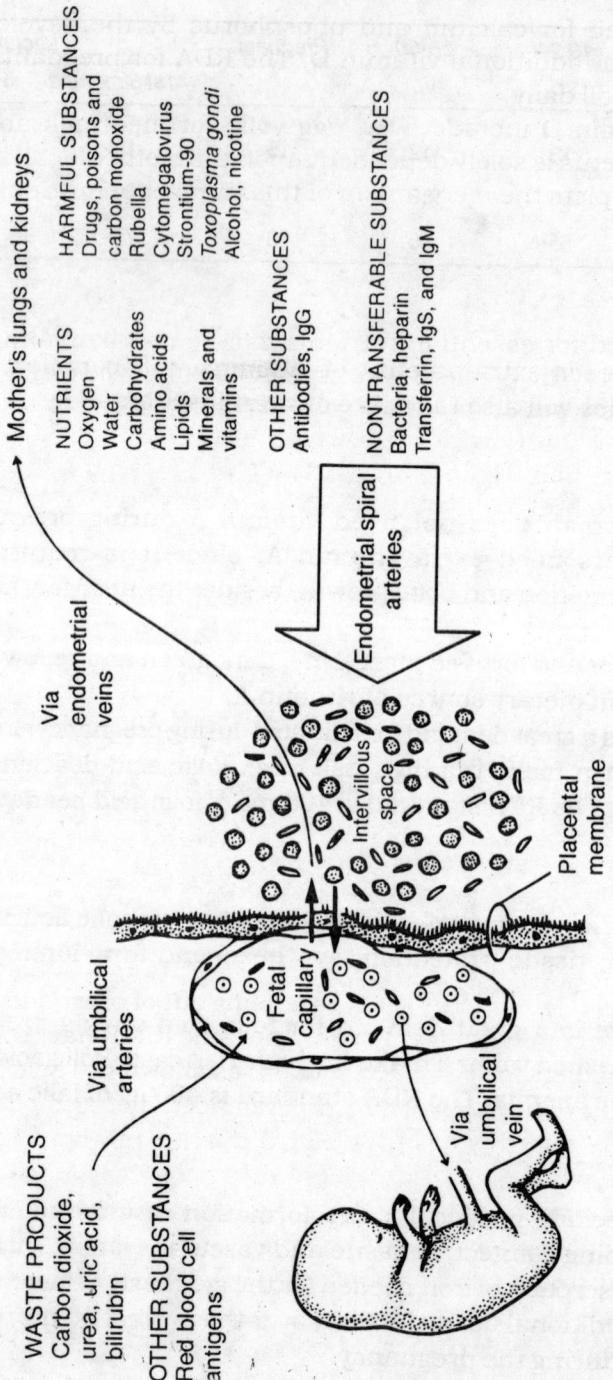

Fig. 10.1: Diagrammatic Illustration of Transfer Across the Placental Membrane

(From Moore KL: *The Developing Human,* 5th ed. Philadelphia, WB Saunders, 1993.)

Vitamin D

The increased demand for calcium and phosphorus by the developing fetal skeletal tissue calls for additional vitamin D. The RDA for pregnant women is 400 IU (15 mg calciferol) daily.

Foods rich in vitamin D include liver, egg yolk, fortified milk and fortified margarine. Since the fetus is solely dependent upon the mother for all its nutrient needs. Figure 10.1 depicts the mechanism of this transfer of nutrients from the mother.

DIET PATTERN

The increased demand for essential nutrients can be met by planning a daily menu using select foods. The Western prescription for enhanced dietary nutrients are 3-5 cups of milk, cheese or ice cream, about two servings of lean meat, fish and poultry, 1-2 eggs, 1-2 servings of vegetables, besides fresh fruits, fruit juices and moderate amounts of butter or margarine.

Table 10.5 gives the Pregnancy diet which provides 1500-2300 kcal for the Western women.

TABLE 10.5: DIET FOR PREGNANT WESTERN WOMEN – VARYING CALORIES

Food	2300 kcal	1800 kcal	1500 kcal
Milk	1 qt (whole)	1 qt (whole)	1 qt (Skimmed)
Meat, Fish/Poultry	4 oz	4 oz lean	4 oz lean
Fruits	Citrus/others	One serving	One serving
Vegetables—GLV incl. potato or yellow vegetables	4 servings	4 servings	4 servings
Butter/Margarine	3 Tsp	3 Tsp	3 Tsp

Since most of the problems/complications arising out of pregnancy take place in the weaker sections of the developing countries, the ICMR has recommended the following low-cost diets for pregnant women, as shown in Table 10.6. In the above stipulation, diet A costs less than the balanced diet and offers more of cereals with moderate quantity of milk. Diet B offers a minimum of milk and hence costs the least, while diet C is meant for the non-vegetarians.

Planning a diet for a pregnant woman that would supply about 2500 kcal of energy and 59 g proteins, the menu in Table 10.7 provides the list of food exchange items in an Indian diet. Of course, this dietary plan permits some regional adjustments.

Hereunder, in Table 10.8, Rekha Sharma gives the detailed diet chart for a pregnant Indian woman. For the sake of a comparison, we also give the menus of Western diet for pregnant women in Table 10.9.

TABLE 10.6: LOW-COST DIETS FOR PREGNANT WOMEN IN INDIA

Diet	Cereals	Oils	Sugar/ Jaggery	Milk	Pulses	Meat	Egg	Fruits	GLV	Other Veg.	Roots/ Tubers
	g	g	g	ml	g	g		g	g	g	g
Balanced diet for a Pregnant women	400	20	30	20	55	—	—	—	150	50	50
Prevalent diet of poor folks	276	20	12	40	20	—	—	25	—	25	—
Nutritious low -cost diets											
A	440	20	25	110	50	—	—	—	150	50	50
B	450	20	25	100	45	—	—	—	150	50	50
C (Non-vegetarian)	440	20	25	100	25	30 or	One egg	—	150	50	100

Source: ICMR: Dietary Recommendations—1990.

In the long run, it is not the foods but the specific nutrients that are the cornerstone of a successful pregnancy. But the two important nutrition principles that should guide a pregnant women are:

1. She must eat sufficient quantity of food.
2. She must eat regularly without skipping meals, especially the breakfast.

TABLE 10.7: FOOD EXCHANGE LIST FOR DIET IN PREGNANCY

	Food Group	No. of Exchanges	Proteins (g)	Energy (kcal)
1.	Milk	4	20	400
2.	Legumes and Pulses	2	12	200
3.	Flesh Foods	1	10	100
4.	Vegetables-A (GLV)	2	—	—
5.	Vegetables-B	2	—	100
6.	Fruits	3	—	150
7.	Cereals	9	18	900
8.	Fats	5	—	500
9.	Sugar	40	—	160
	Grand Total		**60.0**	**2,510**

Source: *Nutrition and Dietetics* by S A Joshi.

TABLE 10.8: MENU FOR A PREGNANT INDIAN WOMAN

7.00 AM	Tea	1 cup with sugar
9.00 AM	Milk	200 ml
	Bread	2 slices
	Porridge	1 bowl or
	Chapattis	2 or
	Idlis	2 (medium)
	Cottage Cheese	30 g or
	Egg	1 or
	Sprouts	25 g—1 bowl
11.00 AM	Buttermilk/Fruit juice	1 glass (medium)
1.00 PM	Fresh Salad	1 bowl
	Fortified	
	Chapattis	4 (80 g) (4 : 1 proportion) or
	Rice	4 dessert spoonfuls (80 g)
	(preferably steamed with pulses or green vegetables)	
	Pulses	2 bowls (60 g) or
	Meat/Fish Poultry	90 g (edible portion)
	Curd	125 g—1 bowl
	Green, cooked	
	Vegetables	250 g—2 bowls
	Cooking Oil	10 g-2 tsp
4.00 PM	Milk	200 ml—1 glass
	Cheese	
	Sandwich	1 small or
	Vada	1 large or
	Poha	1 bowl
	(Puffed rice)	
7.00 PM	Dinner same as Lunch (1.00 PM)	
9.00 PM	Milk	200 ml

Source: Dr. F. P. Antia. *Clinical Dietetics and Nutrition*, Oxford, 1989.

N.B. Fruits, 1-2 servings anytime during the day.
This special diet suppplies

	Proteins	90 g
	Fats	60 g
	Total Calories	2200

For the diabetics, omit sugar and for hypertension cases, restrict salt.

TABLE 10.9: SAMPLE MENU FOR PREGNANCY (WESTERN WOMEN)

	Food	Pregnant Women (Normal wt.)	Pregnant Adolescent Girls (Normal wt.)
Breakfast	Orange juice	4 0z	4 oz
	Scrambled egg	1	1
	Cornflakes/ grits	—	1 cup
	Toast slice	1	1
	Butter/Margarine	2 tsp	—
	Coffee	1 cup	
	Milk	—	½ pint
Mid-morning	Milk	½ pint	½ pint
Lunch	Meat chops or	✓	—
	Peanut Butter sandwich		
	Hamburger on a bun	—	—
	Carrot stick	✓	✓
	Cole slaw	—	—
	Oatmeal cookies	✓	✓
	Milk	½ pint	½ pint
Afternoon	Milk	½ pint	—
	Fruit juice/Milk shake	—	½ pint
	Frankfurter on a bun	—	✓
Dinner	Roasted/Boiled Beef/		
	Pork/Liver/Fish	✓	✓
	Brocolli/Greens	✓	✓
	Baked Potato	✓	✓
	Butter/Margarine	✓	✓
	Green Salad with		
	French Dressing	✓	✓
	Fresh/Canned Fruit	✓	✓
	Coffee/ Tea/ Milk	✓	½ pint
Bedtime	Milk/Coffee	½ pint	—
	Fruit juice/Cocoa	—	½ pint

Source: Mitchel *et al.* in *Nutrition and Health Care*, Pub. Lippincot.

GENERAL DIETARY PROBLEMS

1. Nausea and Vomiting

Almost 50% of the pregnant women show these signs of 'Morning Sickness', usually starting from 5th or 6th week of pregnancy and ending about the 16th week. The factors responsible for these are physiologic, hormonal changes and tension or anxiety. More frequent but smaller meals and snacks which are easily digested and provide energy too are recommended. Liquids are best taken between the meals, rather than with meals. In rare cases, prolonged nausea and vomiting develop into a serious condition known as *Hyperemesis gravidarum*, which calls for hospitalization and parenteral nutrition.

2. Constipation

Placental hormones relaxe the gastrointestinal muscles and pressure exerted by the enlarged uterus often lead to constipation. Herein, increased fluid intake, laxative diet with high fibre, fresh juice or dried fruits like figs and prunes and leafy vegetables are recommended. However, one must avoid the use of laxative pills in pregnant women as it become an addiction.

3. Weight Gain

An average weight gain during pregnancy is about 25-30 lb (11-14 kg). This is accounted for by fetus, placenta and maternal stores, as shown in Table 10.10.

TABLE 10.10: AVERAGE WEIGHT OF PRODUCTS OF NORMAL PREGNANCY

	Product	Weight	
		Grams	Pounds
1.	Fetus	3400	7.5
2.	Placenta	450	1.0
3.	Amniotic Fluid	900	2.0
4.	Uterus (Weight gain)	1100	2.5
5.	Breast Tissue (Wt. gain)	1400	3.0
6.	Blood Volume (Wt. gain)	1800	4.0 (1500 ml)
7.	Maternal Stores	1800	- 4-8
		3600	
	Total Gain	**11,000**	**11-13 kg or**
		13,000 g	**24-28 lb**

There is usually an average weight gain of 2-5 kg (1-2.3 kg) during the first trimester. Thereafter, it is usually 1 lb (0.5 kg) per week. Table 10.11 however, presents a more systematic and phased out weight gain during pregnancy.

TABLE 10.11: ANALYSIS OF WEIGHT GAIN DURING PREGNANCY

Components	Increase in Weight			
	Upto 10 weeks (g)	20 weeks (g)	30 weeks (g)	40 weeks (g)
Fetus, placenta and liquor	53	720	2530	4750
Uterus and breast	170	765	1170	1300
Blood	100	600	1300	1250
Extracellular water	—	—	—	1200
Fat (by difference)	325	1915	3500	4000
Total Weight Gain	**650**	**4000**	**8500**	**12,500**

Adapted from Hytten and Leitch, 1970.

4. Sodium

Sodium is the major mineral required for guarding against the extracellular fluid compartment, which is increased during pregnancy. Usually, 2-3 g sodium intake/day is recommended. Adequate amount of sodium and proteins are required to maintain the needed increase in circulating blood volume.

5. High Risk Mothers

Poor nutrition during pregnancy can lead to high risk and other unwanted complications later on. Hence, it is desirable to avoid these risk factors, as shown in Table 10.12. The adolescent pregnancy carries many social and nutritional risks. Nulligravidas , i.e. women never pregnant, 15 years old or younger girls are high risk cases, owing to their own incomplete growth. On the other hand, Primigravida (over 35 years of age), owing to hypertension, are also high risk pregnancies.

6. Anemia

Anemia in pregnant women is a global problem. Even in the USA, about 10% of all women in prenatal clinics are reported to have hemoglobin concentration of less than 10 g/dL and hematocrit reading below 32%. But this problem assumes gigantic proportions in Asia and Africa.

(a) Iron-deficiency Anemia

This is the most commonly reported anemia in pregnancy. The total iron stores requirement of a single normal pregnancy is 500-800 mg iron. Of this, 300 mg is used by the fetus alone. And the remainder iron is used in expanded maternal blood volume and the increased hemoglobin mass. Such anemias call for prolonged treatment with a therapeutic dose of 120 mg to 200 mg iron/day to be continued for 4-6 months after the anemia has been corrected. This is done to replenish the depleted iron reserves in the body.

TABLE 10.12: NUTRITIONAL RISK FACTORS IN PREGNANCY

Risk Factors at the Onset of Pregnancy	Risk Factors Occurring During Pregnancy
1. Age—15 years or younger 35 years or older	1. Low Hemoglobin and/or hematocrit Hb - less than 12.0 g Hematocrit less than 35.0 mg/dL
2. Frequent Pregnancies	2. Inadequate weight gain Any weight loss Wt. gain less than 2 lb/month after the first trimester
3. Poor Fetal performance	3. Excess Wt. gain More than I kg (2 lb)/week after the first trimester
4. Economic poverty	
5. Food Fads	
6. Alcohol/Drug abuse	
7. Inadequate Weight gain Less than 85% of standard weight More than 120% of standard weight	

(b) Folate-deficiency Anemia

Also called Megaloblastic anemia of pregnancy, it results on account of increased metabolic requirement of folic acid not being met in the body. The RDA for folic acid is stated to be 400 mg of folic acid per day.

(c) Hemorrhagic Anemia

Heavy blood loss occurs during labour and delivery stage. Blood transfusion and iron therapy is recommended to correct hemorrhagic anemia.

(d) Pregnancy-induced Hypertension (PIH)

Also called Toxaemia, pregnancy-induced hypertension is related to protein-deficiency in diet, which may also be poor in calcium and salts. It usually occurs in the 3rd trimester with symptoms of hypertension, excessive edema and albuminuria. In very severe cases (Eclampsia), it shows up in the form of convulsions or coma.

Optimal nutrition with adequate salts, vitamins and minerals are the corrections needed for maintaining the metabolic balance.

7. Diabetes Mellitus

It comes up due to pre-existing insulin deficiency. Routine screening helps detect the incidence of diabetes mellitus, which can, with adequate care and precaution, be brought under control.

8. Maternal Phenylketonuria (MPKU)

The incidence of Maternal Phenylketonuria is attributed to the missing enzyme (phenylalanin) for the metabolism of essential amino acids. However, MPKU responds to corrective diet containing low phenylalanine before conception.

NUTRITION DURING LACTATION

A healthy baby is a matter of deeper satisfaction, both biological and psychological. Hence, the first four to six months' breast feeding lays a very strong foundation for the good health of the new-born. This period of lactation is a great drain on the mother's body. As such, there is an increased need for some of the essential nutrients than that of the pregnancy period. Solid foods are added to the baby's diet at about six months of age. However, exclusive breast-feeding by well-nourished mothers can be adequate for periods ranging from 10-15 months.

Proteins

The average protein content of breast milk of an average Indian women is 1.22 g/dL. An increase of 20 g of proteins over the RDA for non-pregnant women is recommended. This would mean a total of protein allowance of 65 g/day for a lactating mother.

Energy (Calories)

Approximately 130 kcal are required for each 100 ml of milk produced by the nursing mother. Thus, lactation demands an additional 1000 kcal over the normal adult requirement of 2200 kcal. This is based on the fact that average milk production is 850 ml/day (30 oz). Human milk has a calorie range of 20-60 kcal/oz or an average of 24 kcal. That means 30 oz milk has an average value of 700 kcal. The metabolic work to produce this much daily milk requires about 400-450 kcal. Additional energy needed for lactation is drawn from maternal adipose tissue store deposited during the pregnancy.

Minerals

The amount of calcium and iron during lactation period remains the same as during pregnancy. The calcium needed earlier for mineralisation of fetal bones now gets diverted to production of milk. As iron is not a principal mineral component of milk, hence there is no need for increasing it in the diet.

Vitamins

An increase of 35 mg/d of ascorbic acid above the normal pregnancy requirement is recommended for the lactating mothers, *i.e.* a total of 95 mg of vitamin C per day. Besides vitamins A and B complex, especially riboflavin and niacin, involved as co-enzyme factors in energy metabolism, also need to be enhanced.

Fluids

The fluid intake of the lactating mother also needs to be increased. Herein, additional beverages as juice, milk, tea and coffee contribute both calories and fluids.

The ICMR recommends the norms for the lactating mother, as shown in Table 10.13.

As against this Indian menu, the diet chart in Table 11.14 depicts the diet chart for Western women.

Table 10.15 depicts the menu for a lactating women in Indian conditions.

TABLE 10.13: RDA FOR INDIAN LACTATING MOTHERS—ICMR

Nutrients	Unit	Lactating Mothers (0-6 mths) - 27 00 kcal	Lactating Mothers (7-12 mths) - 2600 kcal
Proteins	g/d	75	68
Fat	g/d	45	45
Calcium	mg/d	1000	1000
Iron	mg/d	30	30
Vitamin A-Retinol		950	950
-β-Carotene		3800	3800
Thiamine	mg/d	1.4	1.3
Riboflavin	mg/d	1.6	1.5
Nicotinic acid	mg/d	18	17
Pyridoxine	mg/d	2.5	2.5
Vitamin C	mg/d	80	80
Folic acid	µg/d	150	150
Vitamin B$_{12}$	µg/d	1.5	1.5

TABLE 10.14: DIET MENU FOR A LACTATING WOMEN

7.00 AM	Tea	1 cup
9.00 AM	Suji Porridge	1 bowl
	Boiled egg	1
	Banana/Orange	1
11.00 AM	Methi Laddoo	1 (Fenugreek sweet made with jaggery)
1.00 PM	Chapattis	2
	Rajma/Urad Dal	1 cup
	Methi leaves curry	1 cup
	Pulses	½ cup
	Rice	1 cup
	Curd	1 cup
4.00 PM	Tea	1 cup
	Sapota	1
	Potato Poha	1 cup
5.30 PM	Milk/Fruit shake	1 glass
7.00 PM	Chapattis	2
	Green gram Usal	1 cup
	Pumpkin -Gwar	
	Curry	1 cup
	Pulses	1 cup
	Rice	1 cup
	Egg	1
	Buttermilk	1 glass
9.00 PM	Hot Milk	1 glass

Source: S .A. Joshi in *Nutrition and Dietetics*.

One must not underestimate the intrinsic value or the nutritive quality of mother's milk, simply because it does not appear to be as rich or its consistency as thick as the cow's milk. More so from the immunological considerations, breast milk remains, by far, the best milk for the 'New-born'. This point stands duly vindicated by the fact that in the olden days, Indian mothers would go on breast feeding the baby up to 1-2 years of age. However, the contingencies of the modern age must not allow the discontinuance of breast feeding before six months of age.

TABLE 11.15: DIET CHART FOR WESTERN LACTATING MOTHERS

Breakfast	Orange juice
	Oatmeal/grit with Milk
	Poached egg on toast
	Coffee/Milk (if desired)
Mid-morning	Milk
Lunch	Vegetable soup
	Cottage cheese with fruit salad
	Biscuits with butter/margarine
	Milk/Coffee (if desired)
Afternoon	Fruit juice
Dinner	Green salad
	Baked ham
	Scalloped potato
	Green beans
	Bread with butter/margarine
	Sliced peaches
	Milk/Coffee (if desired)
Bedtime	Milk

Source: Mitchel et al. in Nutrition and Health Care, Pub. Lippincot.

DR. (MRS) JAIN SUPPLEMENT

A Naturopath's Strategy

The pregnant women, if they suffer from too much vomiting, must be kept solely on fruit diet. Table 11.16 gives the special Diet Chart for pregnant women and lays down instructions for the lactating mothers, as per Naturopathy principles.

TABLE 11.16: DR. USHA JAIN'S DIET CHART FOR PREGNANT WOMEN

7.00 AM	Curry leaves juice with lemon and honey	1 glass
	Tea made out of above in winter	—
8.00 AM	Fresh fruit juice/vegetable juice	1 glass
9.00 AM	Overnight soaked	
	Figs	2
	Almonds	5
	Dried Raisin	10
	Seasonal fruit salad	1 cup
	Milk—whole	1 glass
	Dalia/carrot/lauki kheer	1 cup
12.00 AM	Fruit salad	1 bowl
	Seasonal vegetables cooked	1 bowl
	Fortified chapattis	2-3 (25% bran admixture)
	Fortified amla chutney with coriander, ginger, onion and garlic	
	Soaked Ragi	1 tbsp
	Brown (unpolished) rice	1 tbsp
	Rice and ragi mixed together and made into a paste with almonds (5) and the seed liquor and all eaten together	
	*Special Seed Liquor	
	Seeds of cucumber, melon, watermelon and pumpkin	*Soak, grind and drain thru' sieve;
	It is an excellent Restorative for Anemia	Heat with ½ tsp ghee (oil) and one clove
		Decanted liquor boiled with one cup milk, sugar/honey. Take one cup of this liquor morning and evening.
4.00 PM	Milk with fresh fruits	1 glass
7.00 PM	Dalia (wheating)	1-2 cups
	Fresh fruit salad	1 bowl
	Coconut chutney	
	Raita (curd-vegetable admixture)	1 cup
9.00 PM	Special seed liquor (as above)	1 cup

Special Instructions for the Lactating Mothers

1. Add milk preparations with suji kheer, Carrot/ashgourd kheer or milk-dalia, 1-2 cups
2. Milk be given abundantly morning, evening and at night.
3. Asparagus powder, 1 tsp with milk is another very useful item.

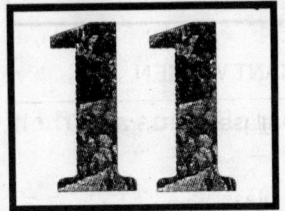

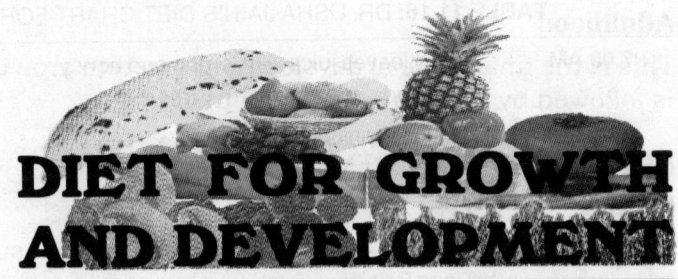

DIET FOR GROWTH AND DEVELOPMENT

NORMAL GROWTH PATTERN

The normal cycle of life follows four distinct stages of growth and development. These stages are

1. Infancy
2. Childhood
3. Adolescence
4. Adulthood

Infancy

This is the very first phase of rapid growth from day one to one year of infant's life, in which there is a slight tapering of rate of growth from 6 months to one year. At the age of 6 months, the infant would have doubled the birth weight and by the end of one year, it would have tripled.

Childhood

This is the intervening or latent period between infancy and adolescence, which is marked by a slackened and often erratic rate of growth. There is an occasional spurt in growth, followed by plateaus. At times, the child may have ravenous appetite, while on other occasions, he shows virtually no appetite.

Adolescence

This is the second period of rapid growth that begins with the onset of puberty. Accelerated by hormones, there is a multiplicity of body changes which include growth of long bones, development of sex characteristics and the growth of fat and muscle tissue.

Adulthood

This is the final stage of development wherein growth almost plateaus and then is followed by a gradual decline into old age.

NUTRITIONAL REQUIREMENTS FOR GROWTH

Infancy

This phase of super-fast growth calls for special support on the following five counts:

1. Energy
2. Protein
3. Water
4. Minerals and Vitamins
5. Milk

1. *Energy*

Since an infant grows rapidly in the first year, hence his energy needs are also very high. The FAO/WHO Committee had recommended the following schedule:

Energy Allowance for Infants	*kcal/kg*
0-3 months	120
3-5 months	115
6-8 months	110
9-11 months	105
Overall average during the first year	112 kcal/kg body weight.

The quantity of breast milk needed to meet these energy levels would be 850 ml up to first 3 months and 1200 ml between 3-6 months of age.

2. *Proteins*

Rapid growth in infancy demands higher intake of proteins. These have got to be simple, easily-digestible proteins foods (fluids). And this is ideally supplied by the breast milk. The ICMR recommends, like the FAO/WHO stipulations, the following protein allowance for the infants.

Age in months	Protein allowance/day
	(g/kg)
0 - 3	2.3 *
3 - 6	1.8 *
7 - 9	1.8 $
10 - 12	1.5 $

*—In terms of milk proteins only
$—Equal parts of milk proteins and vegetable protein supplements with relative NPU of 65.

Beyond six months, liquid or mashed foods and vegetables must be given to supplement the breast milk. In the case of working mothers, it is necessary to wean the child at 3-4 months age and put him on to special formula supplements and bottle feeding.

3. *Water*

Infant's relative need for water is greater than that of the adults. Infant's body content of water is from 70-75% of the total body weight. And most of this water is outside the cells and hence easily lost. Generally, an infant drinks an amount of water equivalent to 10-15% of body weight.

The approximate daily fluid needs are shown hereunder:

0-3 months	120 ml/kg
4-6 months	115 ml/kg
7-12 months	100 ml/kg.

4. *Minerals and Vitamins*

Rapidly growing young bones require calcium and phosphorus. Calcium is also needed for teeth formation, muscle contraction, blood coagulation and heart muscle action. Iron is needed for hemoglobin formation. These must be given as drops initially, but later on, these could be mixed with milk or fruit juice. Enriched cereals and egg yolk also serve the needful.

Iron requirement for infants is 1.0 mg/kg.

The calcium content of the breast milk of Indian mothers varies from 30 mg to 40 mg/100 ml. That way, up to 6 months age, calcium intake of about 300 mg per day would be adequate.

FAO/WHO expert group has categorically recommended a daily allowance of vitamin A 400 mg retinol up to 6 months age. Vitamin D, in doses of 100 IU, has been found to prevent rickets and promote normal mineralisation of bones.

Table 11.1 depicts the recommended dietary allowance for different age groups, till the age of 3 years.

5. *Breast Milk*

To counter the vested propaganda of the multinationals, one must take into account the strong plus points of the mother's milk for the healthy growth of an infant. These scoring points are

1. Breast milk provides the best mix of all the essential nutrients needed by a growing infant.
2. The protein level being lower than cow's milk, it results in very soft flocculi of curd that permit easy digestibility.
3. It contains higher amount of disachharide, lactose, which helps keep low electrolyte concentration.

TABLE 11.1: RECOMMENDED ALLOWANCES FOR CHILDREN, BIRTH TO AGE 3 YEARS

Nutrient	Age (years)		
	0.0-0.5	0.5-1.0	1-3
Energy	kg × 108	kg × 98	kg × 102
Protein (g)	kg × 2.2	kg × 1.6	kg × 1.2
Vitamin A (μg RE) †	375	375	400
Vitamin D (μg) ‡	7.5	10	10
Vitamin E (mg) §	3	4	6
Vitamin K (μg)	5	10	15
Vitamin C (mg)	30	35	40
Thiamine (mg)	0.3	0.4	0.7
Riboflavin (mg)	0.4	0.5	0.8
Niacin (mg NE)"	5	6	9
Vitamin B_6 (mg)	0.3	0.6	1.0
Folacin (μg)	25	35	50
Vitamin B_{12} (μg)	0.3	0.5	0.7
Calcium (mg)	400	600	800
Phosphorus (mg)	300	500	800
Magnesium (mg)	40	60	80
Iron (mg)	6	10	10
Zinc (mg)	5	5	10
Iodine (μg)	40	50	70
Selenium (μg)	10	15	20

† RE = Retinol equivalents; 1 RE = 1 μg Retinol or 6 μg β-Carotene.
‡ As Cholecalciferol; 10 μg Cholecalciferol = 400 IU of Vitamin D.
§ α-Tocopherol equivalents; 1 mg d, α-tocopherol = 1 α-TE
" NE = Niacin equivalent.
Source: Food and Nutrition Board, National Academy of Sciences, *Recommended Daily Dietary Allowances*, revised 1980 (Washington, DC.: National Acedemy Presss, 1980).

4. The fat in the breast milk contains higher levels of PUFA—linolenic acid and α-linolenic acid, both being very good for the infants.
5. Vitamins, both fat-soluble and water soluble, are found in good amount in mother's milk.
6. Breast milk contains antibodies that provide protection against many infections, especially *E. coli*. Other anti-infective agents are lactoferrin, phagocytes, lysozyme, lactoperoxidase and the bifdus factor.
7. Breast milk possesses anti-allergic properties.
8. Breast milk has got specific immunological factors like lymphocytes, which help in the production of Immunoglobulin A (IgA).
9. Breast feeding builds up strong emotional ties between the baby and the mother.

The appendix 1 at the end of this Chapter gives the relative composition of different milks, as compared to the mother's milk.

Supplementary Feeding

Usually, around 6 months of infant's age, some supplementation must be done so that the infant starts getting other important supplementary nutrients. It is done in three stages:

1. Liquid supplements
2. Solid supplements, mashed well before feeding
3. Solid supplements, Lumpy or chopped solids.

Liquid Supplements

Liquid supplements include juice of fresh fruits like orange, grapes, sweet lemon, and tomatoes. To begin with at 6 months of age, juice should be diluted with equal amount of clean boiled water. It should be given a few teaspoonfuls. This amount should be gradually increased, till in a few weeks time, he gets about half a tumbler of orange juice or ¾ tumbler of fresh tomato juice. In case juice is not available, soup of green leafy vegetables can be given. Fish liver oil is also recommended at this stage. Starting with a few drops, it can be gradually increased up to 1 tsp per day.

Solid Supplements

From 7-8th month onwards, supplementation is done with mashed vegetables like potatoes. If cereals are to be given, these should better be mixed with milk and sugar in the form of a gruel. By the end of the first year, a child should be getting 2-4 tsp of cereal or starchy vegetables and 1-3 tsp of mashed green vegetables. A spoonful of ripe mashed banana is an ideal supplement for the weaker sections of the society.

Since eggs contain very valuable protective and blood-forming nutrients, it is advisable to start with egg yolk, say one quarter of an egg. it could be gradually increased to full one egg yolk. Later, by the age of one year, he can be given soft-boiled or poached egg. Minced meat or boiled fish or mashed pulses with little salt can be given later on. The pulses and meat preparation could be given on alternate days.

When the baby starts cutting teeth, he should be given some chopped and lumpy foods and after one year age, he should start getting soft boiled leafy vegetables. A piece of biscuit or toast will serve to exercise his gums and make the teeth stronger. A slice of carrot and fresh fruits will also do the needful.

Table 11.2 shows feed-supplementation for different age groups.

TABLE 11.2: FOOD SUPPLEMENTS FOR THE INFANTS

Foodstuffs	Age When to Introduce	Quantity per Feeding	Special Instructions
1. Fruit juice and soups with a dash of tomato, spinach, carrots, onions and rice	Five months	1-2 tsp twice a day	Increase quantity gradually Soups may be seasoned
2. Seasonal mashed fruits—banana, apple, sapota with cream; stewed papaya	Five months	1 - 2 tsp twice a day	Avoid sour fruits
3. Suji porridge/dalia i.e. wheating, with cereals like ragi, sago, rice powder and custard	Within a week of starting fruits	1-3 tsp twice a day	Increase quantity gradually
4. Half-boiled egg	Within a week of starting porridge	One tsp Egg yolk	Increase quantity gradually, giving one full egg within a month
5. Cooked, mashed vegetables	One week after starting egg	1 - 2 tsp twice a day	Green and leafy vegetables—carrots, potato, pumpkin, green peas, etc.
6. Yoghurt (Curds)	One week after starting vegetables	3 - 4 tsp	Avoid sour curds
7. Cooked rice, pulses and khichdi (rice-pulses mix) and upma	One week after starting curds	2 - 4 tsp	A dash of butter and seasoning permitted

N.B. These figures pertain to well-developed, above-average children.

CHILDHOOD (1-12 years)

Childhood may be divided into three phases:

(*i*) Toddlers, 1-3 years
(*ii*) Preschool, 3-6 years
(*iii*) School age, 6-12 years

(A) Toddlers (1-3 years)

This phase of relatively slow but steady growth follows faster growth period of infancy. It witnesses firm changes in the anatomy of the child. The bone development and muscle formation are the two special features of development in childhood. The legs become longer and there is a progressive depletion of the body fat.

There is a shift in water balance, more water is found in the cells and less body water outside the cells.

The muscle development is steady, since this accounts for nearly one-half of the total gain in body weight in this period. Prominent among the muscles to develop are the big muscles in the back, buttocks and thighs. There is significant skeletal growth, with more mineral deposition, rather than lengthening of the bones. This helps strengthen the bones to enable them to support the growing body weight. From 6-8 teeth at the beginning of the toddler stage, it goes up to full set of deciduous ('Baby') teeth by three years of age.

1. Energy Requirements

The relative slackening in growth rate means not-so-high demand for calories, as is the case in the first year of growth. The child needs about 1000 Kcal every day, which gradually goes up to 1300-1500 kcal by the age of three. Even the eating habits of the child become bit erratic during this stage. The basal metabolism of the children is higher than that of adults. The energy requirement is met mainly through increase in cereals and carbohydrates, so that proteins are spared for more vital tissue building jobs. A moderate amount of fat, preferably avoiding animal fats, should supplement the dietary schedule during childhood. As per FAO/WHO, and also the ICMR recommendations, the energy requirement of children are given in Table 11.3

TABLE 11.3: ENERGY ALLOWANCE FOR CHILDREN

Age Group	RDA for Body Weight (Kg approx.)	Total Allowance (kcal)
A: Childhood		
1 - 3 years	12	1220
4 - 6 years	19	1720
7 - 9 years	26	2050
B: Boys		
10 - 12 years	34	2420
13 - 15 years	47	2660
16 -18 years	56.5	2820
C: Girls		
10 - 12 years	36.5	2260
13 -15 years	45.5	2300
16 -18 years	50	2200

N.B.: These figures pertain to well developed, above average children.

2. Proteins

There is a relatively greater need for proteins during childhood. It should be 1-1.2 g/kg of body weight. At least half of these proteins should be of animal origin, since they have higher biologic value. As the body needs full range of essential amino acids, there should be a judicious blend of different protein foods in the child's diet. Table 11.4 gives a very elborate RDA for children.

TABLE 11.4 RDAs FOR CHILDREN (1980)

Specification	Age, years		
	1-3	4-6	7-10
Weight (kg)	13	20	28
(lb)	29	44	62
Height (cm)	90	112	132
(in)	35	44	52
Nutrients			
Energy (Calories)	1300	1700	2400
Protein (gm)	23	30	34
Vitamin A (RE)	400	500	700
Vitamin D (µg)	10	10	10
Vitamin E (mg α TE)	5	6	7
Vitamin C (mg)	45	45	45
Thiamin (mg)	0.7	0.9	1.2
Riboflavin (mg)	0.8	1.0	1.4
Niacin (mg NE)	9	11	16
Pyridoxine (mg)	0.9	1.3	1.6
Folacin (µg)	100	200	300
VitaminB12 (µg)	2.0	2.5	3.0
Calcium (mg)	800	800	800
Phosphorus (mg)	800	800	800
Magnesium (mg)	150	200	250
Iron (mg)	15	10	10
Zinc (mg)	10	10	10
Iodine (µg)	70	90	120

Source: Food and Nutrition Board, National Academy of Sciences, *Recommended Daily Dietary Allowances*, revised 1980 (Washington, DC.: National Acedemy Presss, 1980).

Computing the children's requirement by the factorial method and based upon the studies made by WHO/FAO, the ICMR has stipulated the following RDA for proteins for the children of different age groups, belonging to the fairly well-off sections in Table 11.5.

3. *Minerals*

Calcium and phosphorus are needed for bone mineralisation. Adequate supply of minerals helps strengthen the bones to keep pace with muscle development.

The RDA for calcium is 400-500 mg/day and that of iron is 0.65 mg/day. Table 11.6 depicts the dietary intake of calcium and iron for different age groups, as recommended by the ICMR.

TABLE 11. 5: RDA FOR PROTEINS FOR INDIAN CHILDREN (ICMR)

Age group	Body weight (Approx. kg)	R D A (g/kg/day)	Total allowance (g/day)
A: Children			
1-3 years	12	1.83	22
4-6 years	19	1.56	29
7-9 years	26	1.35	36
B: Boys			
10-12 years	34	1.24	43
13-15 years	47	1.10	52
11-18 years	56.50	0.94	53
C: Girls			
10-12 years	36.5	1.17	43
13-15 years	45.5	0.95	43
16-18 years	50	0.88	44

N.B. In terms of Mixed Vegetable Proteins of NPU.

For a young child, 2-3 cups of milk are sufficient, but these must be supplemented with cooked or mashed cereals. Excluding solid foods and depending solely on milk deprives the child of minerals and it may lead to a condition—'Milk Anemia'. Table 11.6 gives the RDA for calcium for different age groups.

TABLE 11.6: RDA FOR CALCIUM AND IRON

Age group	Dietary intake (mg/day)	
	Iron	Calcium
Infants	1.0 mg/kg BW	500-600
Children		
1-9 years	20-25	400-500
10-15 years	20-25	600-700
Adolescents		
Boys	25	500-600
Girls	35	500-600

Table 11.7 gives the diet chart for the younger children.

(B) Pre-school Children (3–6 years)

The physical growth in this age group takes place in spurts. Their protein requirements is very high—24 g/day of high quality proteins from milk, eggs, meat and cheese. Calcium and iron is needed for reserve storage. Fresh fruits and vegetables supply the necessary vitamins A and C needed for optimum growth. Cereal supplementation helps improve the quality of diet for the vegetarians. Table 11.8 depicts the important food stuffs in a vegetarian diet for the pre-schhol children.

TABLE 11.7: DIET CHART FOR CHILDREN (2-5 YEARS)

Breakfast	Bread slices	2 large pcs
	Porridge	50 g
	Milk	200 ml-1 glass
	Sugar	2 tsp
	Butter	1 tsp
Mid-morning	Fruit	1 medium
Lunch	Rice	50 g
	Chapattis	2 medium
	Dal (Pulses)	½ bowl
	Curd	½ bowl
	Vegetables	½ bowl
Afternoon	Milk	200 ml
	Sugar	2 tsp
	Roasted gram/Biscuits/	
	Sandwich	
Dinner	Rice	50 g
	Chapattis	2 medium
	Curd/Pulses	½ bowl
	Vegetables	½ bowl or
	Salad	75 g
	Cooking Fat	1 tsp
Bedtime	Milk with sugar	200 ml

The above diet for the children supplies the following nutrients:

Carbohydrates	192 g
Proteins	30 g
Fats	27 g
Calories	1130

Source: Rekha Sharma in Diet Management.

TABLE 11.8: USEFUL SOURCES OF NUTRIENTS FOR PRE-SCHOOL CHILDREN
ON A VEGETARIAN DIET

Nutrient	Sources
Proteins	Soya protein, pulses, baked beans, grains, seeds, soya cheese, groundnuts
Calcium	Fortified soya milk, fortified soya desserts and soya yoghurts, tofu, seeds, green leafy vegetables, nuts, bread, dried fruit
Iron	Fortified breakfast cereals, bread, pulses, green vegetables, dried fruits, nuts, plain chocolate, raisins, curry powder
Zinc	Tofu, fortified cereals, groundnuts, beans and lentils, wholemeal bread, plain popcorn, sesame seeds and tahini
Vitamin B_{12}	Fortified soya milk, some margarines, textured vegetable protein products
Vitamin D	Fortified margarine, fortified soya milk, fortified breakfast cereals, sunshine
Vitamin A	Yellow or orange vegetables (e.g. carrots), sweet potato, yellow or orange fruit (e.g. mangoes and apricots), fortified margarine, red peppers

(C) School-age Children (6-12 years)

The 6-12 years age group is the latent period of growth. It is the proverbial *'Lull before the Storm'*, *i.e.* adolescent stage. Herein, the growth rates vary. It is comparatively faster growth period in the girls.

ADOLESCENCE (12-18 years)

It is the age of Puberty, when the final spurt in growth takes place. These profound body changes result from hormones regulating the development of sex characteristics. In the girls, the amount of subcutaneous fat deposit increases, more so in the abdominal region. The hip breadth increases and the bony pelvis widens considerably in preparation for the reproductive phase that follows later. A pelvic girth of subcutaneous fat results, which sometimes causes anxiety.

In the boys, there is increased muscle mass and growth of long bones, although its growth rate is slower than that of girls. The total period of adolescent growth seldom lasts for more than 2-3 years, when the adult build and stature is reached. However, growth in skeletal muscle mass continues. A further *'lengthening out'* may occur in males and females up to the age of 30 years.

Nutritional Requirements of Adolescents

The stage of adolescence demands more energy, proteins, vitamins and minerals. The girls need 1800-2500 kcal energy per day, as against boys' requirement of

2500-3500 kcal/day. In addition to calcium, proteins and calories, girls also need an iron supplement when menses begins. This higher energy demand often leads to greater consumption of snack-foods, which are usually high in sugar and fat but low in proteins. The protein requirement during puberty is very high, up to 45-55 g per day. Table 11.9 gives the recommended diet allowance for different age groups of adolescents.

TABLE 11.9: RDAs FOR ADOLESCENTS (1980)

Food	11-14 years		15-18 years		19-24 years	
	M	F	M	F	M	F
Energy (Calories)	2700	2200	2800	2100	2900	2100
(MJ)	11.3	9.2	11.8	8.8	12.2	8.8
Protein (gm)	45	46	56	46	56	44
Vitamin A (RE)	1000	800	1000	800	1000	800
Vitamin D (μg)	10	10	10	10	7.5	7.5
Vitamin E (mg α TE)	8	8	10	8	10	8
Vitamin C (mg)	50	50	60	60	60	60
Folacin (μg)	400	400	400	400	400	400
Niacin (mg NE)	18	15	18	14	19	14
Riboflavin (mg)	1.6	1.3	1.7	1.3	1.7	1.3
Thiamine (mg)	1.4	1.1	1.4	1.1	1.5	1.1
Vitamin B_6 (mg)	1.8	1.8	2.0	2.0	2.2	2.0
Vitamin B_{12} (mg)	3.0	3.0	3.0	3.0	3.0	3.0
Calcium (mg)	1200	1200	1200	1200	800	800
Phosphorus (mg)	1200	1200	1200	1200	800	800
Iodine (μg)	150	150	150	150	150	150
Iron (mg)	18	18	18	18	10	18
Magnesium (mg)	350	300	400	300	350	300
Zinc (mg)	15	15	15	15	15	15

Source: Food and Nutrition Board, National Academy of Sciences, *Recommended Daily Dietary Allowances*, revised 1980 (Washington, DC.: National Acedemy Press, 1980).

The boys show great appetite for food during adolescence. Because of physiologic sex differences in girls associated with fat deposits during puberty, they gain more weight, a factor which unwittingly makes many of them to go for semi-starvation diet in order to maintain good form.

The diet regime for adolescent boys and girls is given in Table 11.10

TABLE 11.10: DIET PLAN FOR ADOLESCENTS (16-18 YEAR)

Breakfast	Bread toast with butter	3 slices
	Poached egg	1
	Fruit milk shake	1 glass
Lunch	Potato paratha	2
	Cucumber salad	½ cup
	Rajma (broad beans)/	
	urad (black gram) dal	1 cup
	Rice	1 cup
	Buttermilk	1 glass
Afternoon	Milk	1 cup
	Suji laddoo (sweets)	1
	Banana	1
Dinner	Chapattis	2
	Mixed vegetable curry	1 cup
	Rice	1 cup
	Spinach with pulses	1 cup
	Curd	½ cup
Bedtime	Milk with Protinules (A pro-prietary protein supplement	1 glass

Source: S. A, Joshi in *Nutritution and Dietetics.*

Appendix 2 gives the dietary intake for different age groups as recommended by ICMR.

Composition of Various Milks

Milk	Calories (kcal)	Proteins (g)	Fat (g)	Carbohydrates (g)	Calcium (mg)
Human milk	71	1.2	3.8	7.0	33
Cow's milk	69	3.3	3.7	4.8	125
Buffalo milk	102	3.8	7.5	4.4	200
Sheep's milk	108	5.6	7.5	4.4	200
Goat's milk	71	3.3	4.5	4.4	130

Source: Nutrition for Mother and Child, ICMR Special Report No. 41, National Institute of Nutrition, Hyderabad.

When breast milk is not available or the quantity available daily is not enough or the mother is ill, then the infant needs to be fed artificially.

Cow's milk is the most common food item for artificial feeding. It is rich in most of the body building principles, as compared to the breast milk, as shown in the tabulation above. Hence, cow's milk needs to be suitably diluted with clean boiled water in order to bring its composition as near to the natural milk as possible. Since breast milk is more sweet, hence some sugar must be added to cow's milk when it is to be given to the infants.

The ICMR recommends the following dilution of cow's milk:

First Week   2 parts boiled water to 1 part cow's milk + sugar 1 tsp

As the infant grows, gradually reduce the amount of water, but keep on increasing the quantity of sugar so that by the age of six months, the infant gets:

Cow's milk, Whole—no dilution and
Sugar about 4 tsp per day.

As regards the frequency of feeling, it should be 3-4 feeds per day in the first few days. Till the end of the first month, it goes up to 6 feeds per day. Subsequently, the feeding schedule be reduced to five till about six months age.

Appendix 2 gives milk modification practices followed in UK. For the Western countries, the following weaning plan has been recommended.

EXAMPLE OF A WESTERN WEANING PLAN (0-6 MONTHS)

Age	Solids/drinks to introduce	6.00 am	10.00 am	2.00 pm	6.00 pm	10.00 pm
4 months	1-2 teaspoons of pureed baby food	✔	✔ ●	✔	✔	✔
4½ months	3-4 teaspoons of pureed baby food	✔	✔ ●	✔	✔ ●	✔
5 months	6 teaspoons of pureed baby food	✔	✔ ●	✔ ●	✔ ●	✔

		8.00 am	12.00 pm	5.00 pm	9.00 pm	
5½ months	3-4 tablespoons of pureed baby foods	✔ ●	✔ ●	✔ ●	✔	
6 months	5-6 tablespoons of mashed baby food	✔ ●	✔ ●	✔ ●	✔	

✔ = infant feeds (breast or formula)
● = solids

Since the children in the developing countries are beset with many socio-economic problems, ICMR has given a very comprehensive RDA for different age groups or sex, as shown in Appendix 3.

Modification of Cow's Milk to Infant Formula (UK)

Nutrients	Cow's milk	Whey-based infant formula	Casein-based infant formula
Protein			
Quantity	High	Lowered	Lowered
	3.3 g/100 ml	1.4–1.9 g/100 ml	1.4–1.9 g/100 ml
Type	80% casein	40% casein	80% casein
	20% whey	60% whey	60% whey
Carbohydrate			
Quantity	Low	Increased	Increased
	4.9 g/100 ml	7.0–8.6 g/100 ml	7.0–8.6 g/100 ml
Type	Lactose	Usually all lactose	Usually all lactose, but ocassionally other carbohydrates added
Fat			
Quantity	3.6 g/100 ml	2.6–3.8 g/100 ml	2.6–3.8 g/100 ml
Type	High in butter milk	Vegetable oils and other fats replace buttermilk. Correct quantity and ratio of essential fatty acids added. Some formulae have very long chain fatty acids added	Vegetable oils and other fats replace buttermilk. Correct quantity and ratio of essential fatty acids added
Minerals			
Quantity	High in phosphorus, sodium, Potassium and calcium	Minerals reduced	Minerals reduced
Sodium	3.3 mmol/100 ml	0.65–1.1 mmol/100 ml	0.65–1.1 mmol/100 ml
Calcium	3.0 mmol/100 ml	0.88–2.1 mmol/100 ml	0.88–2.1 mmol/100 ml
Phosphorus	3.2 mmol/100 ml	0.9–1.8 mmol/100 ml	0.9–1.8 mmol/100 ml
Vitamins and Trace Elements	Low in iron, zinc, copper, vitamins C, D, and folic acid	A range of added vitamins and minerals to meet nutritional requirements	A range of added vitamins and minerals to meet nutritional requirements

Source: *Nutriition and Child Health* by Holden, MacDonald and Wharton, Pub: Bailliere Tindall.

Appendix 3

Recommended Dietary Intakes of Nutrients for Indians (revised in 1981)

Group	Particulars	Net calories (kcal)	Protein (g)	Calcium (g)	Iron (mg)	Rational (µg)	or β-carotene (µg)	Thiamine (mg)	Riboflavin (mg)	Nicotinic acid (mg)	Vitamin B6 (mg)	Ascorbic acid (mg)	Folic acid (µg)	Vitamin B12 (µg)	Vitamin D (I.U.)
Women	Sedentary work	1900	45	0.4–0.5	32	750	3000	1.0	1.1	13	2.0	40	100	1	
	Moderate work	2200	45			750	3000	1.1	1.3	15					
	Heavy work	3000	45					1.5	1.8	20					
	Pregnancy (second half of pregnancy)	+300	+14	1.0	40	750	3000	+0.2	+0.2	+2	2.5	40	300	1.5	
	Lactation 06-months	+550	+25	1.0	32	1150	4600	+0.3	+0.3	+4	2.5	80	150	1.5	
	6-12 months	+400	+25					+0.2	+0.2	+3					
Infants	0-6 months	118/kg	2.0/kg	0.5–0.6	1.0 mg/kg	400	—	59µg/kg	71µg/kg	780µg/kg	0.3	20	25	0.2	
	6-12 months	108/kg	1.7/kg			300	1200	54µg/kg	65µg/kg	710µg/kg	0.4				
Children	1-3 years	1220	22.0	0.4–0.5	20-25	250	1000	0.6	0.7	8	0.6	20	25	0.2	
	4-6 years	1720	29.4			300	1200	0.9	1.0	11	0.9				
	7-9 years	2050	35.6			400	1600	1.0	1.2	14	1.2				
Boys	10-12 years	2420	42.5	0.4–0.5	25-30	600	2400	1.2	1.5	16	1.6	40	100	0.2	200
Girls	– do –	2260	42.1					1.1	1.4	15				–1.0	
Boys	13-15 years	2660	51.7	0.6–0.7	25	750	3000	1.3	1.6	18	20				
Girls	– do –	2360	43.3		35			1.2	1.4	15					
Boys	16-18 years	2820	53.1	0.5–0.6	25	750	3000	1.4	1.7	19	2.0				
Girls	– do –	2200	44.0		5			1.1	1.3	15					

Source: Recommended Dietary Intake for Indians, ICMR, Government of India, New Delhi.

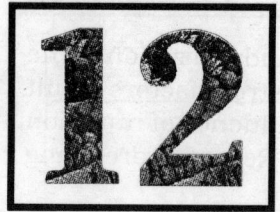

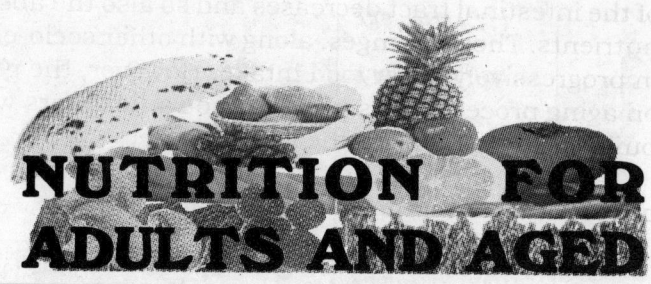

NUTRITION FOR ADULTS AND AGED

In a man's life, adulthood and aging are the last phase of development. In one sense, aging is a positive phenomenon that starts from day one and ends at death, i.e. it encompasses whole of his life and is not merely restricted to the end years, as is commonly believed. Physiologically speaking, aging is a multifactorial process which is the ultimate consequence of several metabolic interactions.

Adulthood may be divided into 3 stages:

1. Young adulthood — 8 to 40 years
2. Middle adulthood — 40 to 60 years
3. Old adulthood — 60 to 80 years onwards

BIOLOGICAL CHANGES

There is a progressive decline in the physiologic functioning of the body as the man advances in years. There is a gradual but steady loss of cells and reduction in metabolic processes which means the performance capacity of his systems goes on steadily deteriorating.

This decline varies in different systems in different persons. However, in general, the body mass becomes leaner. By 65-70 years of age, the kidneys and lungs lose about 10% of their weight. This loss goes up to 18% in case of liver, while the skeletal muscles diminish by approximately 40%. And the bone mass loses as much as 25%.

All this creeping decline results in overall reduction in the body's reserves. An important feature of this aging process is the reduced rate of blood flow through the kidneys, to the extent of 65%. The blood sugar level takes longer time to return to the normal level. But the major role player in aging is the gastrointestinal system. The secretion of digestive juices goes down, the motility of the intestinal tract decreases and so also the absorption and utilization of the nutrients. These changes, along with other socio-economic stress factors result in progressively lower food intake. However, the greatest influence of nutrition on aging process takes place in the earlier years when the 'Reserves' are being built up in the body for the later day life.

Table 12.1 categorically lists the geriatric physio-pathological changes concomitant with the advancing years.

TABLE 12.1: PHYSIO-PATHOLOIGCAL CHANGES DUE TO AGING

	System	Functional changes
1.	Cells and Tissues	Overall shrinking, atrophy and regressive changes manifesting as fibrosis and sclerosis
2.	Skeletal System	Bone loss and decalcification of bones, stiffening of joints, calcification of ligaments and reduced collagen elasticity and osmotic swelling ability
3.	Digestive System	Reduced stomach motility resulting in weakening of peristalsis leading to digestive disorders and intestinal upsets and onset of gastritis
4.	Respiratory System	Overall decrease in lungs and vital capacity, probability of calcification of cartilages and emphysema
5.	Cardiovascular System	Hypertension, coronary sclerosis, irregular heart beats (arhythmia) and decline in heart output
6.	Genito-urinary System	Reduced blood flow in kidneys leading to reduced filtration rate, reduced blood flow in kidneys and water and electrolyte imbalance
7.	Nervous System	Psychiatric problems, break down of brain tissues, insomnia and loss of memory
8.	Senses	Loss of sensitivity to touch, pain, odor, taste and reflex action

NUTRITIONAL REQUIREMENTS

Energy

The reduced metabolic rate caused by deterioration in cell functioning and reduced activity means relatively lesser demand for energy as the age advances. Many nutritionists recommend lesser amount of rich diet—'Under-nutrition without Malnutrition' would help prolong life. The metabolic activity decreases considerably in the middle and later years. Thus, after the age of 30, the calorie requirement diminishes by 7.5% for every 10 years of life. As such, the RDA for energy is 2200 kcal for men and 1900 kcal for women.

Table 12.2 shows the FAO/WHO Committee recommendations for energy for adults and the aged men and women.

Carbohydrates

It is generally recommended that 50-55% of the total kilocalories in the diet must be supplied through carbohydrates, mostly starches. The fasting blood sugar level is a normal feature in the aged. It is essential that their diet contains large amount of soft fibre food which helps maintain the intestinal activity and prevents constipation.

TABLE 12.2: ENERGY REQUIREMENT OF MODERATELY ACTIVE ADULTS

Age in years	Men (55 kg) (kcal)	Women (45 kg) (kcal)	Percentage of reference
40 - 49	2660	2090	95
50 - 59	2520	1980	90
60 - 69	2240	1760	80
70 - 80	1960	1540	70

Impaired glucose tolerance, in association with a delayed insulin response, is a fairly common occurrence in elderly people, specially women. In such cases, total amount of carbohydrates, especially sugars must be curtailed.

Fats

Fats should contribute about 10-15% of the total calorie intake. Serum cholesterol levels increase considerably after the age of fifty. Hence, an old man must avoid rich foods with high cholesterol like egg yolk, whole milk and organ meat. Excess fat must be avoided because of delayed absorption capacity of the elderly people. Fats with higher polyunsaturated fatty acids (PUFA) are to be preferred.

Proteins

The RDA for proteins in older adults is 0.8 g/kg body weight. There is a reduction of about 30% in protein requirement. It is desirable that protein level is brought down to 15-20% of the total calorie requirement.

However, the elderly people, suffering from gastrointestinal infections or others that affect the metabolism, need to consume more protein to sustain themselves. Preferably, 20-25% of these proteins must come from the animal sources.

Vitamins and Minerals

Recent advances in research indicate that antioxidants vitamins like A, E, C and β-carotenes can delay the aging process. They also prevent degeneration in blood vessels, heart, joints and eye lens.

Special attention must be paid to vitamin D, since the decalcification is a common phenomenon in old age. Fat-soluble vitamins A and D need to be provided extra in old age. So also is the case with B group vitamins like thiamine, pyridoxine, cyanocobalamine and folic acid, which quota must be enhanced.

Usually, minerals are not needed in the normal aging process. The RDA for calcium is 800 mg/day. But in case of osteoporosis, this intake must be increased to 1200 mg/day for women over 50 years of age. Calcium is also important for the maintenance of teeth. Iron is essential for the formation of hemoglobin in the blood. Since the amount of iron absorbed from food is very small (*i.e.* 2.5%), hence it becomes necessary to have 20-30 mg iron per day.

Water

Elderly people may suffer from 'Xerostomia'—dry mouth caused by severe reduction in the flow of saliva, which, in turn, affects their food intake. As such, adequate fluid consumption must be ensured. Decreased fluids also result in lower urine output and constipation.

Table 12.3 gives the sex wise RDA for the aged people.

TABLE 12.3: RECOMMENDED DIETARY ALLOWANCES FOR PERSONS AGE 51 YEARS AND OLDER

	Men	Women
Energy (kcal)	2300.0	1900.0
Protein (g)	63.0	50.0
Vitamin A (µg RE)	1000.0	800.0
Vitamin D (µg)	5.0	5.0
Vitamin E (mg a-TE)	10.0	8.0
Vitamin K (µg)	80.0	65.0
Thiamin (mg)	1.2	1.4
Riboflavin (mg)	1.4	1.2
Niacin (mg NE)	15.0	13.0
Vitamin B_6 (mg)	2.0	1.0
Folate (µg)	200.0	180.0
Viamin B_{12} (µg)	2.0	2.0
Biotin (µg)	30-100	30-100
Pantothenic acid (mg)	4-7	4-7

Since minerals play a very important role in preventing many age-related diseases, Table 12.4 gives an elaborate list of RDA for minerals and trace elements in the aged.

HYPOTHESES ABOUT AGING

Although the causes of aging remain a mystery, many hypotheses have been offered to explain this biologic process. These are:

1. Errors occur in copying the genetic blueprint
2. Connective tissue stiffness
3. Toxic products build up in the system
4. Electron-seeking compounds damage cell parts
5. Hormone function changes
6. Immune system loses efficiency
7. Auto-immunity develops

8. Death is programmed into the cell
9. Glycoylation of proteins, *i.e.* chronically elevated blood glucose attaches to various blood and body proteins.

TABLE 12.4: RDA FOR MINERALS OR TRACE ELEMENTS FOR THE AGED

Minerals	Men	Women
Macro Elements		
Calcium (mg)	800	800
Phosphorus (mg)	800	800
Magnesium (mg)	350	280
Iron (mg)	10	10
Zinc (mg)	15	12
Iodine (µg)	150	150
Selenium (µg)	70	55
Trace Elements		
Copper (mg)	1.5-3.0	1.5-3.0
Manganese (mg)	2.0-5.0	2.0-5.0
Flouride (mg)	1.5-4.0	1.5-4.0
Chromium (µg)	50-200	50-200
Molybdenum (µg)	75-250	75-250

Source: Adopted from NRC and NAS, 1989 Reports.

Most likely, aging results from interaction of these events and changes. Because cell aging and diseases like cancer are aggravated by environmental factors, it makes good sense to avoid such risks like exposure to excessive sunlight and hazardous chemicals. That way, a man can have some control over how quickly he ages.

THE AGING SYNDROME

Dr. Ronald R. Watson, in his book: Handbook of Nutrition in the Aged has highlighted the latest research findings in the aging syndrome. These are mentioned below:

1. System Breakdown

Aging can be characterised by a breakdown and loss of coordination between several physiological systems, including endocrine and immune system, all of which lead to dysfunction in cells and organs and the progressive loss of adaptability of the organism.

2. Weight Loss

Weight loss and malnutrition have invariably been cited as common problems in the aged and are associated with adverse health outcome, such as infections, poor wound healing and increased mortality.

3. Lean Body Mass

The body mass slowly declines at a rate of about 0.3 kg/ year, beginning with the third decade. Much of this decline is attributed to the decreased skeletal muscle mass, loss of bone mass and decreased organ size associated with aging.

4. Fat-free Body Mass

A decrease in 'Fat-free Body Mass' (FFM) occurs with age, both in men and women. This transpires as a result of loss of muscle, bone, viscera and skin. The loss of these tissues is accompanied by progressive loss of body water, minerals and proteins. In as much as it contains the body's protein reserves, muscle and Body Cell Mass (BCM), the FFM represents an important correlate of nutrition, functional status and health.

5. Bone Loss

The bone loss is a hallmark of aging. A decline in bone mineral mass and its density occurs in both men and women. This bone loss is attributed to the decline in FFM and when it becomes excessive, leads to osteoporosis, some thing which has now become a matter of great public health concern.

6. Obesity

Obesity is perhaps the most important factor contributing to the development of glucose intolerance in the elderly people. Attenuated glucose intolerance and insulin sensitivity in the aged are an interlinked physical activity.

7. Free Radicals

The acceptance of 'Free Radicals' as a causative factor in the progressive deterioration of physiological function is based largely on their ability to induce damage in biological structure and functioning thereof.

8. Endocrines

Various age-related alterations in endocrine processes pose serious threat with respect to homeostasis and can result in cellular senescence.

9. Glucose Intolerance

The process of aging has been associated with the development of glucose intolerance. Among the most important physiologic and metabolic changes, the most significant one is the impaired ability of the system to maintain glucose homeostasis. As such, proper control of blood glucose concentration is very important, especially for the aged.

10. Fatty Acids

Age-related fatty acid changes suggest two different trends. First, aging is associated with increase in some long-chain polyunsaturated fatty acids, PUFA (20 : 4, 22 : 5 and 22 : 6). Secondly, there is a decrease in linolenic acid in the membranes of live mitochondria and microsomes.

11. T Cells

Aging is closely associated with impairment of cell functions, the most important being the decline in T cell proliferation. This is dependent, to a great extent, on the age-related changes in T cell subsets.

12. Sarcopenia

Poor nutritional status of the aged may lead to 'Sarcopenia', the age-related loss of muscle mass. And sarcopenia is a direct cause of age-associated loss of muscle strength. Herein, inadequate dietary proteins may be an important cause of sarcopenia.

13. Under-nutrition

Under-nutrition in majoring the macrophase-T cell disequilibrium leads to progressive loss of body's nutritional reserves after any stress or disease. This pushes the very healthy aged to frailty, the frail elders to a more progressive frail state, which leads to protein-energy malnutrition (PEM). In turn, the PEM-elderly are pushed down to a more profound state of PEM, which eventually leads to death.

14. Dietary Restrictions

Moderate dietary restrictions (DR) without malnutrition is the primary key that retards the onset of cancer and many other late-life auto-immune diseases, including renal diseases. Thereby, this dietary intervention helps increase the life span.

15. Dietary Restriction Tool

The use of DR, as a toll to retard aging and disease processes, has shown that nutritional intervention helps modulate many processes known to be deleterious to the normal biological functioning, e.g. free radical damage, plasma glucose and glycation of biological systems.

GERIATRIC COMPLICATIONS

The geriatric syndrome and research findings listed earlier apart, there are many broad-ranging complications that are a sequel to the aging process. These are as under:

1. Constipation

Due to greater use of processed foods and other items easy to chew, constipation is a common occurrence in the aged. It is due to lack of enough dietary fibre or roughages in the food. The excessive use of antacids which contain aluminium and carbonates also results in constipation. Obviously, the remedy is consumption of high-fibre diet. This must be supplemented with large intake of fluids.

2. Anemia

Normally, anemia would follow when there is a prolonged or multiple deficiency of proteins, vitamins and minerals, especially iron, vitamin B_{12}, folacin and ascorbic acid. All this results in reduced level of hemoglobin formation in the red blood cells, a precursor of anemia.

3. Malabsorption

The body's inability to absorb nutrients results in malabsorption of nutrients. Another contributory cause is lowered gastric acidity.

4. Hypertension

The incidence of increased blood pressure adds to the risk of hypertension, which could lead to coronary heart disease. By judiciously reducing the intake of sodium, one can bring down the blood pressure and also considerably check the loss of weight in the aged.

5. Dentition Problems

Often, the aged may loose all the teeth, which could lead to serious problem in chewing the food. Sometimes, the ill-fitting dentures prove to be a nuisance and it affects the proper eating of food.

6. Obesity

Overweight an d obesity are a cause of great concern, since these increase the risk of many diseases like heart diseases. The old food habits, if not, properly checked, could lead to accumulation of fat and obesity. Hence, strict diet control is advised in such cases.

7. Bone Diseases

The incidence of arthritis, osteoporosis and osteomalacia adds to the misery of the aged. For joint pains and arthritis, judicious diet control and Naturopathy can be very helpful. Osteoporosis is a common complaint in the elders, owing to hormonal imbalance or lack of adequate dietary calcium. Osteomalacia comes up in the elderly males who use very little milk or are confined to sunlight-devoid environs.

With proper supplementation of calcium and vitamin D, the latter two maladies can be brought under control.

8. Ulcer

Gastric or peptic ulcers in the GI tract occur due to hyperacidity or excessive acid content of digestive secretions. These could be kept in check by the use of antacids and bland foods.

9. Gall Bladder Problems

One of the serious afflictions is the formation of gall stones and the use of high fat diet aggravates the pain syndrome. Initially, low-fat diet helps, but in advanced cases, surgical removal of gall bladder is recommended.

10. Diabetes Mellitus

Diabetes is caused due to excess of sugar in the blood and urine, which is caused due to inadequate insulin in the body. In the not-so-advanced cases, diabetes can be controlled by proper diet intervention, controlling obesity and medication. Insulin therapy is the last-resort treatment.

11. Coronary Heart Disease

Coronary heart disease (CHD) and atherosclerosis often result from the narrowing of blood vessels owing to deposition of cholesterol therein. This leads to reduced supply of blood to the body organs, thus hampering their proper functioning. And when this condition affects the arteries supplying the heart, it leads to CHD or heart attack.

The contributory causes for CHD include obesity, lack of exercise, excessive cholesterol-rich diets, saturated fatty acids and sodium. Too much consumption of alcohol, colas and caffeine also cause these heart problems. Timely diagnosis responds to nutritional intervention, weight loss and medication.

DIET THERAPY

The ICMR has worked out a special 'Balanced Diet' for the elderly as shown in Table 12.5.

The food exchange lists in Table 12.6 are recommended for a man 65 years old, who needs 1750 kcal and 55 g proteins.

TABLE 12.5: BALANCED DIET FOR THE AGED (ICMR)

	Quantity Per Day (raw g)	
	Males	Females
Cereals	350	225
Pulses	50	40
Vegetables, Fresh	200	150
G.L.V.	50	50
Roots and Tubers	100	100
Fruits	200	200
Milk and Milk Products	300	300
Sugar	20	20
Fats and Oils	25	20
Approximate Nutrients Supplied		
Calories	2200	1700
Protein	65 g	50 g
Fat	50 g	40 g
Calcium	1 g	0.9 g
Iron	38 mg	30 mg
Vitamin A (Retinol)	1030 µg	930 µg
Thiamin	1.96 mg	1.45 mg
Riboflavin	1.78 mg	1.51 mg

TABLE 12.6: FOOD EXCHANGE LISTS FOR THE AGED

Food stuffs	No. of exchanges	Proteins (g)	Energy (kcal)
Milk	4	20	400
Legume and Pulses	2	12	200
Flesh Foods	½	5	50
Green Leafy Vegetables	2	—	—
Green Vegetables	2	—	100
Fruits	2	—	100
Cereals	6	12	600
Sugar	25 g	—	100
Fat	2	—	200
Total		**49 g**	**1750 kcal**

The diet chart for the same person is given in Table 12.7.

TABLE 12.7: DIET CHART FOR THE AGED

7.00 AM	Tea	I cup
9.00 AM	Bread with butter	I slice
	Banana	1
	Milk with sugar	1 glass
1.00 PM	Chapatti	1
	Rice	½ cup
	Dal	1 cup
	Spinach curry	1 cup
	Curd	½ cup
	Orange/Sweet Lime	1
4.00 PM	Tea	1 cup
	Biscuits	2
7.00 PM	Chapatti	1
	Dudhi (Lauki) or Pumpkin curry	1 cup
	Curd	½ cup
	Salad	I cup
9.00 PM	Milk	1 glass

Source: Tables 12. 6 and 12.7—*Nutrition and Dietetics* by S. A. Joshi.

DR. (MRS) JAIN SUPPLEMENT

For the aged, one must avoid too much oil/fats, spices.
Give only easily digestible and nourishing foods.

TABLE 12.8: DIET CHART FOR THE GERIATRICS

7.00 AM	Honey squash	1 glass
8.00 AM	Tender coconut water with honey and lemon	1 glass
9.00 AM	Overnight soaked figs	2
	Four Seeds' Liquor in milk	1 glass
	with Brahmi Powder	1 tsp (to improve memory)
	Dalia in milk	1 cup
	Fresh fruit—Papaya	
11.00 AM	Beetroot/Amla/Lemon Juice	1 glass—Tomato if amla not available
	Fresh fruit Salad	
12.00 AM	Seasonal Green Vegetable	
	Salad/Russian Salad	1 bowl
	With Sprouts-	1 tbsp—Alfalfa or moong etc.
	Vegetable Chapattis fortified with bran 25%	2
	Special Amla Chutney and Raita	1 bowl
4.00 PM	Fruit Juice	1 glass
7.00 PM	Dalia	1 bowl
	Vegetable Soup or As lunch	1 bowl
9.00 PM	Milk with dates 3 or figs 2 Boil the dates in milk	1 glass

CHERIE CALBOM SUPPLEMENT

🖎 **Vitamin C and E and the Mineral Selenium** are antioxidants that protect the cells from free radical damage, thus preventing premature aging. In other words, antioxidants gobble up the bad guys before they get your cells.

🖎 **Beta-Carotene and other Carotenoids** (over 500 have been Identified) are antioxidants that are converted by the body to vitamin A as needed. These are some of the most powerful interceptors known to protect the body from a particular free-radical bad guy called singlet oxygen. The carotenoids are also very helpful in preventing shrinkage of the thymus gland, and thus strengthening the immune system.

🖎 **Bioflavonoids** prevent free-radical damage. Like the carotenoids, these nutrients, which are found in plants, are considered antioxidants.

🖎 **Methionine and Cysteine** are sulfer-containing amino acids that may promote longevity. Sulphur is abundant in beans, fish, liver, eggs, brewer's yeast, cabbage, and nuts.

BENEFICIAL JUICES

🖎 Kale, parsley, green pepper, and broccoli—source of vitamin C

🖎 Spinach, asparagus, and carrot—source of vitamin E.

🖎 Red Swiss chard, turnip, garlic, and orange—source of selenium.

🖎 Carrot, kale, parsley, and spinach—source of beta-carotene and other carotenoids.

🖎 Apricot, balck currant, blackberry, broccoli, cabbage, cantaloupe, cherry, grape, grapefruit, lemon, orange, papaya, parsley, plum, prune, sweet pepper, and tomato—source of bioflavonoids.

SUGGESTED JUICING RECIPES FOR AGING

Beauty Spa Express

Small handful parsley
Handful spinach
4-5 carrots, green removed
½ apple, seeded

Bunch up parsley and spinach
and push through hopper with
carrots and apple.

Fresh Complexion Express

2 slices, pineapple, with skin
½ cucumber
½ apple, seeded

Push pineapple through hopper
with cucumber and apple.

High-Calcium Drink

3 kale leaves
Small handful parsley
-5 carrots, greens removed

Bunch up kale and parsley, and
push through hopper with carrots.

Garden Salad Special

3 broccoli flowerets
1 garlic clove
4-5 carrots or 2 tomatoes
2 stalks celery
½ green pepper

Push broccoli and garlic through
hopper, with carrots or tomatoes,
Follow with celery and green
pepper.

Cantaloupe Shake

½ cantaloupe, with skin

Cut cantaloupe in strips, and push
through hopper.

Fruit Salad Cocktail

1 medium bunch grapes
½ apple, seeded
¼ lemon

Push grapes through hopper,
followed by apples and lemon.

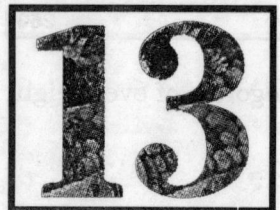

13 NUTRITION AND WEIGHT MANAGEMENT

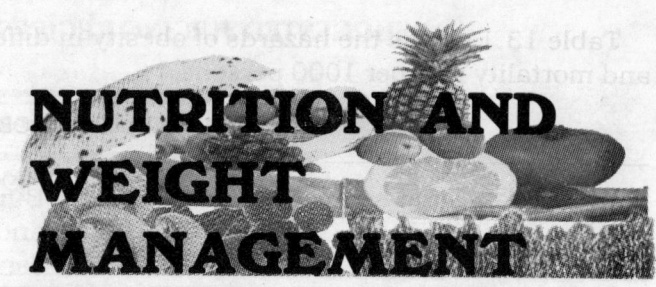

BODY WEIGHT vs BODY FAT

A public health problem of universal concern is weight management—usually over-weight, nay over-fat to be technically correct. Often the common term, 'Obesity' is confused with overweight.

OBESITY

Obesity is a clinical term used for excess body weight—generally 20% more than the 'Ideal Body weight'. The latter is the average weight taking in to consideration a man's height and frame. Obesity is, in reality, a disease condition of excess fat that frequently results in significant impairment of health.

There are a number of health risks and maladies associated with obesity. These disorders are

1. Diabetes
2. Cancer
3. Gall stones
4. Gout
5. High Blood Pressure
6. Heart Disease
7. Infertility
8. Menstrual Problems
9. Intestinal Disorders
10. Joint Stress
11. Pregnancy Problems
12. Respiratory Disorders
13. Skin Problems
14. Stroke

Table 13.1 shows the hazards of obesity in different categories of overweight and mortality rate per 1000 persons.

TABLE 13.1: HAZARDS OF OBESITY

Disease	Normal Weight Mortality	Over Weight Type		
		5 - 15% Mortality	15 - 25% Mortality	>25% Mortality
1. High blood pressure and CVD	23	34	45	51
2. Heart attack	80	115	133	139
3. Renal disease	82	108	202	224
4. Diabetes	14	22	45	117
5. Accidents	60	65	66	87

N.B. The above data pertains to late 1990s. Obviously, the incidence and hazards would have gone up considerably during the last one decade.

When a person is overweight or gains weight, it results in

(a) Increased Blood pressure,

(b) Increased Blood fats (-arteriosclerosis),

(c) Increased Blood sugars and insulin (-diabetes),

(d) Increased likelihood of bone and joint disorders

(e) Increased likelihood of gall stone formation.

All these hazards and consequences have been vividly sketched out in Fig. 13.1

Overweight

Overweight, despite its connotations, is a distinct, though slightly less dangerous situation. It is usually 10% more than the average body weight. From health angle, it is better to call it 'Overweight', because it merely represents percentage of excess fat in the overall body composition.

Body Composition

Body composition refers to how much of the overall share comes from fat and how much is from lean body mass. Based on metabolic activity, body composition has four components.

1. *Lean Body Mass (LBM)*

Lean body mass is the major component of active fat-free cell mass that determines the basal metabolic rate, energy and nutrient requirements of the body. It usually accounts for 30% to 85% of the total body weight.

2. *Body Fat*

Gross body fat reflects the number and size of fat cells that make up the adipose tissue. In a healthy man, fat accounts for 14% to 28% of the total body weight,

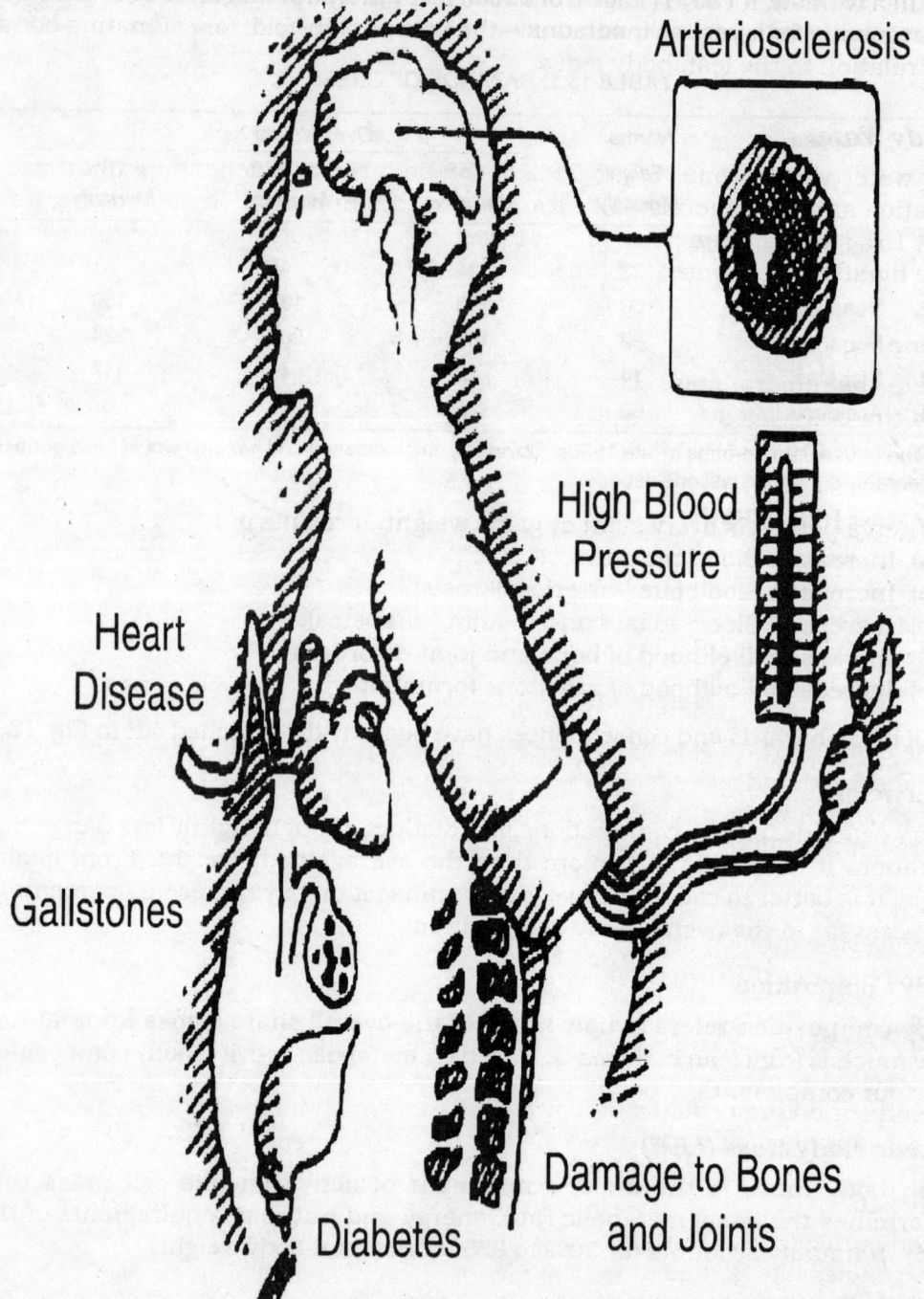

Fig. 13.1: Consequences of Obesity

while in a woman, it could range from 15% to 29%. About half of this fat is in the subcutaneous fat layers as insulation—the triceps skin-fold, for estimating body fat in relation to the lean body mass.

3. *Body Water*

Body water varies from 15% to 25% of the body weight, depending upon age, hydration and the general health standards of an individual. In fat persons, it is about 15%, while in lean persons, it is about 25% of the total body weight, because of the higher water content of the lean muscle tissue.

4. *Bone*

Bone or the mineral mass, largely in the skeletal structure, accounts for about 6% of the body weight. Herein, the main mineral is calcium, which makes up about 2% of the body weight.

Body Mass Index (BMI)

While assessing the risk factors associated with obesity, Body mass index (BMI) gives the measure of relative body fatness. BMI is calculated by the simple formula:

$$BMI = \frac{Weight\ in\ kilograms}{Height\ in\ square\ metres}$$

The desirable BMI range for an adult is 20-25 kg/m^2. From 25-30 kg/m^2, the BMI is considered risky for health, whereas the BMI the BMI above 40 kg/m^2 indicates severe obesity with adverse health effect.

A recent research study by Dr. Satish Kenchaiah of the Framingham Heart Society, Massachusetts (USA) has shown that for every one point increase in the BMI, the risk of heart failure rose by 5% in men and 7% among women.

An overweight woman has a 50% greater risk of heart failure and the obese women had double the risk of heart failure.

Ideal Weight

Ideal weight is more of an ideal concept. In practice, a man's ideal body weight depends upon many factors like age, body shape, metabolic rate, genetic make up, sex and physical activity.

Body Fat

A modicum of body fat is necessary for survival, since it helps provide energy in emergencies like famine or severe disease conditions. A man requires 3% body fat and a woman 20% body fat for mere survival. Menstruation (Menarche) begins when the young girl's body fat reaches this critical proportion of the body weight (20%), which is the amount needed for ovulation, as a precursor to pregnancy.

Causes of Obesity

1. *Genetic (Heredity) Factor*

Genetic inheritance influences a person's chance of becoming fat more than anything else. There is a 40% chance of his becoming fat if one of the parents is obese. And this probability factor goes up to 80%, if both the parents are obese. There does exist an underlying biochemical mechanism of a genetic link, an enzyme that acts as a 'Signaling molecule' to the body's fat metabolism.

Other genetic factors are the spontaneous physical activity and the habits of fidgeting or wriggling which use up calories equivalent to those of jogging.

Some changes result in genetically altered fat tissue to store more fat, rather than burn for energy. These abnormally large fat cells are resistant to insulin that regulates the cells' use of sugar (glucose). A high insulin production, in consequence, triggers further action as

(a) Stimulates hunger and eating.
(b) Stimulates the liver for producing more fat.
(c) Causes the fat cells to multiply.

All these factors have been sketched out in Fig. 13.2.

2. *Environmental Factors*

A man's food habits and eating pattern are reinforced by environmental milieu or any such subconscious pressures. It could be the family situation or influence by media or TV commercials or over-indulgence by kins and the peer pressure. It also happens in persons who lack discipline and will power. The Behaviour Modification approach to weight control is based on this environmental theory.

3. *Social Factors*

People placed high in the economic order tend to maintain a moderate weight despite their rich diet. On the other hand, those in the lower economic strata treat obesity as a common feature. These are the cultural factors that affect our food habits.

4. *Physiologic Factors*

Childhood and puberty are obesity-prone period when there is accumulation of fat tissue deposits. Both men and women tend to gain weight after the age of 50, because of lower BMR and lowered physical exercise.

5. *Glandular Malfunctioning*

Some people suffer from obesity due to some malfunctioning of endocrine glands like pituitary, thyroid and sex glands.

Hypothalamus gland, located in the base of the brain, controls body temperature, emotional state and many other body functions like appetite. When

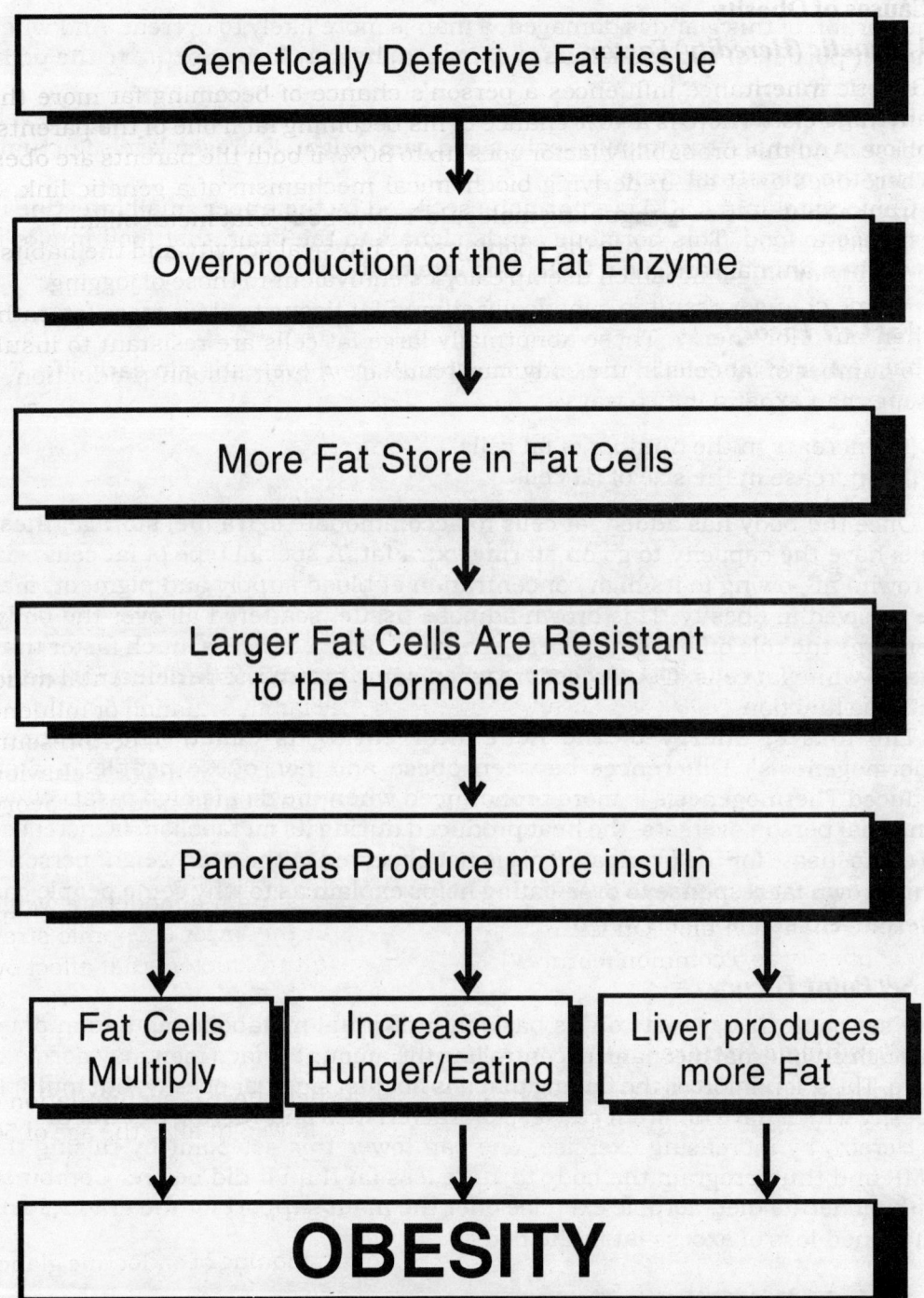

Fig. 13.2: Mode For Genetic Obesity

one portion of this gland is damaged, a man is more likely to overeat. And when another portion of hypothalamus is damaged, he may lose appetite to the point of self-starvation.

Estrogen is another hormone that affects the system. When estrogen levels are low in animals, they resume eating and gain weight. Estrogen levels fluctuate during the menstrual cycle.

Cholecystokinin (CKK) is a hormone secreted by the upper small intestine in response to food. This hormone sends signals to the brain that food intake is low. When animals are given CKK, food intake stops.

6. *Fat Cell Theory*

The number of fat cells in the body may result from overeating in early life. Fat tissues can expand in two ways;

(a) Increase in the number of fat cells.
(b) Increase in the size of fat cells.

Once the body has added fat cells to accommodate extra fuel storage, these cells have the capacity to go on storing extra fat. A special type of fat cells, viz. 'Brown Fat', owing to its high concentration of blood supply and pigment, may be involved in obesity. This brown adipose tissue, scattered all over the body, performs the role off burning excess energy as heat, a process much faster than that of white fat cells. Obesity occurs when some brown tissue defect interferes with the function.

The loss of energy or the heat after eating is called 'Diet-induced Thermogenesis'. Differences between obese and non-obese people in diet-induced Thermogenesis is more pronounced when the diet is high in fat. When a normal person overeats, the heat produced during its metabolism is increased to compensate for the overload. This is not observed in the over-weight persons. This brown fat response to over-eating helps explain as to why some people can overeat and still not gain weight.

7. *Set Point Theory*

The set point theory rests on its basis in individual metabolic regulation of fat through an internal mechanism controlling the amount of fat a man may normally have. Thus, it reinforces the finding that it is not just singular obesity, but multiple obesity which have different causes, characteristics and varying treatments.

Herein, by increasing exercise, one can lower this set point by raising the BMR and thus program the body to store less fat than it did before. Combined with moderate diet, aerobic exercise offer the main support for the gradual and sustained loss of excess fat in the body.

8. *Carbohydrate Balance Theory*

Carbohydrates are often promoted as high-calorie foods that encourage weight gain. But this is not true for all the carbohydrates. According to this theory, the

'Appetite Centre' in the hypothalamus and specialised cells in the liver are sensitive to the level of glucose in the blood. When sugar level is low, messages are sent to the brain: 'It is time to eat'. This explains why some people overeat.

Starches or complex carbohydrates are absorbed slowly. They do not cause the rapid rise in blood sugar, something seen with simple carbohydrates or sugars and so they do not trigger excess insulin secretion and the consequent drop in blood sugar.

A POSITIVE PERSONAL APPROACH TO WEIGHT CONTROL

In proper weight control, the degree of personal motivation counts a lot. A personal weight management program will induce the following steps:

1. Food Behaviour

Consume only small quantity of food and it should be eaten slowly. One must choose a variety of foods, preferably those having high dietary fibre. Avoid the processed foods. There should be an even distribution of foodstuffs each day.

2. Exercise Regime

A progressively increasing exercise regime helps. Start with simple walking exercise and then go on to aerobics for about half an hour. Other activities like swimming can be added later on.

3. Relaxation Exercises

Progressive muscle relaxation and stress reduction exercises should be followed regularly. Starting with 10 minutes activity, it can be gradually increased. The Indian system of Yogasanas can help reduce fat selectively from some parts of the body. These have synergistic effect on the reducing diets. As such, permanent weight loss program (precisely fat reduction) must equally incorporate exercise with diet. The benefit of exercise may be summarized as

1. Increased Muscle Mass
2. Increased Basal Metabolic Rate
3. Reduced fat stores
4. Increased energy level
5. Suppressed appetite
6. Increased overall stamina and fitness
7. Reduced Blood Pressure
8. Decreased anxiety and hypertension
9. Increased use of calories
10. Normalised Blood Sugar
11. Lowered Set Point

Examples of aerobic and anaerobic exercises are

Aerobic	**Anaerobic**
Walking	Tennis
Cycling	Badminton
Swimming	Sprinting
Cross-country Skiing	Down-hill Skiing
Jogging	Weight lifting
Trampsoline	Racketball.

PRINCIPLES OF A SOUND FOOD PLAN

A healthy and sound food plan involves following components:

1. Energy Balance

The calorie intake is adjusted to meet individual weight-reduction requirements. *It is necessary to reduce 1000 kcal per day from the normal diet, if one has to lose 2 lb/week and 500 kcal for one pound loss to be effected.* This gradual weight loss would go for long time success of the program. For men and women of heavy build, this reduction level would go up to 1500-1800 kcal/day.

2. Nutrient Balance

(a) **Carbohydrates:** About 50% of the total kilocalories should come from complex carbohydrates with fibre. The use of sugar should be restricted.

(b) **Proteins:** Greater amount of lean foods should be consumed to cut down on fat. This should provide 20% of the total calorie intake.

(c) **Fat:** It should constitute about 25-30% of total kilocalories, with greater emphasis on vegetable fats, rather than animal fats.

Table 13.2 gives the usefulness of different exercises in weight management. Providing vitamin-rich green leafy vegetables, fresh fruits, whole grain cereals and sprouted legumes will take care of minerals and vitamins essential for the body. Regular exercise in a regime of reducing diet helps considerably. One must exercise longer, but not too much or too hard to strain the heart muscles.

Food Guide

The food exchange system provides some choice to fulfill the basic needs. Diverse food items can be judiciously combined into different dishes. Using alternate seasonings, such as herbs and spices, onion and garlic, lemon juice, vinegar and wine does help. Table 13.3 shows the exchange lists.

TABLE 13.2: ENERGY EXPENDITURE ON EXERCISE

	Exercise	*Calories/minute*	*Calories/hour*
1.	Walking briskly on level ground		
	(a) - Weight 100 lb	3.6	216
	(b) - Weight 140 lb	4.6	276
	(c) - Weight 180lb	5.4	324
2.	Walking briskly uphill		
	- Weight 155 lb	8.9	534
3.	Climbing Stairs		
	- Weight 140 lb	6.2	372
	- Weight 140 lb	8.6	516
3.	Climbing on slope with light weight	10.7	642
5.	Cycling		
	- Speed 8 Kph	4.5	270
	- Speed 15 Kph	7.0	420
6.	Marathon - Cross country	10.6	636
7.	Swimming	5-11	330- 660
8.	Jogging	5-5.8	300-350
9.	Tennis	4.4-5.6	270-400
10.	Gardening		
	- Weeding	4.5 -6.6	264-336
	- Digging	8.6	516

Source: Passmore, R and Durin, JVGA—*Physiology Review*, **35**: 801, 1955.

An illustrative dietary guideline for weight loss is shown in Table 13.4.

Since the reduction of fat is a major point of action, the following practical tips for fat reduction can go a long way in ensuring better weight management.

1. Bake, broil, steam or poach foods. Do not saute, fry or use gravies/sauce.
2. Always cook meats at low temperature to help remove complete fat.
3. Skim froth from broth before making gravies or soup stock.
4. Do not bread or flour meats. The flour will absorb excess fat.
5. Avoid using oil or butter. Prefer non-stick pans for cooking.
6. Saute in defatted chicken stock, rather than in oil or butter.
7. Prefer non-fat milk, over whole milk or cream in cooking.
8. Reduce the oil by one-half in recipes.
9. Prefer jam or marmalade instead of butter on toast.

TABLE 13.3: FOOD EXCHANGE LISTS AND VALUES

	Food Group	Carbohydrates (g)	Proteins (g)	Fat (g)	Kilocalories
1.	Starch on bread	15	3	Trace	80
2.	Meat				
	- Lean meat	—	7	3	55
	- Medium fat	—	7	5	75
	- High fat	—	7	8	100
3.	Vegetables	5	2	—	25
4.	Fruits	15	—	—	60
5.	Milk				
	- Skimmed milk	12	8	Trace	90
	- Low fat milk	12	8	5	120
	- Full cream milk	12	8	8	150
6.	Fat	—	—	5	45

Source: Franz M. J. *et al.* Exchange Lists Revised, 1986; *Am. Diet Assoc.,* **87**(1): 28, 1987.

TABLE 13.4: DIETARY GUIDELINES FOR WEIGHT LOSS

	Food	Portion	Portions per day	Calories/ portion
1.	Fruits	½ cup, 1 medium	3	40
2.	Vegetables	½ cup cooked, 1 cup raw	3	25
3.	Whole grain bread, cereals, rice or pasta	1 slice; ½ cup cooked cereal, ½ cup rice/pasta	5	70
4.	Lean meat, chicken, fish, dried beans and peas	3 oz meat, chicken, fish or ½ cup dried beans and peas	2	130
5.	Low fat or no fat milk or yogurt	8 oz milk or yogurt	2	90
6.	Fats	1 tsp butter/margarine/oil 1/8 avocado, 1 tbsp oil and vinegar dressing	2-3	45

Source: Weight Loss and Nutrition, Pub. CBS.

Based on the degree of overweight, the weight reduction exercises can be:

(a) Mild, *i.e.* 20-40% overweight. It calls for moderate calories restriction.

(b) Moderate, *i.e.* 41-100% overweight—reported in about 10% of the US women. It calls for medically-supervised, very low calorie formulae and re-feeding diets.

(c) Severe, *i.e.* more than 100% over weight calls for special surgical procedures like liposuction.

Total Calories   1120
Share of Fats   31%
Share of Carbohydrates 49%
Share of Proteins   20%

Table 13.5 advises greater variation in the Food Exchange that makes for 1000-1800 kcal reduction in weight.

TABLE 13.5: WEIGHT REDUCTION FOOD (EXCHANGE) PLAN

	Food exchange group	1000 kcal	1200 kcal	1500 kcal	1800 kcal
1.	**Total number of exchanges/day**				
	Non-fat Milk	2	2	2	2
	Vegetables	3	3	4	4
	Fruits	3	3	4	4
	Bread	4	5	7	9
	Meat	3	4	5	7
	Fat	4	4	5	5
2.	**Meal pattern of foods exchanges**				
	Breakfast				
	Fruits	1	1	1	1
	Meat	—	—	1	1
	Bread	1	1	2	2
	Fat	1	1	1	1
	Milk	0.5	0.5	0.5	0.5
	Lunch				
	Meat	1	1	1	1
	Vegetables	1	1	2	2
	Bread	1	2	2	3
	Fat	1	1	2	2
	Fruits	1	1	1	1
	Milk	0.5	0.5	0.5	0.5
	Dinner				
	Meat	2	2	2	3
	Vegetables	2	2	2	2
	Bread	1	1	2	3
	Fat	2	2	2	2
	Fruits	–	–	1	1
	Milk	0.5	0.5	0.5	0.5
	Snacks				
	Meat	2	2	2	3
	Vegetables	2	2	2	2
	Bread	1	1	2	3
	Fat	2	2	2	2
	Fruit	—	—	1	1
	Milk	0.5	0.5	0.5	0.5

Source: Sue Rod Williams: *Essentials of Nutrition and Diet Therapy.*

The people with sedentary habits and retiring nature must learn to strike a proper balance between energy expenditure and food intake, otherwise it would lead to a 'Creeping Obesity' developing unnoticed over a period of time. In the overall analysis, what really counts is early nutrition education and positive food habits. The whole weight management regime has to be a 'Preventive Regime', before the obese conditions actually start manifesting.

AVOID

Hereunder, we give a very comprehensive list of foodstuffs that one must religiously avoid in order to ward off any lurking risk of obesity in any of its subterranean manifestation. Better avoid the foods:

1. Sugar, jaggery, sweets jams, chocolates
2. Bakery products—cakes, cream—biscuits and pastries
3. Concentrated milk products like 'Barfi', Shrikhand, Basundi
4. Fried foods and fried or roasted snacks
5. Fatty meat cuts, organ meats and shell fish
6. Butter, ghee, oil and cream dressings
7. Alcohols, beverages and soft drinks
8. Dried fruits, nuts and beans.

Table 13.6 gives the diet chart for a moderately obese person, while Table 13.7 gives the diet regimes for both vegetarians and non-vegetarians.

TABLE 13.6: DIET CHART FOR A MODERATELY OBESE PERSON (1500 KCAL)

7.00 AM	Tea with sugar	1 cup
9.00 AM	Skimmed milk without sugar	200 ml
	Bread slices without butter	2
	Orange	1
1.00 PM	Capsicum soup	1 cup
	Green salad	1 bowl
	Spinach curry	1 cup
	Chapattis	2
	Rice	½ cup
	Pulses thin	½ cup
	Curd	½ cup
4.00 PM	Tea with sugar	1 cup
7.00 PM	Tomato soup	1 cup
	Cabbage curry	1 cup
	Usal	1 cup
	Chapattis/bhakri	1
	Rice	½ cup
	Curd	½ cup

Source: S. A. Joshi: *Nutrition and Dietetics.*

TABLE 13.7: DIET CHART FOR OBESITY

7.00 AM	Tea with sugar	1 cup
9.00 AM	Skim milk	1 cup
	Toast	2
	Sweet lime	1
	(Scrambled egg for Non-veg.)	
12.00 Noon	Mixed vegetable/cucumber	
	and celery soup	1 cup
	Thin dal/curd curry	1 cup
	Green vegetable salad	1 bowl
	Cooked pumpkin or	
	Steamed lady finger	1 bowl
	Chapattis	2
	Custard apple	
	(Chicken roast/grilled fish for Non-veg.)	
4.00 PM	Tea with sugar	1 cup
6.00 PM	Orange	1
8.00 PM	Tomato soup	1 cup
	Skim milk	½ cup
	Cooked carrot/spiced stuffed	
	Thin dal	1 cup
	Steamed cauliflower	1 cup
	Chapattis	2
	Baked apple	
	(Minced meat or fish for Non-veg.)	

Dr. F. P. Antia: *Clinical Dietetics and Nutrition*, Oxford University Press, 1989.

NATUROPATHY

Special mention needs be made of a few very helpful steps recommended in Naturopathy. These are:

- Yoga exercises
- Magnet therapy
- Massage
- Acupressure
- Steam/Sauna bath

Fasting has very limited effect on weight reduction, which is more if a person continues to eat some (moderate) amount of food than when he fasts.

Drs. Blondheim, Kaufman and Bortz claim that in the long run, total fasting and subsisting on 800 kcal diet yielded about similar results. As regards exercise, when energy worth 3500 kcal is burnt, the weight is reduced by half a kg. Into the figures given earlier in Table 13.1, the additions can be made (kcal/hour):

Light Yogasanas	350-400
Household chores	150-250
Dancing	400-500
Skipping	650-700

NUTRITION FOR UNDERWEIGHTS

While obesity may be a major health concern in the West, the developing countries continue to suffer from a high degree of underweight incidence. Herein, besides the erratic eating habits of the economically weaker sections, it is very active, tense and nervous people who are the unwitting victims of loss of weight. This may also occur in cases of severe infections, hyperthyroidism and gastrointestinal diseases.

After scrutinising and removing the contributing causes of weight loss, a high calorie diet is to be recommended under the following guidelines.

1. Energy

Normally, an extra dose of 500 kcal/day will lead to the addition of one pound to the body weight. For effective weight gain, the RDA for a moderately active person is 2500-3000 calories per day.

2. Proteins

For an ideal body weight, one gram protein is recommended for each one kg body weight. This would call for an intake of 60-80 g protein every day.

3. Vitamins and Minerals

A diet rich in legume sprouts, fresh leafy green vegetables and fruits would serve the purpose and save on any unnecessary vitamin-mineral supplements.

4. Exercise

Moderate regular exercise stimulates appetite and thus helps in the overall improvement of the body systems.

Table 13.8 gives a high calorie, high protein diet for the undernourished and the underweights, as recommended by Rekha Sharma, the Chief Nutritionist of the All India Institute of Medical Sciences (AIIMS).

Alongside in Table 13.9, for the sake of wider choice, as also for comparative analysis, we give the eminent Naturopath and Practising Dietician: Dr. (Mrs) Usha Jain's Special Diet Chart for obesity and other relevant guidelines, based solely on Bio-Nutrition.

TABLE 13.8: HIGH CALORIE, HIGH PROTEIN DIET

7.00 AM	Tea with sugar	1 cup
9.00 AM	Milk	200 ml—1 glass
	Bread slices with butter or parathas or Idlis	2
	Cheese	50 g or
	Eggs	2
11.00 AM	Fruit Juice/ cold drink/milk	1 glass
1.00 PM	Vegetable soup	1 cup
	Chapattis	4-6
	Rice	150 g
	Vegetables	1 serving
	Curd	125 g
	Pulses	1 bowl
	Chicken	1 serving
	Fruits	2 medium
	Cooking oil	20 g—4 tsp
4.00 PM	Milk	200 ml
	Sandwich/Samosa	1
7.00 PM	Same as Lunch	
9.00 PM	Milk	200 ml

Source: Rekha Sharma—*Diet Management.*

The above diet provides

Calories	3055
Proteins	110 g
Carbohydrates	395 g
Fats	115 g

DR. USHA JAIN'S DIET CHART FOR OBESITY

TABLE 13.9: SAMPLE MENU FOR MODERATE OBESITY

6.00 AM	Lime juice with honey (1 tbsp)	1 glass
8.00 AM	Seasonal fresh fruits	
	Buttermilk	1 glass
10.00 AM (Brunch)	Raw Green Vegetable Salad	1 bowl
	Seasonal Vegetables—steamed	300 g
	Oat/Wheat porridge	1 cup or
	Wheatflour chapattis, without oil	2-3
12.00 Noon	Buttermilk or Vegetable soup	1 glass
4.00 PM	Fruit juice or fresh juicy fruits	1 glass
7.00 PM	Seasonal fruit salad—2-3 varieties	100 g each
	Steamed Vegetables	200 g
	Sprouts—Bengal gram or Alfalfa	1 tbsp
	Seasonal Vegetable soup	1 cup
10.00 PM	Soaked Figs	2 plus
	Amla (Gooseberry) powder with	1 tsp plus
	Honey	1 tbsp
	Drink the soak (figs) water	

SPECIAL GUIDELINES

Dr (Mrs) Jain advises special steps as under:

1. Excessive Over-weight

1. Use exclusive Juice diet for the first three days
2. From the 4th day onwards follow the above sample diet. This should be continued till 8th day.

But the conditions of abnormal or extreme obesity demands special attention and prolonged treatment. Rather, it has got to become a new way of life, which calls for new habits and new mores of thinking.

2. Extreme Obesity

1. For the first seven days, tender coconut water to be taken every three hours. This should not be gulped down, but sipped very slowly.
2. Alternatively, take ashgourd (Petha vegetable) juice—250 g (raw) at a time and repeat every three hours.
3. Eat green salad first and rest of the sample diet follows. Chew these thoroughly well.
4. Eat very slowly. Avoid diversions like reading newspapers or watching TV, else too much chatting during the meals, as these could inadvertently lead to overeating.
5. One must keep a proper record of one's activities, as also of the food taken at different times. This would make for more regularity in eating habits.
6. Do not drink water in between the meals. Water should be taken only half an hour before or an hour after the meals.
7. Keep a regular note of your progress.
8. Better visualise every day the desired impact in weight loss. This has a positive psychological effect. It also hastens the process of recovery.
9. Yoga-nidra (sleep) does help positively.
10. More equanimity and regularity should become a way of life.

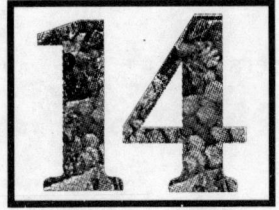

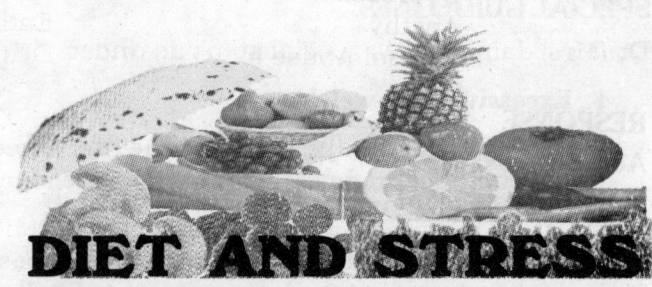

DIET AND STRESS

Stress is a normal part of life. All events, even the most positive ones, do cause some stress!

Stress is a force that pushes a person to an 'Altered Response'—to change, to grow, to fight, to adapt or to yield. It was the Canadian physician, Hans Selye, who first showed in 1956 the close relationship between stress and disease. In the modern era of stress and strain, for a large majority in the urban areas, it is too much stress and restricted or limited ability to cope with this 'On-going Rush of Stressful Sentiments'. The physical and psychological stress of day-to-day life ultimately leads to physiologic stress with serious consequences in the long run. In all such cases, good nutrition is a very important tool to fight stress. This extra nutritional support or defence helps in three ways:

1. Nutrition fortifies an individual to overcome the physical and mental demands of stress.
2. Poor nutrition, *per se*, causes additional stress on the body and mind.
3. Stress situation automatically increases the demand for extra nutrients.

Stress Disorders

Stress-related disorder include:

Heart disease	Ulcers
Allergies	Asthma
Rashes	Hypertension
And possibly cancer	

The above serious maladies apart, stress can also cause life-long psychological problems like:

Depression	Anxiety
Apathy	Eating Disorders
Alcohol Abuse	Drug Abuse.

RESPONSE

Acute Stress

Acute stress occurs suddenly and is usually quite severe in its intensity. It markedly raises the body's metabolic rate (BMR) and so upsets the internal balance ('Homeostasis').

Conditions that lead to stress are:

Infections
Surgery
Burns
Fractures
Deep penetrating wounds, e.g. gunshot and fistula wounds.

In response to acute stress, the body alters blood flow to the site of injury or infection so that the spread of invading organism is halted. The metabolic rate speeds up (Hypermetabolism) to mobilize nutrients into glucose and amino acid pools. It is from these reserves that the body synthesizes the special factors needed to limit and repair the damage and further, to help restore homeostasis. Immune systems and hormones mediate this response, which ultimately affects the body systems. Herein, special proteins: Cytokines direct changes in cardiovascular and nervous systems that, in turn, stimulate the production of cells necessary to destroy the foreign organisms.

Clinical Stress

Herein, the duration of exposure to stress is prolonged. This happens in the case of inflammatory bowel disease, congestive heart failure, cancer and HIV infections.

Dietary Stress

Notwithstanding the corrective role that nutrition plays in combating stress, certain diets can either create or aggravate the stress in a man's life. These stress-producing items include coffee, alcohol, sugar and rigid dieting.

Caffeine

The morning cup of coffee is indeed a booster to start off the day—the boost being provided by caffeine. Caffeine stimulates the central nervous system and is found in tea, coffee, soft drinks (colas), cocoa, chocolates and some medications. But an excess of caffeine can cause problems. It stimulates the stress hormones which cause an increase in the rate of heart beat and blood pressure. Drinking more than 5 cups of coffee can lead to many such conditions. Caffeine is a diuretic and causes increased urinary excretion of the vitamins B and C. This stimulant action may also increase the risk of cancer, specially of colon, bladder and pancreas. A dose of 200 mg caffeine, equivalent to 1-3 cups of coffee (depending upon brewing) may cause undesirable effects. However, decaffeinated coffee is a good substitute for those people, who suffer from stress.

Sugar

One-fifth of the calories of an average American's diet comes from refined sugar. These excess calories can lead to overweight and obesity. Sugar, a carbohydrate, supplies energy to the body. Several members of vitamin B group, viz. thiamine, riboflavin, niacin and vitamin B_6 are likely to be deficient in a high-sugar diet, since these are required to digest carbohydrates and process these for energy. That leaves very little vitamins for other body processes. Sugar can add to mental and physical stress by its effects on blood sugar. Consuming large amount of sugar causes rapid release of insulin, which removes sugar from the blood, leading to very low blood sugar levels. Herein, the symptoms are fatigue, hunger, nausea, mental cloudiness and blurred vision.

Dieting

Drastic reduction of calories threatens to disturb the body equilibrium, thus leading to stress. A diet of less than 1000-1200 calories can create problems by slowing down the metabolism. At the same time, the proportion of body fat increases. Such prolonged nutrient deficiency can impair the immune system.

Alcohol

Alcohol has been called the 'Anti-nutrient Nutrient', since it provides only calories but no vitamins or minerals. Thus, it depletes the body of several nutrients.

Normally, the liver burns fat. However, when alcohol is present, fat is not burnt for energy, but can cause damage to the liver. Consumption of alcohol breeds a sense of euphoria, which decreases appetite and the desire for food. Excess of alcohol produces irritation in the stomach, which results in reduced nutrient absorption.

Alcohol metabolism demands a steady supply of B vitamins, especially of thiamine and niacin. Their depletion can lead to low blood sugar. Alcohol is a diuretic and can dehydrate the cells of the body. Many vitamins like vitamin B and C and minerals—Mg, Ca and Zn are lost with water. In the long run, this alcohol stress can affect liver, heart, brain and other organs.

Nutrition Stress

The immune system defends the body against infections, chemicals and gases and other environmental stress. It has been shown that stress might alter the immune system, making it less capable of resisting infections and disease.

Several vitamins and minerals effect immunity. A deficiency of zinc in protein-calorie malnutrition cases causes destruction of tissues in the immune system.

Inadequate iron also impairs the immune system. Copper deficiency increases susceptibility to bacteria and increases the risk of infection. The deficiency of selenium, along with low vitamin E diet, also lowers the immune system. So also with vitamin B deficiency. But an excess of vitamin A can cause toxicity, which shows up as skin problems, liver damage, abdominal pains and bone deformities.

Disease Stress

As stated earlier, many diseases are related to the stress factor. This list of stress diseases includes:

Cardiovascular Disease	Coronary Heart Disease
Cancers	Hypertension
Migraine	Ulcers
Allergies	Asthma

Cardiovascular Disease (CVD)

Diseases of the heart and blood vessels are a major cause of death and disability. And psychological stress of modern day life greatly contributes to CVD. The stress hormones accelerate this liability factor by increasing blood pressure. The increased pressure in the arteries damages artery walls and encourages the formation of fat deposits and also increases the cholesterol level. This leads to atherosclerosis, i.e. hardening of the arteries. The arteries get clogged, blocking the flow of blood which can lead to a heart attack.

Reducing the intake of saturated fats and cholesterol is the best means to prevent CVD. Increased intake of foods high in fluorides, copper, magnesium and chromium helps in preventing heart diseases.

Of the dietary fibre, pectin, found in apples and other fruits, lowers the cholesterol level by binding the cholesterol in small intestine and thus leading to its greater excretion.

The following list gives different types of fibre-rich foods:

Cellulose	*Hemicellulose*
Whole Grains	Whole Grains
Bran	Bran
Fruits	Fruits
Vegetables	Vegetables

Lignin	*Pectin*
Whole Grains	Apples
Vegetables esp.	Citrus Fruits
Cabbages	Nuts
Broccoli	
Strawberries	
Apples	

Gums and Mucilages
Grains
Fruits
Vegetables

Cancer

Psychological stress is associated with some forms of cancer, including breast cancer, cervical cancer, leukemia and lymphoma. Excess fat intake, whether saturated or unsaturated, might contribute to cancer, more so the colon cancer.

To reduce the risk of cancer, nutritionists recommend diet containing low-fat meats, low-fat dairy products, whole grain bread, dried beans and peas and fresh fruits and vegetables. Adequate intake of dietary fibre also helps, as fibre might dilute and speed up the passage of cancer-causing substances through the intestines.

A diet high in vitamin A or β-carotenes reduces the risk of cancer, specially of skin, breast and bladder cancer. Some vitamins and minerals act as antioxidants to prevent cell damage and possibly cancer. These include vitamins A, C and E, acting along with selenium. Vitamin C inhibits the activity of cancer-causing nitrites in processed meats and thus helps prevent stomach cancer. Cruciferous vegetables like cabbage, broccoli, Brussels sprouts and kohlrabi are the most preferred vegetables for cancer prevention. Herein, the non-nutrient substance, indole is the major preventive factor that helps in significantly reducing the incidence of cancer.

IMMUNE RESPONSE

Immune system is the body's natural system of defence against the pathogens. It enables the body to fight infectious agents. Serious infections generally tax the body and if the immune response is not adequate, it can even lead to death.

The inflammatory response, the natural reaction to tissue damage, helps repair the tissue by inactivating and removing foreign organisms. As a result, the blood flow to the injured area is re-routed to seal it off from the rest of the body, while repair is under way. Alongside, the immune systems disarm any foreign invaders that might have gained entry to the site. As such, these two mechanisms acting together protect the body from the spread of stress or infection. However, acutely ill people may develop sepsis, which could lead to greater complications later.

HORMONAL RESPONSE

Adrenaline, the stress hormone, is released from the adrenal glands. This hormone travels through the body, increasing blood pressure and heart rate, speeds up the breathing rate and alters other body processes. Blood sugar also increases and the fat cells release fat into the bloodstream. All this leads to extra alertness and a tense state of the body.

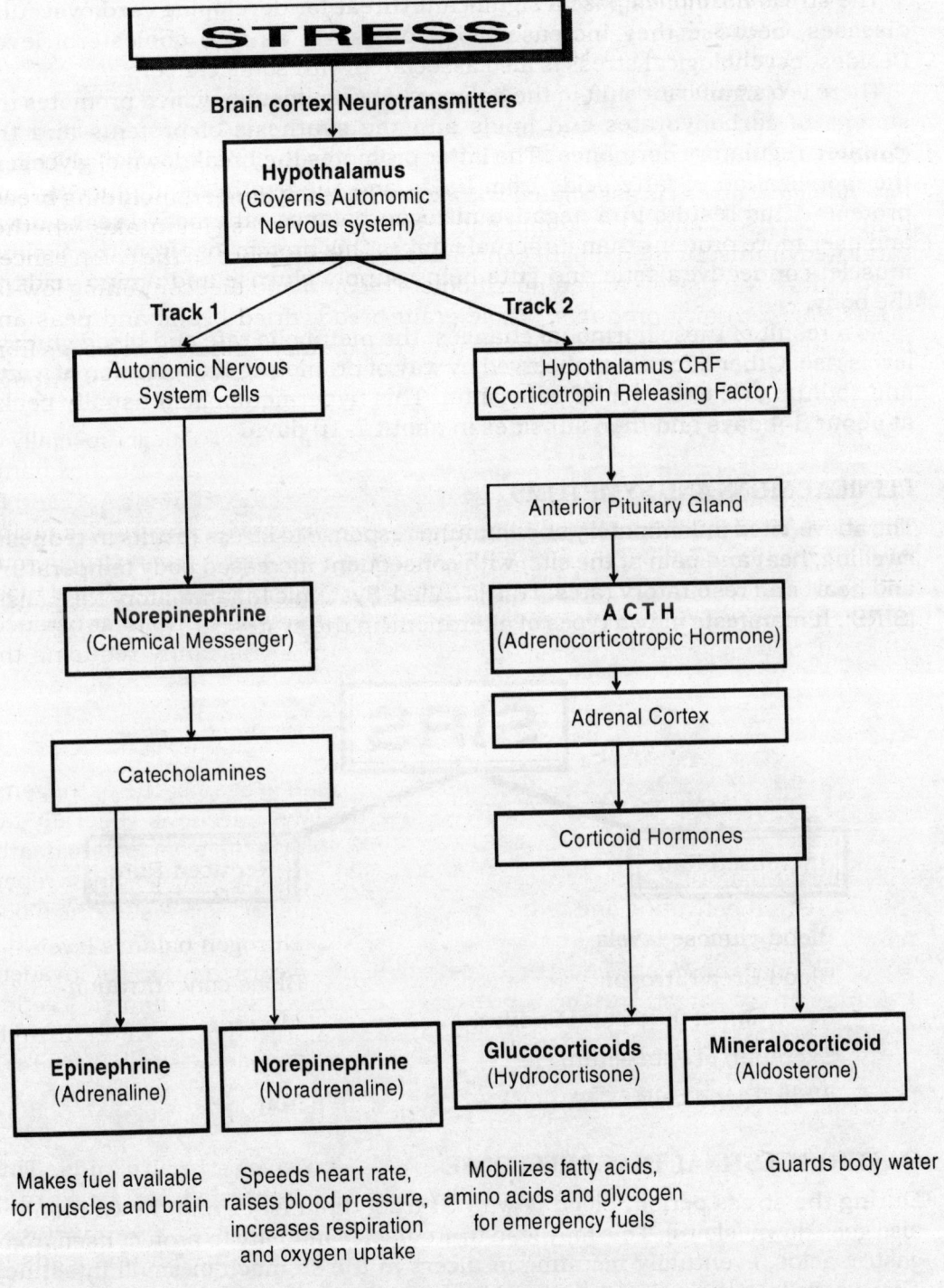

Fig. 14.1: Progressive Sequence of Physiologic Events in Response to Stress

The stress hormones pose a significant threat for developing cardiovascular diseases, because they increase blood pressure, as also cholesterol level. Besides, psychological stress is also associated with some cancers.

There is a significant shift in the balance between insulin, which promotes the storage of carbohydrates and lipids and the synthesis of proteins and the 'counter-regulatory hormones'. The latter promotes the breakdown of glycogen, the mobilization of fatty acids from lipids and the synthesis of glucose from proteins. This results in a negative nitrogen balance—the body breaks down and uses more proteins than its actual intake. This protein loss from the skeletal muscle, connective tissue and guts helps supply glucose and amino acids to the body.

As a result of these hormonal changes, the metabolic rate and blood glucose levels rise. Other effects are observed by way of promoting the retention of water and sodium and excretion of potassium. This hypermetabolism usually peaks at about 3-4 days and then subsides in about 7-10 days.

CLINICAL SIGNS AND SYMPTOMS

The above-cited inflammatory and immune response to stress results in redness, swelling, heat and pain at the site, with consequent increased body temperature and heart and respiratory rates. This is called 'Systemic Inflammatory Response' (SIRS). It manifests in two types of alterations in the system:

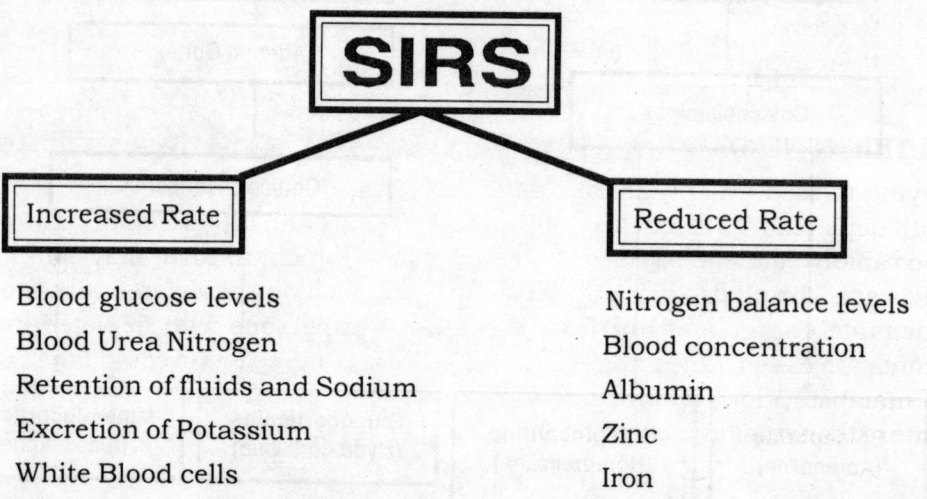

SIRS

Increased Rate

Blood glucose levels
Blood Urea Nitrogen
Retention of fluids and Sodium
Excretion of Potassium
White Blood cells

Reduced Rate

Nitrogen balance levels
Blood concentration
Albumin
Zinc
Iron

GASTROINTESTINAL TRACT RESPONSE

During the stress period, blood flow to GI tract diminishes and the GI motility also goes down (slows). This may lead to stomach's inability to protect itself from gastric acids, eventually resulting in ulcers in the stomach or small intestine. These cells lose their absorptive and immune functions.

EFFECTS ON NUTRITION STATUS

If a person is well-nourished, the short term stress of negative nitrogen balance is tolerable, since sufficient protein remains to support defence systems and also help maintain other vital body functions. But in acute cases, the elevated metabolic rate rapidly depletes energy reserves and breaks down protein tissues. This could lead to acute malnutrition, or worse still, extreme protein-energy malnutrition. Prolonged stress leads to loss of lean body mass, depletion of vital proteins that could affect heart, lungs, kidneys and GI tract. The overall system begins to fail and the recovery process is seriously compromised.

Optimum nutrition support following stress conditions helps to minimise nutrient losses, preserve organ function and also maintain immune defences. All these help in speedier recovery.

Table 14.1 records the consequences of stress that leads to malnutrition.

TABLE 14.1: CAUSES OF MALNUTRITION DURING ACUTE STRESS

Reduced Nutrient Intake	Excessive Nutrient Losses	Enhanced Nutrient Demand
Anorexia	Blood Loss	Fever
Emotional Stress	Immobility	Hypermetabolism
Immobility	Malabsorption	Infections
Location Injury	Urinary Losses	Medication
Medication		
Nausea/Vomiting	Vomiting	Pressure Sores

NUTRIENT NEEDS

Trying to feed an acutely stressed person is a cumbersome job. For persons with depleted nutrient reserves, both overfeeding and underfeeding, else feeding too rapidly can lead to serious complications, which, in turn, may compromise recovery. The physiologic and metabolic complications associated with providing adequate energy and nutrients too rapidly in persons with depleted nutrient stores are called 'Refeeding Syndrome'. These complications could take the form of malabsorption, respiratory distress, cardiac insufficiency, congestive heart failure, convulsions, coma and in extreme cases, even death.

Energy Requirements

Supplying too little energy would further compromise the nutrition status and this would lead to the risk of infections, and it also interferes with wound healing and lung functions. On the other hand, if the energy supplied is higher than what is needed, it could further elevate the metabolic rate which, in turn, increases oxygen use and carbon dioxide production. This would impose additional burden on the already overworked heart and lungs in order to keep the body's gases in proper equilibrium. And if these vital organs are already weakened by the pre-existing malnutrition, then the magnitude of stress will be still greater. As such, these energy needs for most stress cases range from 100 - 120% of the basal energy expenditure. It means 30 kcal/kg body weight, which figure goes upto 45 kcal/kg in severe stress.

Proteins and Amino Acids

The people exposed to stress, but having normal kidney and liver functions, need between 1.2 and 1.5 g proteins/kg body weight per day. But the severe stress cases need more proteins, about 1.5-1.7 g/kg body weight.

Glutamine, which is normally considered as a non-essential amino acid, becomes an essential element in such cases. It provides the fuel for intestinal cells and also plays an important role in maintaining the immune systems and promoting wound healing.

Carbohydrates and Lipids

Carbohydrates provide a ready source of energy, but the body can metabolize only about 500 g/day of glucose during stress. Excess glucose, serving no useful purpose, contributes to hyperglycemia, which can adversely affect fluid and electrolyte balance and the increased risk of infections. It is recommended that non-protein calories be supplied through a mixture of 70% carbohydrates and 30% lipids.

Micronutrients

The requirement of many group B vitamin members goes up when the intake of proteins and energy increases. Many micronutrients act as co-factors in other metabolic functions. Others contribute to speedy wound healing and repair of broken bones. During stress, blood iron level may fall as iron moves from blood into the liver for storage. However, iron is not given to compensate this because the shift robs the invading organisms of the iron they need to grow. Thus, it indirectly helps prevent the spread of infections.

Hormones

Growth hormones and Insulin-like growth factor-1 (IGF-1) are reported to stimulate the growth of intestinal cells and thus may play an important role in protecting the intestinal tract during the stress period.

Fluid and Electrolyte Balance

It is critically important that we prevent dehydration and electrolyte imbalance. Without adequate blood volume, oxygen, nutrients and medications cannot be delivered to the cells, the organ system cannot function properly and toxic wastes cannot be eliminated from the body. On the other hand, providing excess fluids puts extra stress on the heart, which must pump much greater volume of blood. Without adequate precautions, blood levels of these electrolytes can plummet to very low levels, resulting in serious complications.

REPLENISHING NUTRIENTS

Oral Diets

Mild stress cases would need IV solutions to maintain fluid and electrolyte balance and provide minimal calories. However, when the GI tract motility returns, oral diet can be resumed, starting with clear liquids to soft foods and then moving on to regular food.

Tube Feeding and Parenteral Nutrition

In severe cases or those with high nutrient needs are put on tube feeding or parenteral nutrition. One must wait for gastric motility to be restored, otherwise abdominal distension, nausea and vomiting complications may arise. Since peristalsis return more quickly to small intestine, feeding formulas directly into small intestine through a tube is more advantageous than parenteral nutrition. Early feeding, within 48 hours of stress, stimulates intestinal blood flow and adaptation, thus preventing hypermetabolism. Once oral feeding is possible, then both tube feeding and parenteral nutrition must be discontinued.

STRESS FORMULAS

There are available special formulations designed to meet the nutrient needs during stress. Many of these formulas have high nutrient density. Some contain extra vitamins A and C and zinc designed to promote wound healing. Others contain glutamine, argininie, nucleotides and omega-3 fatty acids. Arginine may help minimise negative nitrogen balance, improve wound healing and stimulate the immune system. Nucleotides are nitrogen-containing components of RNA and DNA that are important to the structure and functions of intestinal cells and may help improve the immune system.

NUTRITION DURING STRESS

The incidence of stress, marked by extensive tissue damage and hyper-metabolism, places heavy demands on the body system. Then the body uses its internal defence mechanism to survive and regain health. In the overall analysis, recovery depends upon replenishment of energy and nutrients, which would subsequently help mount a defence, repair the damaged tissue, and also restore the depleted reserves of nutrients in the body.

Adequate dietary protein is an important step during stress. The day's protein quota can be had from two servings of lean meat or chicken or fish. And for the vegetarians, two servings of low-fat dairy products or several servings of whole grain bread and cereals combined with vegetables, dried beans or peas would suffice.

Carbohydrate foods are particularly important, because the calories they provide prevent the dietary proteins from being used for the production of energy. Instead, these proteins can be used to maintain a healthy immune system and adequate muscle size. One must avoid salty foods. To supplement the dietary intake of vitamins, vitamin and mineral supplements or tablets may be used with advantage.

One must consume foods rich in vitamin C like citrus fruits, berries, broccoli and tomatoes, as also potassium. The latter include dark green leafy vegetables, bananas, tomatoes and dates. Low-fat milk/curds and cheese might help prevent loss of calcium from bones. One must take regular meals and avoid dieting.

In order to counter the threat of Cancer, owing to prolonged stress conditions, many nutritionists recommend high fibre diet. This diet offers the dual benefit:

(a) To counter the effect of high dietary fat
(b) To dilute and speed up the passage of cancer causing substances through the intestines.

Table 14.2 gives the menu for a high fibre diet for safeguarding against cancer.

EXERCISE

Physical exercise has two-pronged impact on stress. Firstly, it alleviates the physical and mental tensions and the physiological changes that accompany stressful conditions. Secondly, exercise itself acts like a stress on the body, changing patterns of nutrient use and creating a greater demand for additional nutrients. This means an increased need for water, calories, minerals and vitamins. But the most crucial factor is fluids. One must drink lots of water to provide the cells with ample fluids and to aid kidneys in flushing out the waste products from the body.

Regular exercise positively helps in relieving stress. Vigorous exercise also releases special compounds called 'Endorphins' from the brain—their effect resembles that of morphine and promotes a feeling of well-being. Three sessions a week of aerobic exercises of 20-30 minutes duration are a minimum requirement to provide improvement in cardiovascular fitness.

YOGA AND SKP

Yoga is the Eastern way of exercise that is moderate and well-regulated. Yoga asanas prevent the build up of chronic psychological stress, which is the root cause of high blood pressure and heart diseases. Yoga causes healthful physiological changes in the heart and circulatory system. The rate of blood flow increases and the heart becomes stronger and beats more rhythmically to pump blood in to the body. This way, the oxygen and nutrients reach body cells and waste products are carried away more efficiently. Elasticity of lungs increases, thus enabling more air being breathed in. Hence, greater amount of oxygen reaches the body cells, which would help delay positively the degenerative changes that accompany the process of aging.

TABLE 14.2: MENU FOR 45 g FIBRE DIET FOR STRESS-CANCER

	Item	Amount	Fibre (g)
Breakfast	All bran	1/3 cup	7.9
	Banana	1 medium	1.3
	Milk 1%	1 cup	—
	Orange juice	6 oz	0.6
	Whole wheat bread	2 slices	5.4
	Jelly	1 tsp	—
	Total fibre		**15.2 g**
Lunch	Salad:		
	Spinach	1 cup	2.2
	Carrots	¼ cup	0.8
	Lima beans	¼ cup	1.8
	Tomato	¼ cup	0.5
	Cheese	2 oz	—
	Dressing	1 tbsp	—
	Whole wheat roal	1	5.4
	Orange	1	3.8
	Total fibre		**14.5 g**
AN Snacks	Tangerine	1	1.8
	Rye crackers	2	1.5
	Total fibre		**3.3 g**
Dinner	Salmon fish	4 oz	—
	Baked potato with skin	1 medium	5.2
	Yogurt dressing	2 tbsp	—
	Broccoli	2/3 cup	3.2
	Dinner salad	1-1½ cup	2.0
	Dressing	2 tsp	—
	Total fibre		**10.4 g**
Bedtime Snacks	Graham Crackers	2	1.3 g
	Grand Total of Fibre Content		**44.7 g**

Source: David Heber *et al.* in *Stress and Nutrition*, Pub. CBS, Delhi.
One may profitably refer to the Chapter on Cancer for more such menus.

There are quite a large number of yogic exercises listed for relaxing the body. *Shishasan* (Dead man's pose) totally relaxes all the body muscles and nerves. But it is the *Pranayam* (breathing exercises), which have the maximum impact on countering or preventing stress.

Recent studies conducted at the Ali India Institute of Medical Sciences (AIIMS), Delhi have conclusively proved the link between rhythmic breathing exercises and a state of relaxed alertness. Dr. Kochu-pillai, Head, Rotary Cancer Hospital at AIIMS says that whatever affects the mind affects the body and vice versa and that stress could aggravate any disease, if not induce it. Herein, *Sudarshan Kriya* and *Pranayam* (SKP) impact was recorded on electro-encephalogram. Significant increase in beta activity (a measure of a person's state of alertness) was observed in the left frontal, occipital and mid-line regions of the brain, all of this indicative of heightened alertness. The SKP also had beneficial effect on the immune system; it reduced depression and also reduced the cholesterol levels.

Hence, exercise in the form of regular Yogic asanas provides the most efficacious mechanism to tackle and manage the negative effects of stress.

GUIDELINES FOR ANTI-STRESS DIET

1. Two-three servings of low-protein foods, say fish, poultry, lean meat, dried beans and peas.
2. Half the protein serving must come from plant foods, say fried beans, pea soup with a whole grain muffin.
3. Six servings of bread, cereals, pasta or grain and at least 50% of these should be whole grains.
4. Two to four servings of low-fat milk, buttermilk, yogurt, low-fat cottage cheese; also green leafy vegetables, ground sesame seeds to provide calcium.
5. Four servings of fruits and vegetables.
6. One vegetable serving high in folic acid, viz., spinach, broccoli, lettuce, green beans and chard.
7. One-two vitamin C-rich fruits and vegetables, viz., orange juice, grapefruit juice and broccoli.
8. Iron-rich foods, such as meats, legumes, grains and vegetables.
9. PUFA—vegetable oil 1 tbsp with seeds or nuts about ¼ cup.
10. High Fluid intake, about 6 to 8 glassfuls every day.

Avoid

- High Fat Meats
- Processed or Fast Foods
- Foods with artificial coloring and added salts
- Hydrogenated Oils
- Sugar, Salt, Coffee—very restricted
- Alcohol.

Environmental

Food Contamination

Water Pollution

Air Pollution

Virus

Bacteria

Noise

Cigarette Smoke

Medication

Nutritional

Sugar

Alcohol

Salt

Cholesterol

Caffeine
Colas
Chocolate
Tea
Coffee

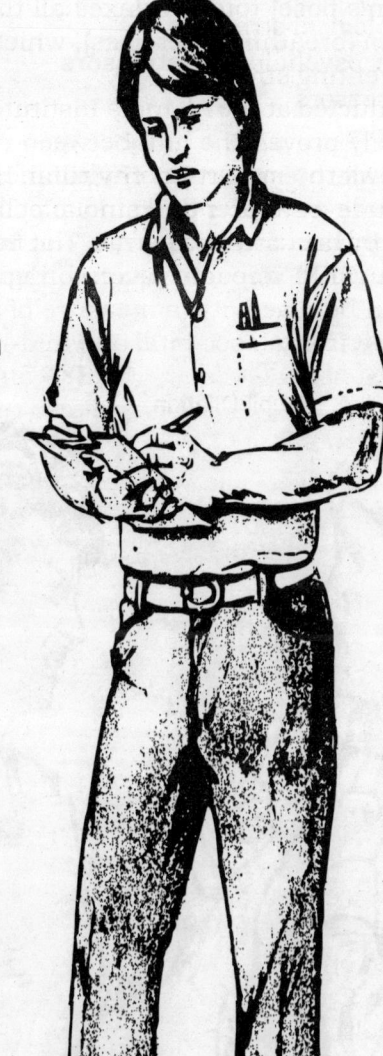

Fig. 1: Environmental Stressors

In day-to-day existence, the common life **stressors** can be of the following types:

1. Physical or physiological stressors
2. Socio-economic or psychological **stressors**
3. Environmental stressors
4. Nutritional stressors

The earlier Fig. 1 shows the important environmental and nutritional stress factors. The former include air, water and smoke pollution, food contamination and also contamination by bacteria and germs. The nutritional stressors include excessive use of salt, sugar, coffee and alcohol. Fig. 2 shows the social stress factors.

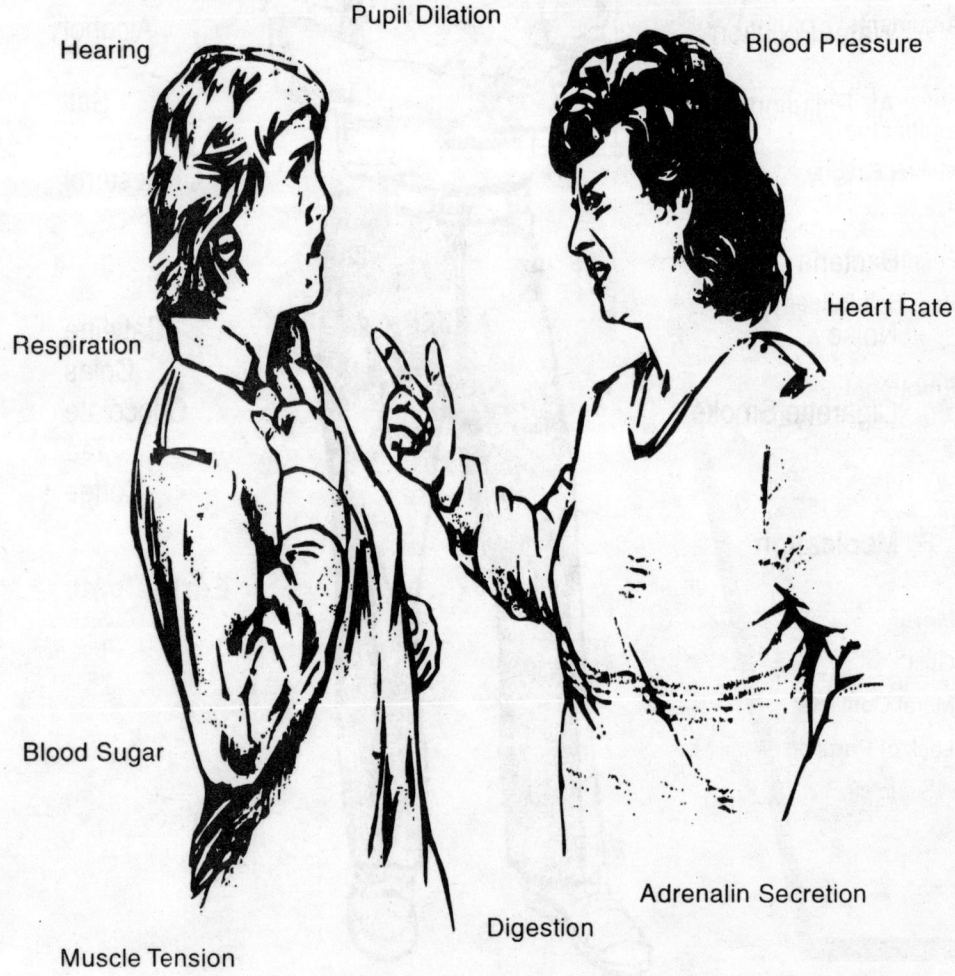

Fig. 2: The Fight or Flight Response to Stress

Howevers, it is the psychological factors listed in Appendix 1 which create the maximum havoc in a man's life.

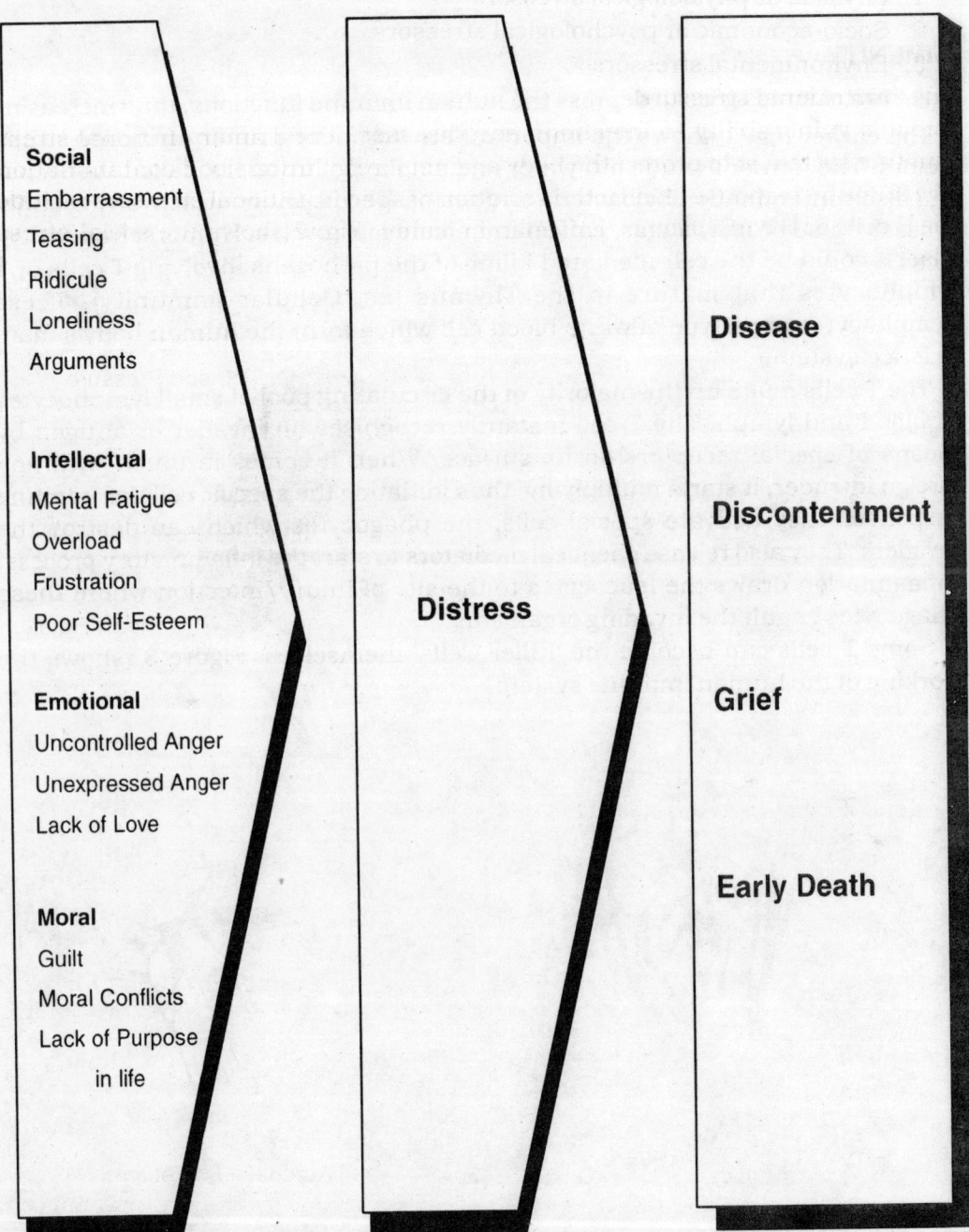

Social

Embarrassment

Teasing

Ridicule

Loneliness

Arguments

Intellectual

Mental Fatigue

Overload

Frustration

Poor Self-Esteem

Emotional

Uncontrolled Anger

Unexpressed Anger

Lack of Love

Moral

Guilt

Moral Conflicts

Lack of Purpose
    in life

Distress

Disease

Discontentment

Grief

Early Death

Psychological Stress Factors

APPENDIX 2

IMMUNITY

Any form of stress goes to depress the human immune functions, thus increasing a man's vulnerability to infections and diseases. The primary function of the immune system is to protect the body against foreign invaders, called 'Antigens'. The immune response leads tothe secretion of specific antibodies involving either the B cells or B lymphocytes derived from bone marrow (*i.e.* Humoral Immunity). Else, it could be the cell-mediated kiling of the pathogens involving T cells or T lymphocytes that mature in the Thymus (*i.e.* Cellular Immunity). These Lymphocytes are a type of white blood cell which form the human body's main defence system.

The T cells make up the majority of the circulating pool of small lymphocytes in blood and lymph. The T cell instantly recognises an invader or antigen by means of special receptors on its surface. When it comes in touch with any foreign intruder, it starts multiplying, thus initiating the specific cellular immune response. They activate special cells, the phagocytes which can destroy the invaders. They also release chemical mediators to start the inflammatory process. Inflammation draws the leucocytes to the site of injury/infection where these phagocytes engulf the invading organisms.

Some T cells can become the 'Killer Cells' themselves. Figure 3 shows the working of the human immune system.

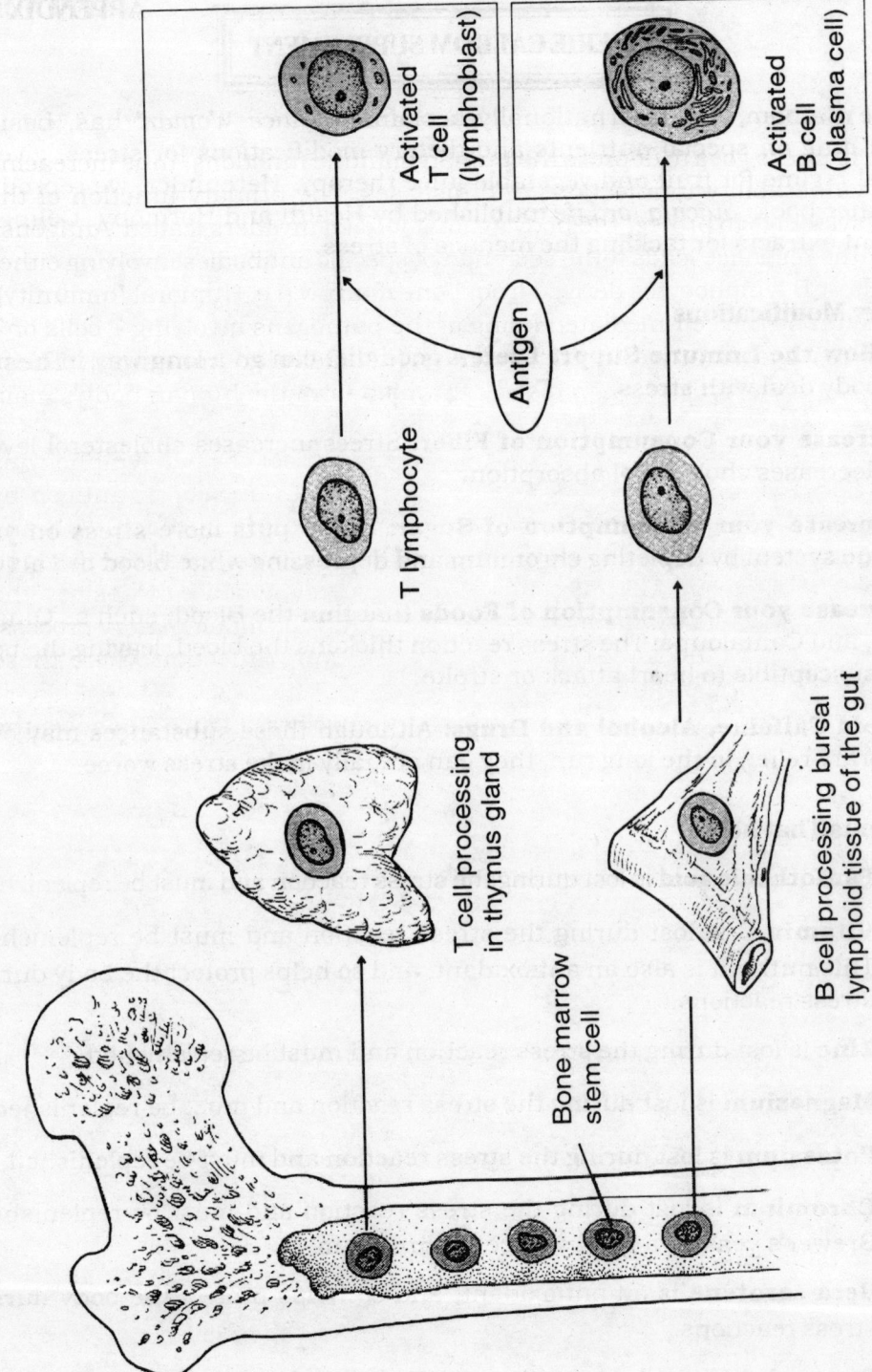

Fig. 3: Development of the T and B Cells, Lymphocyte Components of the Body's Immune System

Activated
T cell (lymphoblast)

Activated
B cell (plasma cell)

Antigen

T lymphocyte

T cell processing
in thymus gland

B cell processing bursal
lymphoid tissue of the gut

Bone marrow
stem cell

┌─────────────────────────────────┐
│ **CHERIE CALBOM SUPPLEMENT** │
└─────────────────────────────────┘

Cherie Calbom, the internationally-acclaimed '*Juice Woman*' has, besides elaborating on special nutrients and dietary modifications for stress, given a special regime for fruit and vegetable juice therapy. Hereunder, we reproduce from ther book: *Juicing for Life* (published by Health and Harmony, Delhi) the relevant extracts for tackling the menace of stress.

Dietary Modifications

1. Follow the Immune Supprt Diet: A good diet can go a long way in helping your body deal with stress.

2. Increase your Consumption of Fiber: Stress increases cholesterol levels: fiber decreases cholesterol absorption.

3. Decrease your Consumption of Sugar: Sugar puts more stress on your immune system by depleting chromium and depressing white blood cell action.

4. Increase your Consumption of Foods that thin the Blood, such as Ginger, Garlic, and Cantaloupe: The stress reaction thickens the blood, leaving the body more susceptible to heart attack or stroke.

5. Avoid Caffeine, Alcohol and Drugs: Although these substances may offer temporary relief, in the long run, they can actually make stress worse.

Nutrients That help

- **Pantothenic acid** is lost during the stress reaction and must be replenished.

- **Vitamin C** is lost during the stress reaction and must be replenished. This nutrient is also an antioxidant, and so helps protect the body during stress reactions.

- **Zinc** is lost during the stress reaction and must be replenished.

- **Magnesium** is lost during the stress reaction and must be replenished.

- **Potassium** is lost during the stress reaction and must be replenished.

- **Chromium** is lost during the stress reaction and must be replenished. Brewer's yeast is a good source of chromium.

- **Beta-carotene** is an antioxidant, and so helps protect the body during stress reactions.

- **B-complex Vitamins** are known as Antistress Vitamins.

Beneficial Juices

- Broccoli and kale—sources of pantothenic acid.
- Red pepper, kale and collard greens—sources of vitamin C.
- Ginger, parsley and carrot—sources of zinc.
- Collard greens and parsley—excellent sources of magnesium.
- Parsley, Swiss chard and spinach—sources of potassium.
- Carrot, collard greens and parsley—excellent sources of beta-carotene.
- Garlic, cantaloupe, and ginger—sources of blood-thinning compounds.

SUGGESTED JUICING RECIPES FOR STRESS

Ginger Hopper

¼-inch slice ginger root
4-5 carrots, greens removed
½ apple, seeded

Push ginger through hopper with carrots and apple

Magnesium Drink

1 garlic clove
Small handful parsley
4-5 carrots, greens removed
2 stalks celery
Parsley sprig for garnish

Wrap garlic in parsley, and push through hopper with carrots and celery. Pour juice into glass, and garnish with sprig of parsley.

Strawberry Shake

1 pint strawberries
½ firm pear
1 ripe banana
1 tsp. brewer's yeast

Push strawberries and pear through hopper. Place juice, banana, and yeast in blender or food processor, and blend until smooth

Spicy Cantaloupe Shake

¼-inch slice ginger root
½ cantaloupe, with skin

Push ginger through haooper with cantaloupe.

Super-Eight Stress Reliever

1 kale leaf
1 collard leaf
Small handful parsley
1 stalk celery
1 carrot, greens removed
½ red pepper
1 tomato
1 broccoli floweret
Celery stalk for garnish

Bunch up leaves and parsley, and push through hopper with celery and carrot. Follow with red pepper, tomato and broccoli. Garnish with celery stalk.

Garlic Express

Handful Parsley
1 garlic clove
4-5 carrots, greens removed
2 stalks celery

Bunch up parsley and push through hopper with garlic, carrots, and celery.

Traditional Sleep Potion

3-4 lettuce leaves
1 stalk celery

Bunch up lettuce and push through hopper with celery. Drink 30 minutes before bedtime.

Potassium Broth

Handful parsley
Handful spinach
4-5 carrots, greens removed
2 stalks celery

Bunch up parsley and spinach leaves, and push through hopper with carrots and celery.

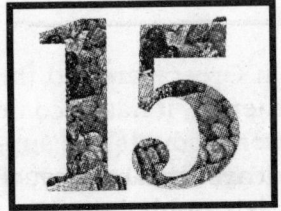

15

DIET AND ATHLETICS (Sports Nutrition)

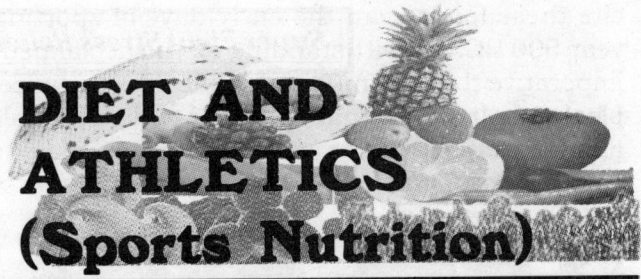

The modern world of sports makes high demand on the nutritional resources of the athletes, sportsmen and sportswomen. There has been a renewed interest amongst both sports authorities and nutritionists about the direct influence of gastronomic issues on physical, rather '*Peak Performance*' and well-being of the players and the athletes. Unlike the conventional norms and RDA for heavy physical work, mainly miners and the lumberjacks, there is a sudden spurt in energy and nutrient requirement of the athletes at a particular moment, since their relative work intensity shoots up out of all proportion to any physical activity. Research in nutrition laboratories in the West have unequivocally proved that dietary manipulation positively leads to improved physical performance. As such, many extraordinary sports food, nay fads, guided solely by commercial considerations, have invaded the market. Special mention needs be made of Carbohydrate Electrolyte Solutions (CES) being concertedly promoted in the sports field. At the same time, there is a steadily growing interest in the Functional (Organic) Foods, which have a definitive effect on the body functions in a positive manner.

Several new elements and compounds classified as 'Other Substances in Foods' have been reviewed for their added physical performance. Wolinsky, Ira, Driskell and Judy have scrutinised the Sports Nutrition as regards vitamins and trace elements are concerned. Herein, newer elements are Co-enzyme Q10, vitamin B_{15}, glandulars, herbs, ginseng and bee pollen. These products are mainly exploited for various healing properties or ergogenic aids, particularly for the athletes.

Reindeer Milk

Remember the introduction of Reindeer milk during the Montreal Olympics or the Special Chinese Herbals during the Barcelona Olympics. We may as well cite these foods from the early days of sporting activity in Greece around the year 500 BC. Notwithstanding all the acclaimed benefits thereof, it has become imperative that one must scientifically scrutinise these newer products and supplements. It is time that we learnt to discriminate between the factual relevance and the exaggerated hype and fantasies created calculatedly around these 'New Sports Utopias'.

FUEL SOURCES

The phosphate bonds form high-energy compounds in body metabolism. The main high-energy compound of the body cells is *Adenosine triphosphate (ATP)*, whch is also designated as the '*Energy Currency*' of the cell. Different forms of energy are called on for the successive energy needs of the body, as under:

1. Immediate Energy

For high-powered needs, the ATP is readily available within the muscle cells. It is used up rapidly and a back-up compound, *Creatine Phosphate* is made available. But these compounds will sustain all-out exercises only for 5-8 seconds.

2. Short-term Energy

For events lasting longer than 30 seconds and up to 2 minutes, muscle glycogen supplies' the short-term needs. Although the amount of available glycogen is small, it is an important rapid source for brief muscular effort.

3. Long-term Energy

The exercises lasting for more than 2 minutes call for an oxygen-dependent or *Aerobic* energy system. Thic can ensure a constant supply of glycogen in the blood. Special cells organelles, *Mitochondria*, located within each cell, produce large amount of ATP. The ATP is produced mainly from the glucose and fatty acids and supplies continued energy to the body for events or exercises for longer duration.

ENERGY FOR PHYSICAL PERFORMANCE

Energy is the prime need for optimum physical performance in the sports field. Normally, a sedentary adult has an energy expenditure between 8.5 and 12.0 MJ per day. As against this, in the athletics the physical activity, whether for training or competition, goes by minutes or hours. This energy expenditure amounts to 2-4 MJ per hour. An average physical activity of 2 to 3 hours would mean almost doubling up the normal energy expenditure.

For example, a Marathon race means expending 10-12 MJ energy. This works out to 3.2 MJ/hour in a recreational athlete and 6.3 MJ/hr in the most intensive phase. In a cross country cycling race, as in France, this figure goes up to 27 MJ/day and further shoots up to 40 MJ when cycling over the mountains. Such inordinately heavy expenditure of energy cannot be easily compensated by the ingestion of normal solid meals, since digestion and absorption process will be impaired during intense physical activity. Hence, there comes the imperative of Energy-rich snacks and 'In-between Meals', which may contribute up to 40% of the total energy required. But these snacks being low in proteins and micro-nutrients could lead to an imbalanced diet.

For maximal muscle performance, the muscle cells depend completely on carbohydrate (CHO) as a substrate. As such, the diet selected for the athletes must provide not only the immediate energy, but also for substrate sources, especially CHO and fat. But the athletes, despite their very high energy expenditure, are required to maintain a low body weight, which poses a ticklish problem.

Carbohydrates

Carbohydrates are the most important fuel for high-intensity exercise and physical performance. But the limited store of glycogen in liver and muscles (Endogenous CHO) lasts barely 60-90 minutes of moderately intense exercise. The body carbohydrate reserve is limited to 400 g only, 100 g as glycogen in the liver and 300 g in the muscles. The muscle biopsy techniques have brought out the fact that muscle/liver glycogen concentration plays a pivotal role in the onset of fatigue. These reserves help maintain a constant plasma glucose level between meals or during exercise, thereby ensuring appropriate substrate supply for those organs like brain, which depend solely upon glucose for their energy needs.

The muscle fibres recruited during anaerobic exercises like sprinting and weight lifting rely heavily on the cellular content of high-energy phosphates (ATP, phospho-creatine) and glycogen-derived glucose, for which purpose fatty acids are not so suitable.

Table 15.1 shows the rate of High-Energy Phosphate (HEP) formation in the muscles, as also the rate of their utilization.

TABLE 15.1: HIGH-ENERGY PHOSPHATE (HEP) PRODUCTION AND UTILIZATION

	Substrate Utilized	Max. Rate of Formation (mol HEP/min.)	Type of Exercise	Rate of Utilization (mol HEP/min)
1.	Endogenous Glycogen (Anaerobic)	2.4	Rest	0.07
2.	Endogenous Glycogen (Aerobic)	1.0	100 metres Sprint	2.06
3.	Blood-borne Glucose	0.37	1500 metres Sprint	1.70
4.	Blood-borne Fatty acids	0.40	Marathon	1.0

Source: Human Nutrition and Dietetics, Pub. Churchill Livingstone

The endogenous muscle energy stores of glycogen and triglycerides are very important when the demands are higher with the increasing power output. In case of glycogen depletion in the muscles, exercise intensity is limited, since ATP production will slow down due to reliance on fats as the substrate. In case there is no CHO intake, the HGP depends entirely on liver glycogen and hepatic gluconeogenesis to produce a constant outflow of glucose and to prevent Hypoglycemia, which is indeed a very serious situation. The liver usually does not allow an increase in glucose output and thus the muscle uptake greater than about one gram per minute.

Glycogen Loading

To keep the body saturated with carbohydrates in order to maximise tissue glycogen levels, an athlete must consume 60-70% of dietary energy as carbohydrates, i.e. 600-800 g CHO daily. This works out to about 3 loaves of bread or 15 cooked potatoes or 15 cups of rice daily. To train for a special event, the exercise is tapered; it usually starts just a week before the event. Every second day, the amount of exercise is halved, until no exercise is performed on the last day. The high-carbohydrate diet is consumed throughout the week. This technique, called 'Glycogen Loading' or 'Super-compensation', yields tissue glycogen level that definitely improve the performance. Sports authorities recommend this Glycogen loading for events that would last up to 2 hours or longer. Detailed analysis of glycogen loading is shown in the Appendix 1 at the end of Chapter.

The nutritionists generally recommend that the endogenous carbohydrate intake should be around 1-1.2 g/min. during the exercise period. Glucose, sucrose and maltodextrins help maintain the blood glucose concentration, CHO oxidation and also help in improving performance. On the other hand, fructose, galactose and amylose result in lower carbohydrate oxidation.

Both climatic conditions and quantitative sweat loss determine the priorities for water and carbohydrate ingestion. Besides, gastric emptying and intestinal absorption also count in this matter.

Optimal carbohydrate sources for high-intensity endurance exercises are processed carbohydrates low in dietary fibre, such as glucose, sucrose, maltose and maltodextrins or soluble starch like the corn starch. Diet must be strongly hypertonic with dissolved mono-/di-sachharides, but not containing maltodextrins/polymers or starch.

The rate of 'Muscle Glycogen Re-synthesis', following exercise, is an important factor in recovery. It is usually restored at a rated of 3-7%, thus requiring about 20 hours to recover fully. This rate of resynthesis is higher during the first two hours after exercise has taken place. As such, an athlete should start eating carbohydrates as soon as possible after the exercise is over.

Fats

Large amount of fats are stored as triglycerides (TG) within the muscle fibres (IMTG, Intramuscular triglycerides). But the rate of fat mobilization from these stores is limited. In the circulation, free fatty acids are bound to albumin, while TGs are transported within low-density lipoproteins.

Another important fact about fat is the adaptation to increased reliance on fat as a substrate during endurance training. The increase in fat oxidation is accompanied by a reduction in glycogen use at a given sub-optimal intensity.

Several studies have shown that fat oxidation during exercise is very sensitive to dietary carbohydrates in the hours before exercise even in relatively small amounts. The medium-chain triglyerides are oxidized almost as rapidly as glucose, and even better when these are combined with glucose.

Creatine and Phosphocreatine

Creatine is another food-ingredient of great importance in high-intensity, short duration exercises like sprinting. Fatigue during short duration exercise has been associated with the depletion of phosphocreatine. By helping reduce the muscle ATP degradation, the creatine level increase can result in significant increase in work output of about 5%.

Proteins

Most RDA agencies do not provide for additional allowance for proteins for active individuals. However, regular exercise does increase the protein needs of the body. In general, the increased protein needs are covered by an increased fat intake. In case of very intense activity the cycling marathon in France, it is found to go up to 3g/kg per day.

The use of amino acids like Arginine and Ornithine is gaining considerable ground. Ingestion of glutamine has been proposed as a means to support the immune competence of athletes engaged in intense daily training. It has been suggested that Branched chain amino acids (BCAA) like valine, leucine and isoleucine are more important, since they are taken up by active muscles during exercise, while most of the other amino acids are released by active muscles.

The current view is that the sport athletes should take 1.2-1.7 g proteins/kg body weight every day and further that the endurance athletes take 1.2-1.4 g/kg body weight per day.

There is a physiological need for higher protein intake as there is a greater breakdown and turn-over of the proteins during heavy exercise and loss of amino acids in sweat. As commented upon by Dr. Narasingha Rao (Ex-Director, NIN, Hyderabad) the protein levels suggested above can take care of all the physiological and metabolic needs of the sports persons. Table 15.2 shows the nutrients needed for male and female athletes.

Fluid Balance

Each one litre of oxygen consumed during intensive endurance exercises will contribute about 20 kJ energy. Of this, only 25% is used for mechanical work, while the remaining 75% is released as heat. Heat loss by convection can be increased considerably, by streaming air (wind) or water. Evaporation of sweat is an important way of eliminating heat in warm environment. At maximal sweat rates, a 70 kg male athlete may lose more than 30 ml/min or 1800 ml/hr of sweat. Without appropriate 'Rehydration', blood flow through the extremities and the skin will decrease and the sweat response diminished. This may cause hypothermia, along with many other associated health risks.

TABLE 15.2: COMPARISON OF NUTRIENTS IN MIDDLE AGE MALE AND FEMALE ATHLETES

Nutrients	Male	Female
Calories (kcal/d)	2959	2386
Proteins (g/d)	102.1	82.2
Proteins (%)	13.8	14.2
Fats (g/d)	134.4	110.7
Fats (%)	40.8	41.1
Carbohydrates (g/d)	294.6	234.3
Carbohydrates (%)	39.8	39.5
Cholesterol (mg. 1000 kcal^{-1})	190.0	205.0
Saturated Fat (g. 100 kcal^{-1})	16.8	16.5
Polyunsaturated Fat (g. 1000 kcal^{-1})	8.5	7.9

Source: Blair S. N. *et al.,* Comparison of nutrient intake the middle aged athletes. *Med. Sci. Sports Excerc.,* **13**: 310,1981.

Therefore, in most exercises/events of 3-4 hours duration, one must ensure that fluid and glucose is made available to prevent exhaustion and heat stroke. When the athletes are dehydrated, *i.e.* fluid loss exceeds 4% of the body weight, there is a higher frequency of gastrointestinal distress symptoms. Hence, restoration of fluid balance after exercise can only be achieved if sweat electrolyte losses as well as water are promptly replaced. As such, the restoration of fluid balance after exercise is an important part of the recovery process.

There is evidence that the limiting factor in long, strenuous exercise is muscle glycogen. Karlson and Satten (1971) showed that it was possible to raise the mean value of glycogen in a biopsy specimen of muscle from 17 g to 35 g/kg by feeding a high carbohydrate diet for 3 days after preliminary exhaustion of the muscle glycogen by hard exercise. This helped improve performance when running a distance of 30 km.

During long athletic performance, some food should be taken. Sugar is easily assimilated and can be safely recommended. It is better to take small quantity, say 50 g sugar each hour. It is also necessary to replace fluids and salt losses in sweat at regular intervals.

Special Supplements

Nutritious diet apart, sportsmen and athletes do need special *'Performance Enhancers'*, as listed in Table 15.3.

TABLE 15.3: SPECIAL SUPPLEMENTS FOR BOOSTING PERFORMANCE

1. **Additional Nutrients**
   - (*a*) Carbohydrate loading to enhance the glycogen storage level before competition.
   - (*b*) Additional vitamins and minerals to help optimize utilization.
   - (*c*) Glucose-electrolyte to be given during the event.
   - (*d*) Extra protein supplementation.

2. **Antioxidant Supplements**
   Antioxidant supplements protect from free radical damage. These could be:
   - (*i*) Nutrient antioxidants, e.g., tocopherols, ascorbic acid, β and α carotenes, riboflavin, glutathione, selenium, vitamin A.
   - (*ii*) Non-nutrient antioxidants, e.g. carotenoids, flavours, polyphenols. Isothiocyanates and terepenes.

3. **Other Non-specific Supplements** like ginseng etc.

OTHER SUBSTANCES AFFECTING ATHLETIC PERFORMANCE

Ginseng

Animals studies on various extracts containing ginsenosides have been shown to spare glycogen and increase fatty acid oxidation. Others have reported increasing endurance and reduction of fatigue. All these have encouraged the use of ginseng as an ergogenic aid in athletes. Appendix 4 at the end of the chapter gives a very comprehensive picture of these Ergogenic aids.

Wheat Germ Oil

Wheat Germ oil contains an active component: 'Octacosanol', which is a long-chain waxy alcohol. It has reported improvement in endurance, which is attributed to increased oxygen transport. Some other researchers have reported improved conditioned reflexes.

Bee Pollen

Bee pollen is a compound containing many vitamins and minerals. And these participate in the energy cycle as Co-factors. Hence, Bee pollen is believed to have ergogenic properties.

Caffeine

Caffeine ingestion increases plasma free fatty acid concentration, as also glycerol. It is reported to take longer time to exhaustion or total work. This time too exhaustion appeared in several studies.

Other Compounds

Because of the biological functions of choline, its supplementation has been promoted as an ergogenic aid. Similar is the case with Carnitine. Ubiquinone (CoQ_{10}) is involved in the oxidative phosphorylation process. Bicarbonates have been reported to have beneficial effect on physical performance. Vitamin B_{15} (DMG) lowers lactic acid levels and increases oxygen utilization in humans. Other compounds with ergogenic and anabolic benefits are Oryzanole, ferulic acid, glandular, smilax and yohimbine.

Vitamins and Minerals

Nearly 40-50% of the American athletes use supplements with vitamins and minerals for enhancing their performance, the vitamin level occasionally going up to 10-100 times the RDA levels. Vitamin C, in doses of 100-500 mg appears to produce ergogenic effect. Thaimine contributes to neuromuscular functioning. It is also needed for carbohydrate and amino acid metabolism. Riboflavin and Niacin improve respiratory metabolism. Vitamin B_6 is involved in the protective effect of exercise on cardiovascular diseases. Pantothenic acid and biotin contribute to better energy metabolism.

Similarly, fat-soluble vitamins A, D, E and K too help in the overall improvement and consequently better physical performance. β-carotenes have antioxidant functions.

Amongst the minerals, iron deficiency leads to diminished physical capacity. Zinc plays a positive role in carbohydrate, lipid and protein metabolism and so it is needed for optimal physical performance. Copper functions as a component of the antioxidant system. Chromium (-picolinate) is a well-acclaimed ergogenic product, which increases lean body mass and decreases body fat. Selenium, acting as an antioxidant, may protect tissues from oxidative stress induced by exercise.

Other compounds that are often used as ergogenic agents are:

- Boron
- Coenzyme Q10
- Inosine
- Aspartates
- Bicarbonates
- Phosphate salts.

However, there does not exist much data to support the claim of most of these compounds and supplements. Probably it is their overall *'Feel good'* effect that psychologically influences the athletes to resort to these ergogenic agents. In that respect, it does help in the improvement of physical performance.

GLYCOGEN LOADING TECHNIQUES

The athletes often resort to Glycogen Loading in three stages, as shown in Appendix Table 15.1, in order to build up their glycogen reserves for strenuous endurance events. However, it is advisable not to adopt this practice frequently, since it carries potential side effects. A modern less taxing strategy consists of a *'Depletion-Tapering'* sequence, as indicated in Appendix Table 15.2. This tapering technique is preferred by the athletes now-a-days.

APPENDIX TABLE 15.1: GLYCOGEN-LOADING PROGRAM BEFORE ENDURANCE EVENTS

Stage	Time Period	Exerices	Diet	Nutrient Schedule (% Total kcal)
Stage 1:				
Muscle Glycogen Depletion	4-7 days before the event	Exhausting exercise of same type in event in the first half of period; general training during diet changes in the second half of period.	Second half—high protein, high fat and low carbohydrate diet	Carbohydrates 6% Proteins 54% Fat 40%
Stage 2:				
Muscle Glycogen Super-saturation	1-3 days before the event	None	High CHO, Low fat, Normal proteins	CHO 80% Proteins 15% Fat 5%
Stage 3:				
Muscle Glycogen Use	On the day of the event	Endurance Event Exercise	Regular	CHO 50% Proteins 20% Fat 30%

Adapted from Forgac: Carbohydrate Loading—A Review, *J. Am. Diet Ass.*, **75**(1): 42, 1970.

APPENDIX TABLE 15.2: DEPLETION-TAPERING GLYCOGEN LOADING TECHNIQUE

Days	Exercise	Diet
1	90 minute period at 70-75% VO_2 max.	Mixed diet—50% CHO (350 g)
2-3	Gradual tapering of time and intensity	Same as above
4-5	Tapering of exercise time and intensity continues	Mixed diet—70% CHO (550 g)
6	Complete rest	Same as above
7	Day of competition	High CHO pre-event diet

Adapted form Wright: Carbohydrate Nutrition and Exercise. *Clin. Nutr.*, **7**(1): 18, 1988.

MARATHON

Marathon is a classic endurance sport run for 42 km. There are two basic pre-requisites for this:

(1) Sufficient glycogen stores to meet their needs throughout the race and

(2) Large aerobic capacity to enable them to "spare" glycogen by burning fatty acids at a high rate.

When the marathoner runs out of glycogen, exercise cannot continue. This is a classic phenomenon known as 'Hitting the wall.' In the mid-1960s, Bergstrom and Hulman explored this glycogen relationship by subjecting their athletes to exhaustive exercise, feeding them for 3 days on a low-carbohydrate diet with continued exercise, feeding them for the next 3 days on a high-carbohydrate diet with little exercise, and then having them perform the exercise again. Needle biopsies showed an increase in muscle glycogen stores in this regimen. The athletes' subsequent performance was nearly twice the prior work load.

This became known as 'Carbohydrate Loading,' or 'Glycogen Supersaturation.' The initial exhaustive exercise and 3 days of low-carbohydrate diet ensures a depletion of glycogen stores. In the absence of exercise but the presence of a high-carbohydrate diet, the body is able to pack away more glycogen than it stored before depletion. If done too frequently, it takes a large toll. The phase of glycogen depletion through a low-carbohydrate diet is physically and psychologically taxing. The athelete becomes nauseous, weak, irritable and depressed. Exhaustive exercise at this point may be counterproductive to preparation for the event.

Others have recommended a modified regimen that eliminates the depletion phase. By simply reducing the level of exercise to minimal, and eating a high-carbohydrate diet for 2 to 3 days before competition, the athlete's glycogen stores may be increased to levels comparable to the classic method of 'Loading'.

Each one gram of glycogen is stored with 3 g of water. Glycogen loading thus leads to an increase in weight and sometimes to a sensation of muscle stiffness. However, added water is important in the prevention of dehydration during a long-distance effort.

Glycogen-loading will benefit performance only if the exercise is of extended duration, in excess of 1.5 to 2.0 hours. The procedure is specifically designated for 'Endurance Sports'. The classic approach does carry dangers, and to prevent possible trauma to muscle tissues, most experts recommend that this more strennous procedure not be practiced more than 2 or 3 times a year. However, the newer, more modified depletion-taper approach does not carry these dangers and may be used more often. And, in the long run, it is more productive.

SPORTS ANEMIA

Athletes occasionally report anemia with endurance exercise. Reduced hemoglobin in a runner's blood means reduced oxygen-carrying capacity, with obvious implications for aerobic capacity and ability to sustain an excessive workload.

Anemia means hemoglobin (Hgb) level less than 12 g% for women (normal 14) and less than 14 g% for men (normal 16). So far, very little is known about the relative influence on athletic performance of Hgb levels within the normal range. Some suggest that athletes' Hgb levels should be higher for optimal performance although excessive concentrations of Hgb lead to increased blood viscosity, resulting in decreased rate of blood flow. Maintenance of Hgb levels at least at the normal levels for women and men have been proposed.

Anemia is rare among competitive athletes. Heavy exercise may induce transient anemia during the initial weeks of training, with Hgb stabilizing in the long run at the low end of normal. But strenuous continued exercise is also associated with low iron stores in athletes, which could pose long-term problems.

The possible causes of sports anemia include:

(1) A diet inadequate in iron
(2) Decreased iron absorption
(3) Increased iron losses

Few studies have revealed a diet low in iron, decreased absorption and increased loss are more probable causes. Women athletes have cyclic menstrual loss of iron, unless they have amenorrhea. Recent studies have shown that significant amounts of iron is lost in profuse sweating. Another possibility is occasional *intravascular hemolysis,* the rupture of red blood cells (RBC) as a result of the stress of heavy exercise. This effect could be transient or chronic. It is manifested as free Hgb in the urine but it is a rare occurence.

Another factor in athletes' low-normal Hgb levels may be *hemodilution.* Strenuous training leads to an increase in both plasma volume and absolute quantity of Hgb, but the increases may not be proportional, plasma volume increases more than Hgb. Hemodilution with increased iron loss and increased red blood cell turnover could account for the prevalence of low normal values among athletes. Obviously, this situation is complicated if the diet is inadequate in bioavailable iron.

EROGOGENIC AIDS FOR ATHLETES

Aid	Description	Claim	Adverse Side Effects/Caution
Bee Pollen	Mixture of bee saliva, plant nectar and pollen	Increases energy levels, enhances physical fitness	Reports anecdotal; not proven; allergic reactions in bee-sensitive individuals most common adverse side effect, because of content of nucleic acids, should be avoided by those with gout
Brewer's Yeast	Byproduct of beer brewing; rich source of B vitamins and bioavailable chromium	Increases energy levels	Claims of blood glucose improvement due to chromium content are documented
Carnitine	A compound synthesized in the body from lysine and methionine	Improves cardiovascular function and muscle strength; delays fatigue; decreases muscle pain; decreases body fat	Although necessary for fat metabolism, the body syntheizes adequate amounts
Choline	Precursor of the neurotransmitter acetylcholine	Improves performance	
DNA/RNA	Deoxyribonucleic acid, ribonucleic acid	Tissue regeneration	Should be avoided by athletes with gout
Gelatin	Obtained from collagen	Improves muscle contraction	
Ginseng	Extract of ginseng root	Protects against tissue damage	Ginseng products (teas, powders, extracts, teas) are of variable quality and strength because of expense of the authentic product
Glycine	An amino acid that is a phospho-creatine precursor	Improves muscle contraction	
Kelp	Seaweed	Vitamin/mineral source	

Lecithin	Phosphatidylcholine	Decreases triglyceride and cholesterol levels	
Octacasanol	Alcohol isolate extracted from Wheat germ oil	Supplies energy and improves performance	
Pangamic acid	Also referred to as vitamin B_{15}; varied composition depending on the supplier	Increases delivery of oxygen	
Royal Jelly	Substance produced by worker bees and fed to the Queen bee	Increases strength	
Spirulina	Microscopic blue green algae; excellent source of β-carotene	Protein source	Probably does not function as protein source, but supplies β-carotene, a powerful antioxidant for which athletes may have increased need
Superoxide dismutase	Antioxidant enzyme system	Protects body against oxidative cell damage incurred from aerobic metabolism	Antioxidant protection provided may affect recovery from athletic endeavors
Amino acid Supplements	Arginine, ornithine, glycine plus lysine, predigested amino acids, branch-chain amino acids	Promote muscle development	

Source: Krause's *Food, Nutrition and Diet Therapy.*

PART 3

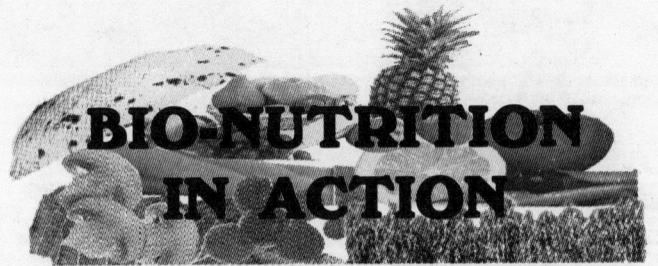

BIO-NUTRITION
IN ACTION

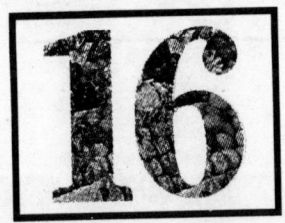

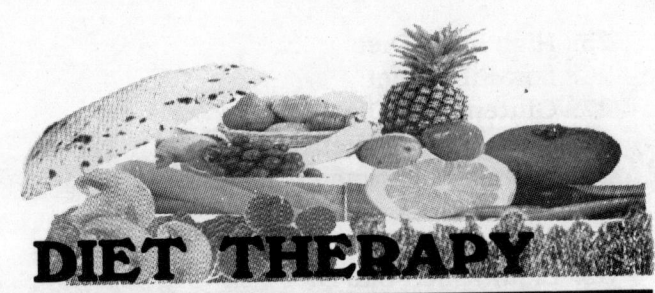

DIET THERAPY

THERAPEUTIC DIETS

1. Acid-Ash Diet
2. Alkali-Ash Diet
3. Aspartame-Restricted Diet
4. Bland Diet
5. Brat Diet
6. Calcium-modified Diet
7. High Calcium Diet
8. Low Calcium Diet
9. Low Calorie Diet
10. Moderate Calorie Diet
11. Very Low Calorie Diet
12. High Calorie Diet
13. Restricted Carbohydrate Diet
14. High Carbohydrate Diet
15. Cholesterol-Restricted Diet
16. Low Cholesterol, Fat-Controlled Diet
17. Copper-Restricted Diet
18. Elemental Diet
19. Diabetic Diet
20. Fat-Controlled Diet (Low Fat Diet)
21. High Monounsaturated Fat Diet
22. Liberal Fat Diet
23. MCT Fat Diet
24. Moderate Fat Diet

25. High Fibre Diet
26. Low Fibre Diet
27. Gluten-Free Diet
28. High Altitude Diet
29. Lactose-Restricted Diet
30. Liquid Diets, Blendeized
31. Liquid Diet, Clear
32. Liquid Microbial Diet
33. Oxalate-Restricted Diet
34. Potassium (High) Diet
35. High Protein Diet
36. Protein Minimal Diet
37. Prudent Diet
38. Purine-Restricted Diet
39. Sodium-Restricted Diet
40. Soy-Restricted Diet

DIET THERAPY

Diet Therapy is that branch of Bio-Nutrition which is concerned with the use of food for therapeutic purposes.

Be whatsoever the phase of human development, else the state of his health, dietetic intervention is invariably called for so that his system performs at the most optimum level. In fact, diet is an essential pre-requisite for the success of any medical treatment.

Medication alone is not always supposed to cure any health disorder, unless it is accompanied by good nutritional management alongside. As Sue R. Williams has aptly summed up,

'*Frequently, Diet is the Primary Therapy itself.*'

Clinically speaking, Diet Therapy may be reckoned as the '*Quintessential Shield*' that protects a person from further attack of a disease, while at the same time, it helps restore the normal health.

Normally, the experts refer to a 'Balanced Diet'. It is the meticulous blending and modification of all the nutrients, nay their 'tailoring' to specific deficiencies (or excess) that forms the core of diet therapy.

Objectives of Diet Therapy

The main objectives of diet therapy are

1. To maintain optimal nutrition status
2. To correct any deficiency or abnormality
3. To afford rest to the body or select organs affected by the disease
4. To alter and adjust the food intake to suit a particular metabolic status
5. To bring about desired changes in the body weight, where necessary.

Types of Food

Dietetic Foods

These are the processed foods specifically meant for therapeutic usage. In the West, quite a large range of dietetic foods are commercially available.

The most common Dietetic Foods are the non-nutritive, albeit artificial sweeteners like low-calorie soft drinks, canned fruits and juices, gelatin desserts and baked foods, plus confectionary. Others may be low in sodium, cholesterol, fats and calories.

Medical Foods

Medical foods are special formulations that are administered under strict medical supervision and are meant selectively for dietary management of a disease. These medical foods are used for the primary treatment of metabolic and genetic disorders.

Basic Concepts of Diet Therapy

1. Normal Nutrition Balance

A Therapeutic diet is usually based on the normal nutritional requirement of a particular patient. It has been modified to suit a special health contingency or a specific need of a person. For example, it is indeed gratifying for the parents to be told of the food plan that is based on the growth and development needs of the child and further that the formulation has been designed to make use of the regularly available foods.

2. Disease Application

The changes herein include:

(a) Modification of one or more basic nutrients like proteins, fats, carbohydrates and vitamins etc
(b) Modification in energy value, expressed as kilocalories
(c) Modification in texture, such as liquid diet or low-residue diet.

3. Individual Adaptation

A therapeutic diet, though theoretically correct, if not accepted by the person, will not mean anything. Hence, it must, as far as possible, conform to his habits, tastes and local customs too. Individual adaptation of the diet to meet particular needs are indeed imperative for any successful therapy.

When and Why

Therapeutic diets may be required in the following situations:

1. When the food intake is altered, as in impaired appetite, gastrointestinal and nervous disorders, conditions of pregnancy, anorexia and alcoholism, besides psychiatric problems.

2. Mal-absorption, as in gastrointestinal hypermotility or in impaired mucosa and drug abuse, leading to interference with absorption.
3. When utilization or storage is interfered with, as in impaired liver function, gastric ulcers and hypothyroidism and after radiation therapy.
4. In cased of increased nutritional requirements, as in athletics, lactation, pregnancy and drug therapy.

MODIFICATIONS IN DIET

The progressive therapeutic diet may be:

    (a) Liquid diet
    (b) Soft Diet
    (c) Light Diet

Certain nutrients need to be adjusted or modified, say carbohydrates, proteins, fats, electrolytes, vitamins and minerals. A few illustrations of modified diets are:

1. Acid-ash diet
2. Alkali-ash diet
3. Aspartame-restricted diet
4. High and low calcium diet
5. High-calorie diet
6. Carbohydrate-restricted diet
7. Cholesterol-restricted diet
8. Diabetic diet
9. Fat-controlled diet
10. Liberal fat diet
11. MCT fat diet
12. High-fibre diet
13. Gluten-free diet
14. High altitude diet
15. Lactose-restricted diet
16. Oxalate-restricted diet
17. High potash diet
18. High protein diet
19. Minimal protein diet
20. Prudent diet
21. Purine-restricted diet
22. Sodium-restricted diet

In this chapter, 40 types of Therapeutic Diets have been exemplified. To make it more beneficial for the Third world denizens, appropriate illustrations have been provided, as recomended by the Indian Council of Medical Research (ICMR). Without anyway implying a diet's extra merit or significance, these are being presented here in an alphabetic order.

1. ACID-ASH DIET

Acid-forming diets are specially recommended when excretion of kidney stones (comprising of calcium, magnesium, phosphorus, carbonates and oxalates) is desired. And also in medication of urinary tract infections.

These acid-forming foods are:

Fruits (except plums, prunes and cranberries).

Vegetables and cereals (except corn and pulses).

Milk, Meat, Fish, Poultry and Eggs.

Cereal and Grain products.

2. ALKALI-ASH DIET

The alkali-forming diets are recommended for patients with uric acid and cystic stones in kidneys. An alkaline urine helps in keeping these stones in solution, thus making it easy for excretion.

These alkali-forming foods are:

Fruits and vegetables, as above

Milk and milk products

Meat, eggs, fish and cereals being acid-forming foods, their usage are restricted.

Note: Foods in Nos. 1 and 2 are used as an adjunct with acidifying or alkalinizing drugs.

3. ASPARTAME-RESTRICTED FOODS

Aspartame, the low-calorie sweetener (it is 200 times more sweet than sucrose) is contraindicated in conditions like Phenylketonuria (PKU).
FDA has set a limit of 40-50 mg aspartame per kg of body weight.
One can of diet soda contains about 200 mg aspartame.

4. BLAND DIET

Bland Diets are used in treating gastric and duodenum ulcers, since they restrict the use of substances that can cause gastric irritation and excessive gastric acid secretion.

The substances to be avoided include:

Black pepper,   Brans and coarse grains
Raw vegetables   Skins and Seeds of Fruits
Red pepper and chillies   Fried foods
Pickles and chutneys   Meat extracts and soups
Coffee and Caffeinated Drinks   Chocolates and puddings
Soft Drinks   Beer and alcohol

Avoid drinking too much milk (A serving of 12 oz milk produces as much gastric juice as 12 oz beer).

TABLE 16.1: ICMR SAMPLE OF A BLAND DIET

Foodstuffs	Quantity of raw material (g)
Rice	100
Wheat Bread	40
Pulses	40
Potatoes	75
Vegetables	100
Milk	1000 ml
Curd	300
Skimmed Milk Powder	15@
Orange juice	150 ml
Banana	50
Sugar	25
Butter	7
Oil/Fat	25**

**This amount is meant for cooking purpose only.
@In case of non-vegetarians, it can be replaced by one half-boiled egg.

These Indian formulations provide:

Calories	2000
Proteins	75 g
Fat	90 g
Carbohydrates	220 g

TABLE 16.2: BLAND DIET CHART

7.00 AM	Milk	1 glass
	Sugar	1 tsp
	Half-boiled egg	1
	Skimmed milk	
	Powder	3 tsp
10.00 AM	Toast	2
	Butter	1 tsp
	Milk	1 glass
	Sugar	1 tsp
1.00 PM	Soft boiled rice	2 cups
	Sieved cauliflower and carrots	1½ cup
	Curd	1 cup
	Sieved green gram	
	Dal (dehusked)	1½ cup
4.00 PM	Milk	1 glass
	Sugar	1 tsp
	Biscuits	2
	Banana	1/2
7.00 PM	Soft boiled rice	2 cups
	Sieved dal	¼ cup
	Mashed potato	½
	Curd	1 cup
	Sieved orange juice	½ glass
10.00 PM	Milk	1 glass
	Sugar	1 tsp

Source: Some Therapeutic Diets, National Institute of Nutrition, Hyderabad.

5. BRAT DIET

This is a special diet to be served with tea and yogurt. It is prescribed in simple diarrhoea in the case of infants and children.

The abbreviation Brat stands for:

> **B** for banana
> **R** for rice
> **A** for unsweetened apple sauce
> **T** for toast.

Being nutritionally not so adequate, Brat diet should not be used for more than just one day.

6. CALCIUM-MODIFIED DIET

The calcium content of a diet that contains a variety of foods, but no milk is estimated as 200 mg/100 kcal per day. This equals to 300-500 mg of calcium per day.

One cup of milk has got 300 mg calcium, while cheese and milk products have 150-200 mg Ca per serving. This can supply about 50-55% of the total daily calcium intake.

7. HIGH CALCIUM DIET

This High calcium diet is recommended in traumatic stress or calcium deficiency cases.

Normal diet is supplemented with additional 400-600 mg Ca/day, derived mainly from milk and dairy products.

Other sources of Ca are green leafy vegetables such as broccoli, kale, mustard, spinach, turnips, tofu, dried fruits and quick-cooking cereals.

8. LOW CALCIUM DIET

This diet is recommended in Renal Hypercalciuria and Type II Absorptive Hypercalciuria. These diets restrict milk and yogurt.

Other foods which contain calcium should be given in a very restricted manner. These are vegetables like spinach, rhubarb, canned fish with bones, tofu and dried beans.

These low-calcium diets (500-600 mg Ca) must be supplemented with multivitamins and minerals. In contrast, a medium Ca diet contains 800 mg Ca for men and 1200 mg for pregnant women.

9. LOW CALORIE DIET

Low calorie diet is recommended for reducing weight, while maintaining good health. A reduction of 500 kcal/day from the normal intake should bring about a weight loss of 1 lb/week. Usually, ½-1 lb weight loss is considered satisfactory. Weight loss of more than 2 lb/week is not advisable, save under strict medical supervision.

When the low calorie diet is combined with regular exercise, it results in greater loss of weight. In weight loss exercises, a liberal intake of proteins is essential for its satiety value and also to prevent negative nitrogen balance.

The foods to be avoided in low calorie diets are:

Gravies   Nuts and dried fruits
Fried foods   Sweets and chocolates
Sauces and desserts   Cream and free fat
Honey and pudding   Alcohol and soft drinks
Fruits like banana,   Custard apple, dates and sapota.

However, extra dietary fibre is recommended to reduce caloric density and to promote satiety.

The ICMR recommends the following sample diet that contains:

Calories	1200
Proteins	60 g
Fat	30 g
Carbohydrates	170 g

TABLE 16.3: LOW CALORIE DIET

Foodstuffs	Vegetarians (g)	Non-vegetarians (g)
Group A:		
Wheat flour	60	60
Rice	30	60
Other vegetables	200	200
Green leafy vegetables	200	200
Pulses	70	50
Citrus fruits/tomatoes	200	200
Group B:		
Cow's milk	600 ml	250 ml
Skimmed powder milk	20	—
Oil/ghee (fat)	7	12
Lean meat/fish	—	50
Egg	—	One

Source: Some Therapeutic Diets, National Institute of Nutrition, Hydedrabad.

10. MODERATE CALORIE DIET

A moderate calorie diet regime is a well-balanced and mixed diet that is prescribed for reduction of weight or for maintaining weight loss already achieved. This diet is nutritionally adequate and can be continued for months, without calling for supplementation, except in cases of pregnant/lactating women or children under 10 years of age.

This moderate calorie diet usually contains 30% lower energy levels than the normal intake. About 20% of the total calories are derived from proteins, preferably lean meats. Carbohydrates provide 50% and fats 30% or less of the total energy intake.

The foods to be avoided or restricted are:

Alcohols	Sugars
Sweets	Calorie-dense foods

11. VERY LOW CALORIE DIET (VLCD)

This VLCD regime is required when planning for weight loss of 2-4 lb/week for women and 3-5 lb for men. This would happen when a patient is at last 30% over-weight and has a minimum body mass index (BMI) of 32. Owing to the potential risk in this rapid weight loss plan, very strict supervision is necessary. Further, the VLCD regime is contra-indicated in the following:

Children	Aged
Pregnancy	Lactation
Cardiac Dysfunction	Hepatic Diseases
Renal Failure	Protein-wasting Diseases
Psychological Disorders	

Herein, one must supplement the VLCD with vitamins and minerals upto 100% of the RDA.

A VLCD may be a liquid or powder mixed with liquid. This 800 Kcal/day diet is preceded by a well-balanced 1200 Kcal diet for 2-4 weeks—to allow the body to adjust to low calories and to promote diuresis. After the VLCD schedule of 12 weeks, a period of gradual 'Re-feeding' follows for 2-4 weeks. This is the normal practice in commercial weight reduction programs.

Potential side-effects with VLCD are alopecia, dry skin, diarrhoea, fatigue, irritability, depression and nausea.

12. HIGH CALORIE DIET

The high calorie regime is prescribed in cases of severe under-nutrition, weight loss, febrile conditions, convalescence, athletics and hyperthyroidism. The calorie intake in high calorie diets can go up from 30% to 100% of RDA, depending upon individual cases. As such, it is better to decide each case on individual basis.

Observations made in the West show certain preferences for extra consumption, as under:

(a) Men consuming additional calories through extra portion of the usual foods at meals

(b) Children and adolescents preferring snacks between the meals,

(c) Women preferring more concentrated diet.

In case of patients convalescing or those having high fevers, fried foods, dry fruits and nuts should be avoided.

The following tabulation gives the ICMR sample diet with a high calorie regime (2700 kcal). It has got proteins 80 g and fats 70 g.

TABLE 16.4: HIGH CALORIE DIETS

Foodstuffs	Vegetarians (g)	Non-Vegetarians (g)
Cereals	250	300
Pulses	100	50
Roots and tubers	50	75
Other vegetables	50	50
Green leafy vegetables	100	100
Bread	60	60
Butter	10	20
Milk	750 ml	300 ml
Curd	100	—
Sugar	50	50
Oil/Fats	30	30
Banana	150	250
Meat/fish	—	100
Egg	—	One

13. RESTRICTED CARBOHYDRATE DIET

The NRC recommends 50% of energy to be provided by carbohydrates (CHO), specially complex CHO. Normally, in a 2000 kcal diet, it should be 250 g CHO/day. But an intake of less than 100 g/day can lead to ketosis and excessive breakdown of tissue proteins.

Restricted carbohydrate is recommended when CHO metabolism is impaired, as happens in the following conditions:

Hypoglycemia   Epilepsy
Vagotomy   Gastrectomy

This low-carbohydrate regime permits restricted use of simple CHO like sugars, cookies, pastries and concentrated sweets like *Barfi*.

In case of specific sugar intolerance, sucrose, maltose, lactose and galactose have also got to be restricted.

14. HIGH CARBOHYDRATE DIET

High carbohydrate diets allow for glycogen formation, ensuring adequate calorie intake for body requirements, thus sparing proteins and minimizing tissue catabolism. This diet regime is indicated in the following conditions:

Fasting Hypoglycemia   Uremia
Toxemia of Pregnancy   Pernicious Vomiting
Acute Glomerulonephritis

Herein, emphasis is laid on the easily available carbohydrates, such as sugar, syrups, jams and jellies.

A high carbohydrate diet is also used by the athletes in pre- and post-game meets, all the more so in endurance events lasting an hour or more. Table 16.5 gives the sample menu for high carbohydrate diet.

TABLE 16.5: SAMPLE MENU FOR HIGH CARBOHYDRATE DIET (2500 kcal, 350 g)

Breakfast	Bran cereal	1 cup
	Low fat milk	8 oz
	English muffin	1
	Margarine	1 tsp
	Orange juice	4 oz
Lunch	Lean roast beef	3 oz
	Hard roll	1
	Mayonnaise	2 tsp
	Cole slaw	½ cup
	Fresh Plums	2
	Oatmeat Cookies	2
	Seltzer Water with lemon	8 oz
Afternoon Snacks	Popcorn	3 cups
Dinner	Chicken, stir-fry	3 oz
	with diced vegetable	1 cup
	Oil	1 tsp
	Rice	2 cups
	Orange or Grapefruit section	1 cup
	Vanila yogurt	1 cup
Bedtime snacks	Hot tea with lemon	1 cup
	Apple Cider	8 oz

Source: *Sport and Exercise Nutrition*. Pub Lippinicof Williams and Wilkins.

15. CHOLESTEROL-RESTRICTED DIET

Low cholesterol diets are prescribed in:

> Hypercholesterolemia
> Atherosclerisis
> Gall Bladder Stones.

Normally, when a person is taking one or more egg per day and is also consuming organ meat regularly, he is ingesting 1000 mg/day or more of cholesterol. Limiting the use of eggs to alternate day and avoiding organ meat can bring down the cholesterol level to 300 mg/day. This figure can be further reduced by avoiding butter and substituting skimmed milk for the whole milk. Omitting eggs altogether will reduce the cholesterol intake to 200 mg/day.

16. LOW CHOLESTEROL, FAT-CONTROLLED DIET

The NIH (USA) recommends double restricted diet, both cholesterol and fats, for lowering high blood total cholesterol count in coronary heart disease. This special diet regime is a two-step graded program. Step one is prescribed for 3 months. In case there is no significant reduction in blood cholesterol, then step two diet is introduced.

In step one diet, cholesterol is restricted to 300 mg or less per day. The total fat is 30% or less of the total calorie intake, with saturated fats less than 10%, PUFA 10% and the remaining 15% provided by monounsaturated fats (MUFA).

In Step two diet, cholesterol is further restricted to 200 mg/day or less, saturated fat to 7% and the protein intake is 12-15% of the total calorie intake.

Diet Restrictions

(A) **Step One:** In this diet include meat, fish, poultry but limit these to 2 servings (2-3 oz) per day. Eggs are restricted to three per week and very lean meats and low-fat milk is taken. Herein, only liquid vegetable oils rich in MUFA and PUFA like soya oils, corn, cottonseed, safflower, canola and olive oils should be used for cooking.

(B) **Step Two:** In this diet, omit egg yolk. And red meats are to be substituted with fish and poultry and very lean meats are only permitted.

Apart from these above steps, additional measures that help are the physical activity and weight control.

ICMR (India) has given the following sample diet:

Foodstuff	Quantity (g)
Cereals	300
Pulses	50
Green leafy vegetables	50
Other vegetables	100
Roots and tubers	100
Fruits	100
Skimmed milk	400
Sugar	30
Oil	30

This double-restriction diet provides

Calories	2400
Proteins	70 g
Fat	55 g
Carbohydrates	400 g

The foods to be avoided are

Butter/Fat	Whole milk and cream
Hydrogenated Fat/Lard	Fatty Meats
Chocolates	Ice creams
Cheese	Organ meats
Prawns	Eggs (twice a week only)

Coconut and coconut oil and all the foods cooked with coconut oil and hydrogenated fats must be avoided.

17. COPPER-RESTRICTED DIET

Copper-restricted diet is a regime that is recommended solely for Wilson's disease. This disorder of Cu metabolism is characterized by a decrease in plasma ceruloplasmin concentration and excessive accumulation of copper in the liver, brain, cornea and kidneys.

The dietary intake of copper must be restricted to 1-2 mg Cu per day. Large quantities of the following copper-rich diets must be avoided.

Liver and organ meats	Shellfish
Mushrooms	Oysters
Nuts	Dried beans
Lentils and peas	Dried fruits
Bran breads	Sweet potatoes
Avocado	Tofu
Soyabeans and soy milk	Chocolates.

18. ELEMENTAL DIET

The elemental diets use monomeric solutions for Enteral feeding, which contain protein as peptides and/or amino acids and carbohydrates as partially hydrolyzed maltodextrins and glucose oligosachharides. The fats are used in the form of medium chain and long chain triglycerides (MCT and LCT).

This diet requires very little digestion and is completely absorbed by upper small intestine. It is also very low in residue.

The elemental diets are prescribed in the following conditions:

Inflammatory bowel disease	Mal-absorption
Short bowel syndrome	Pancreatitis
Pre-operative nutrition.	

19. DIABETIC DIET

The diabetic diet is basically a high carbohydrate, high fibre diet that reduces insulin requirement and improves glycemic control.

The calorie requirements in the Indian conditions are 25 kcal/kg of the ideal body weight (IBW). But it does permit certain adjustments as under:

(1) For moderate activity, add 5 calories/kg IBW.

(2) For over-weights, decrease 5 calories/kg IBW.

(3) For over-weights and the sedentary types, decrease 10 calories/kg IBW.

(4) For the under-weights, increase 5 calories/kg IBW.

(5) For the under-weights engaged in moderate activity, increase 10 calories per kg ideal body weight.

Generally, carbohydrates in the form of complex polysaccharides should provide about 55-60% of energy, with sucrose and other sugars accounting for only 10-15% share. Fibre, especially water-soluble fibre, should account for 25 g/1000 kcal, *i.e.* 40-50 g fibre per day. For proteins, the RDA of 0.8 g/kg body weight for adults will do, with the elderly persons needing 1.0 g/kg. Fats provide 30% energy, of which PUFA accounts for 10% and MUFA 10-15%. The cholesterol intake must be limited to 300 mg/day.

The quality of food is determined by the 'Glycemic Index' (GI), which is a measure of the blood glucose response of a particular food. The lower the GI, still lower is the blood glucose response and hence, such foods are to be preferred. As such, foods with higher amylose content are recommended, e.g. Bengal gram with 33% amylose content is better than wheat which is only 25% and potatoes with 23% amylose content.

Sucrose and sucrose-containing foods, when used, must be substituted for other carbohydrates and not simply added to the meal plan.

Due to impaired insulin secretion in Type II patients, smaller meals and snacks spaced more frequently throughout the day would help prevent high post-meal hypoglycemia.

Additional measures like regular exercise can promote improved metabolic control and weight management.

Thus, by taking all these proper measures, Diabetes could be easily controlled.

The ICMR has recommended the following sample diet that provides:

Calories	1600
Proteins	65 g
Fat	40 g
Carbohydrates	245 g

Foodstuffs	Vegetarians (g)	Non-Vegetarians (g)
Cereals	200	250
Pulses	60	20
Green leafy vegetables	200	200
Other vegetables	200	200
Fruits	200	200
Cow's milk	400 ml	200 ml
Fat/oil	20	20
Fish/chicken without skin	—	100

The foods to be avoided by the diabetics are:

    Roots and tubers

    Dried fruits and nuts

    Fried foods

    Sweets

    Sugars

    Puddings and chocolates

    Fruits such as Banana, custard apple, sapota.

20. FAT-CONTROLLED DIET (LOW FAT DIET)

In this 'Proportioned Diet', it is planned to provide about 30% of the total calorie intake from fat. It is reduced to 15-20% in low-fat diet prescribed for pancreatitis and cholecystitis. And this total amount of fat is then controlled (rationally proportioned) as under:

    Saturated Fatty acids (SFA)   <10%

    Monounsaturated Fatty acids (MUFA)   10-15%

    Polyunsaturated Fatty acids (PUFA)   10%

This helps increase the intake of unsaturated fatty acids so as to bring about a decrease in serum cholesterol and triglycerides.

The desired foodstuff which supply these fatty acids are:

(1) PUFA—Corn, soyabeans, cottonseed and safflower oils

(2) SFA—Palm oil, hydrogenated fats and animal products

(3) MUFA—Vegetable oils such as Olive oil and canola oil.

It is recommended that poultry and meats should be lean and dairy products low-fat or non-fat and skimmed milk.

TABLE 16.6: MENU FOR LOW FAT DIET

Breakfast	Bran Cereal with Raisins	½ cup
	Bagel	1
	Cream Cheese	1 tsp
	Skimmed Milk	1 cup
	Grape fruit	½
Lunch	Wheat bread	2 slices
	Turkey breast	2 oz
	Mayonnaise	1 tsp
	Small Banana	1
	Lettuce salad with 3 cup of fresh vegetables such as Broccoli, cauliflower, carrots, cucumber, tomatoes	
	Fat free salad dressing	3 tsp
Dinner	Large baked potato	1
	Steamed broccoli	1½ cup
	Dinner rolls	2
	Margarine	1 tsp
	Fresh Strawberries	1½ cup
	Skimmed Milk	1 cup
Bedtime	Grapes	30
	Skimmed Milk	1 cup
	Total calories	**190**
	Total fat	**21 g (10% of fat)**

Source: Mcardle and Katch. *Sports and Exercise Nutrition*. Pub. Lippincott Wiliams and Wilkins.

ICMR recommends the following sample diet, which provides:

Calories	2100
Proteins	75 g
Fat	30 g
Carbohydrates	385 g

TABLE 16.7: ICMR-RECOMMENDED LOW FAT DIET

Foodstuffs	Vegetarians (g)	Non-Vegetarians (g)
Cereals	200	250
Pulses	100	75
Other vegetables	100	100
Green leafy vegetables	100	50
Potatoes	50	50
Bread	60	60
Butter	10	20
Cow's Milk	—	100 ml
Skimmed Milk powder	50	—
Curd	200	—
Sugar	50	50
Oil/fats (for cooking)	17	15
Banana	75	75
Meat/Chicken/Fish	—	100
Egg	—	One

Foods to avoid:

Fried Foods	Sausages
Heavily marbled Meats	Nuts
Margarine	Butter
Canned Fish in oils	

Herein, the use of MCT Oil, as source of energy, may be necessary.

21. HIGH MONOUNSATURATED FAT DIET (HMF)

The HMF diet limits the amount of saturated fats and cholesterol. Herein, the protein-rich foods that contain saturated fats are also limited. Monounsaturated fat-rich foods such as canola oil, olive oil, nuts and avocado, are used as replacement for a portion of starch and other carbohydrate-rich foods in diet.

HMF diet is prescribed in the management of non-insulin dependent diabetes mellitus. This diet helps improve glycemic control and lipoprotein profile.

22. LIBERAL FAT DIET

In conditions like under-nutrition, burns and ulcerative colitis, a high fat diet, 35% to 40% of the total calorie intake, is prescribed along with high protein, high calorie diet. It is also used in dumping syndrome, uremia and hyper-insulinism.

The foods rich in high fat diet are:

Butter   Margarine,
Cream   Salad dressing
Vegetable oils.

TABLE 16.8: MENU FOR HIGH FAT DIET

Breakfast	Apple pastry	1
	Orange rice	½ cup
	Whole milk	1 cup
Lunch	Wheat Bread	2 slices
	Turkey breast	2 oz
	Swiss Cheese	1 oz
	Mayonnaise	1 tsp
	Small Banana	1
	Potato chips	15 pcs
Afternoon Snacks	Vanila Ice cream	1 cup
Dinner	T-Bone steak	4 oz
	Large baked Potato	1
	Steamed Broccoli	1½ cup
	Dinner roll	1
	Margarine	1 tsp
	Sour cream	2 tbsp
	Fresh Strawberries	1¼ cup
Bedtime Snacks	Grapes	15
	Chocolate chip cookies	2
	Total Calories	1990
	Total Fat	84 g (38% of fat)

Source: Mcardle and Katch. *Sports and Exercise Nutrition*. Pub. Lippincott Wiliams and Wilkins.

23. MCT FAT DIET

The medium chain triglycerides (MCT) are used in place of ordinary cooking oils and fats. These triglycerides are easily hydrogenated and quickly absorbed, as compared to long chain triglycerides present in the normal fat.

The MCT diet is specially prescribed for the following conditions:

Pancreatitis   Cystic Fibrosis
Chyluria   Celiac Spruce
Intestinal Resection   Deficient Bile Secretion
Biliary Obstruction

Since the MCT does not provide essential fatty acids, hence supplementation with 10 g/day of vegetable oil (sunflower/safflower oil) and margarine is recommended.

24. MODERATE FAT DIET

Herein, fat contributes 25-30% of the total calorie intake.

If found necessary, additional calories may be provided by sugar, sweets and other carbohydrate-rich foods or lean meats and emulsified fats.

This diet is prescribed for the following conditions:

Hepatitis   Cirrhosis of liver
Pancreatitis   Chronic gall bladder

It is also recommended in weight reduction to lend palatability and satiety value to diet.

Foods to be avoided are:

Fried Foods   Nuts
Sausages   Gravies

TABLE 16.9: MENU FOR MODERATE FAT DIET

Breakfast	Bagel	1
	Cream Cheese	1 tbsp
	Orange rice	½ cup
	Milk 1%	1 cup
Lunch	Wheat bread	2 slices
	Turkey breast	2 oz
	Mayonnaise	1 tsp
	Small Banana	1
	Lettuce salad with 2 cup of fresh vegetables such as broccoli, cauliflower, carrots, cucumber, tomatoes	
	Reduced-calorie salad dressing	3 tbsp
Afternoon Snack	Low fat Yoghurt	1 cup
	Fresh Peach	1
	Popcorn, airpopped	6 cups
Dinner	Grilled/boiled sirloin	4 oz
	Long baked Potato	1
	Steamed Broccoli	1½ cup
	Dinner roll	1
	Reduced calorie Margarine	1 tbsp
	Sour cream	2 tbsp
	Fresh Strawberries	1½ cup
Bedtime Snacks	Grapes	30
	Total Calories	**1971**
	Total Fat	**63 g (29% Fat)**

Source: Mcardle and Katch. *Sports and Exercise Nutrition.* Pub. Lippincott Wiliams and Wilkins.

25. HIGH FIBRE DIET

This diet usually contains 20-35 g fibre/day, *i.e.* 10-13 g fibre/1000 kcal.
High fibre diet is prescribed for the following conditions:

Atonic Constipation
Diverticulosis
Diabetes Mellitus
Irritable Bowel Syndrome
Hypercholesterolemia
Colon Cancer.

Good sources of high fibre foods are:

Whole Grain Cereals
Unrefined Breads
High fibre Vegetables
Raw Fruits
Legumes.

26. LOW FIBRE DIET

These diets contain minimum indigestible carbohydrates and dietary fibre. Fibre content is reduced by removing tough connective tissue in meats, removing seeds and skin from fruits and vegetables and using refined cereals and breads.
These low fibre diets are prescribed for:

Gastroparesis
Narrowing of intestines
Small bowel obstruction
Acute diverticulosis
Inflammatory bowel disease

27. GLUTEN-FREE DIET

Also called *Gliadin-free diet*, it is prescribed for:

Dermatitis herpetiformis
Gluten-sensitive celiac disease.

Foods to be avoided are:

Wheat   Oats
Rye   Barley

However, products made from the following can be used as substitutes:

Corn	Rice
Tapioca	Arrow root
Soyabeans	

28. HIGH ALTITUDE DIET

This high altitude diet contains high carbohydrates—65% and low fats—20% liquids, which are prescribed, prior to rapid ascent to high altitudes.

This diet is found beneficial in controlling emphysema and other conditions normally associated with high altitude sickness.

29. LACTOSE-RESTRICTED DIET

Lactose intolerance shows up as bloating, cramping and diarrhoea after ingestion of lactose-rich foods. But many patients can tolerate moderate levels of lactose, say 4-8 oz milk/day. Similarly, cottage cheese and fermented milk products are tolerated by most people.

Calcium supplementation is indicated with these diets in growing children, post-menopausal women and those prone to osteoporosis.

Many lactose-free formulae are available in the Western markets. A commercial lactose enzyme, when added to milk, can sufficiently hydrolyze lactose to allow the use of milk in the diet.

30. LIQUID DIETS, BLENDERIZED

These are diets consisting of fluids and foods blenderized to a liquid puree consistency. This consistency may vary from fruit nectar thickness to that of creamy soup.

The blenderized liquid diet is prescribed in the following conditions:

Dysphagia

Wired jaw (surgery)

Inadequate oral control

Patients unable to use straw or open their mouth would need a syringe for liquid feeding.

31. LIQUID DIET, CLEAR

These diets leave no residue and are recommended in:

    Pre- and post-operative bowel surgery
    Partial paralytic ileus
    Acute inflammatory conditions of GI tract.

Herein, the main object is to relieve thirst and also maintain water balance. The liquid diets used are:

Tea	Black coffee
Ginger ale	Fat-free broth
Plain gelatin	Glucose solution.

Besides, fruit juice and soft drinks are also used to provide additional calories.

Liquid diet should not be used for more than 24 hours. For longer periods, it needs to be supplemented with high-protein broth and high-protein gelatin.

32. LIQUID MICROBIAL DIET

The microbial diets are used after organ transplantation, which help reduce the risk of food-borne infections in immune-suppressed patients.

Raw or uncooked foods must be avoided. Other foods excluded are:

Butter milk	Whipped sour cream
Cheese and yogurt	Dried fruits, juice
Dried meats	Potato salad

One of the most important preventive step is the food sanitation guidelines.

33. OXALATE-RESTRICTED DIET

This diet regime is meant for urinary calcium oxalate stones.

Oxalate-rich foods to be avoided are:

Spinach	Rhubarb
Endive	Beets
Green beans	Sweet potato
Berries	Nuts
Tea	Cocoa

One of the important but simple measure is to take 3-4 litres of fluid throughout the day. This would ensure consistently high dilution of urine.

ICMR has given the following diet chart for this regime:

MENU FOR OXALATE-RESTRICTED DIET (ICMR)

Foodstuffs	Vegetarians (g)	Non-Vegetarians(g) (g)
Rice	200	200
Wheat flour	200	200
Pulses—red gram dal	50	50
Black gram dal	20	20
Other vegetables	100	100
Green leafy vegetables—cabbage	100	100
Potatoes	75	75
Mango	75	75
Bread	60	60
Butter	10	20
Oil / fats	35	40
Sugar	30	30

This oxalate-restricted diet provides:

Calories	2400 kcal
Proteins	65 g
Fat	50 g
Carbohydrates	425 g

34. POTASSIUM (HIGH) DIET

This diet provides 4000-6000 mg potassium/day and is designed to prevent Hypokalemia as a result of drug therapy with potassium-wasting diuretics and steroids. The potassium-high diet is also beneficial in Hypertension.

Increased amount of fruits and vegetables that are good source of potassium are included in the diet. Salt substitutes that contain potassium chloride are very useful in such cases. One may look up Chapter 19 on cardiovascular diseases for such foods.

35. HIGH PROTEIN DIET

An allowance of 1.5-2.0 g/kg protein for adults is recommended in severe stress, hepatitis, long bone fractures and depletion of protein reserves. Increased protein intake is needed in fever, hyperthyroidism, severe burns, nephritis, liver failure and celiac disease.

A liberal protein diet (1.2-1.4 g/kg or 75-100 g/day) is recommended in moderate stress, chronic obstructive pulmonary disease, peritoneal dialysis, as also in surgery.

A very high protein diet has an allowance of 2.5-3.0 g/kg body weight.

It is better to divide the high protein diet into three meals and three between-the-meals snacks.

36. PROTEIN MINIMAL DIET

This diet allows 0.2-0.3 g/kg or approximately 20-25 g proteins per day. It is prescribed for the following conditions:

Acute renal failure   Hepatic coma
Gout (arthritis)   Acute glomerulonephritis

Herein, extra calories are provided by liberal use of sugar and starchy foods. The following tabulation gives different grades of protein levels:

	RDA (g/kg BW)	Daily Allowance (g/day)
Minimal proteins	0.2 - 0.3	20 - 25
Low proteins	0.5 - 0.7	30 - 40
Normal protein	0.8 - 1.0	50 - 65
Liberal proteins	1.2 - 1.4	75 - 85
High proteins	1.5 - 2.0	90 - 110
Very high proteins	2.5 - 3.0	120 - 150

37. PRUDENT DIET

This is the diet recommended by the American Heart Association as a safe and prudent norm to prevent or reduce the incidence of coronary heart disease and other atherosclerotic diseases. Herein, fat is reduced to 30% of the total calorie intake, with PUFA providing 10% and MUFA 10-15%, while the share of saturated fats does not exceed 10% of the total daily calories.

Special recommendations are to choose margarine made from liquid vegetable oils. Cholesterol intake is to be limited to 300 mg/day. Other recommendations are:

Eggs   Thrice per week
Low fat milk   2 cups a day
Cooked lean meat   2-3 oz twice a day
Carbohydrate intake   55-60%
Sodium intake   <3 g/day
Cereals and legumes   4 servings/day
Fresh fruits and vegetables   ad lib.
Restricted use of tea/coffee, alcohol and refined sugars.

In all these combinations, the total calorie intake must be sufficient to maintain the desired body weight.

38. PURINE-RESTRICTED DIET

This is a supplementary diet, given as an adjunct to drug therapy for gout and other purine metabolism disorders. Herein, the purine levels are reduced from the normal 600-1000 mg/day. This purine-restriced diet is indicated to lower uric acid level in the body.

Purine-rich foods to be avoided are:

Sardines and anchovies
Glandular and organ meats
Meat extracts

Restricted use be made of the moderately-rich purine foods like:

Fish and sea foods   Meat and poultry
Peas and beans   Asparagus
Mushrooms   Cauliflower
Spinach   Chocolates, cocoa

(But these are altogether disallowed during acute gout attacks.)

Desirable foods recommended are:

Cereals and bread   Milk and dairy products
Fruits   Eggs
Sugars   Beverages

There must be liberal use of fluids (2-3 lit./day), which would help dilute the urine and promote the excretion of uric acids.

Following sample diet is recommended:

	Quantity (g)
Rice/wheat flour	200
Bread	50
Cow's milk	400 ml
Vegetables	500
Fruits	200
Sago	100
Egg	One
Oil	10
Sugar	30
Tea/coffee	7

This diet provides:
Calories   2100
Proteins   55 g
Fat   36 g

39. SODIUM-RESTRICTED DIET

In this regime, sodium is restricted to specific levels for the prevention/control of the following conditions:

Edema in congestive heart failure
Cirrhosis of liver
Toxemia of pregnancy
ACTH therapy
Nephritis and nephrosis
Hypertension

About food in general, the animal products are high in sodium and plant foods relatively low. The RDA for sodium is 0.5 g/day, but the average American diet contains an average of 3-6 g of sodium, *i.e.* 7.5-15 g of sodium chloride/day. The American Heart Association has provided the following levels of sodium restriction:

3000 mg Sodium   No added Salt
2000 mg Sodium   Medium sodium restriction
1000 mg Sodium   Moderate sodium restriction
500 mg Sodium
and 250 mg sodium

The last case restricts meat intake to 5 oz/day and low-sodium milk is substituted for the whole milk.

ICMR has given the following recommendations for a low sodium diet:

Foodstuffs	Vegetarians (g)	Non-vegetarians (g)
Rice	250	300
Dal	100	75
Fruits	200	200
Vegetables	200	200
Potatoes	100	125
Cow's milk	600 ml	200 ml
Meat/fish	—	50
Egg	—	One
Oil/fat	30	30
Sugar	30	30

This diet provides:

Calories   2200
Proteins   70 g
Sodium   0.5 g

40. SOY-RESTRICTED DIET

Allergy conditions call for very limited soyabean diet. Although soyabean is the most allergenic legume food, other foods of legume groups that may be safely used are:

Beans	Chickpean
Lentils	Peanuts
Peas.	

The soyabeans and soy products that need to be guarded against are:

Tofu	Miso
Tempeh	Soy Extenders
Soy Sauce	Soy Flour
Soy Milk	Soy Oil
Textured Vegetable Products	
Hydrolyzed Soy Proteins	

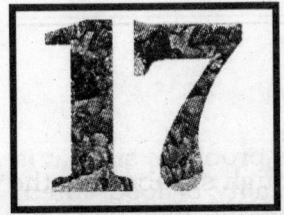

DIET FOR GASTROINTESTINAL DISORDERS

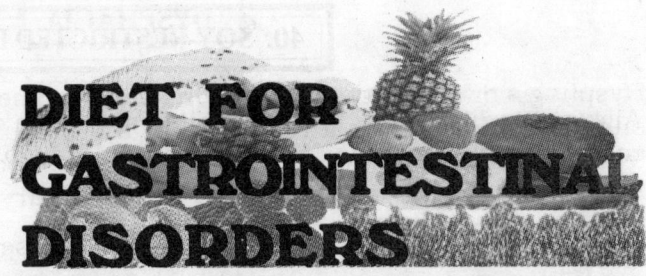

The Gastrointestinal tract is a very sensitive mirror of the individual human conditions. The physiologic functioning and disorder of some of its parts reflect both physical and psychologic conditioning that guides a man's well-being. As such, it is a sheer truism to say that:

'Surrounding every stomach, there is a person'!

The gastrointestinal tract and its optimum functioning serves as the foundation for all the body systems. Any disease or problem of this system can trigger a chain reaction, with repercussions being felt in other systems or the body as a whole. In such cases, *Diet Therapy aims at promoting reversal of the affected parts to their normally observed physiological state.*

Normally, the gastrointestinal tract diseases may be classified as:

(a) Functional diseases, wherein some mechanical causes have affected or altered the digestive functions,

(b) Organic diseases, wherein pathogenic lesions are to be found in some organs.

The common diseases of the gastrointestinal tract are:

1. Dysphagia
2. Dyspepsia or indigestion
3. Hyperacidity
4. Gastric ulcers
5. Colitis
6. Diarrhoea
7. Constipation

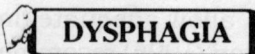

DYSPHAGIA

Dysphagia or difficulty in swallowing can become a serious problem, since it is often accompanied by a reduction in the amount and quality of food eaten, leading rapidly to loss of weight. It my be a temporary phase or a more serious phenomenon if caused by a stroke or head injury, mechanical impairment and diseases of the nervous system.

Causes

The causes of the dysphagia include aging, nervous system diseases, injuries or strokes. In the oropharyngeal phase, the food passes from mouth via the pharynx to the upper oesophagus. In the oesophageal dysphagia, the food passes from pharynx to stomach.

Symptoms

The symptoms include facial drop, drooling, pouching or pocketing of food in the mouth, choking or coughing when eating or drinking. There may be pain on swallowing, weight loss and fear of eating certain foods. Dysphagia may result in aspiration if food enters the respiratory tract.

Diet Therapy

The mechanical soft diet for dysphagia leaves little room for experimentation. Some patients tolerate mildly spiced food or moderately sweet food served at room temperature. Thickened liquids or smooth solids such as milk shakes or puddings are good choice. Commercial thickeners, yogurt, pudding and baby cereals can be used to thicken the liquids. With time, the swallowing function may improve, thus permitting general variation in diet. In early stages, tube feeding is recommended. Avoid sticky foods that adhere to the roof of the mouth.

Depending upon the severity of swallowing dysfunction, the diet is divided into four levels:

Level I: Pureed foods with thick liquids, e.g., yogurt, creamed cottage cheese, strained soup (thickened) and puddings.

Level II: Lumpy pureed food with thick liquids, soft moist cake/pancake, cooked leafy greens, noodles, sliced ripe banana.

Level III: Soft fish, eggs, soft chopped vegetables, finely ground meat bound with thick sauce and drained canned fruits.

Level IV: All regular chopped foods, pureed foods (thickened). Thick liquids, e.g., fruits, nectars, milk and ice creams.

Always feed in small spoonfuls, allow adequate time for complete swallowing.

The American Dietetic Association (1996) recommended a four level Dysphagia Diet plan, as shown in Table 17.1.

TABLE 17.1: DYSPHAGIA DIET PLAN

Phase/Level	Condition	Recommendation
Level 1	For patients who need maximum restriction and cannot swallow	Avoid coarse cereals, nuts and fruits. Water and raw vegetables not allowed. All liquids thickened with a commercial thickening agent.
Level II	Those who can tolerate a minimum amount of chewable foods, but can not swallow liquids.	Advised juice or milk products. No coarse grains/materials allowed. Thickened liquids permitted. Fluid intake to be monitored.
Level III	For patients having difficulty in chewing, manipulating and swallowing certain foods	Meat must be minced. Soft drinks allowed and liquids as and when tolerated.
Level IV	For patients who chew soft foods and swallow liquids safely	Soft diets that do not require chopping. No nuts or deep-fried foods allowed. Liquids as and when tolerated.

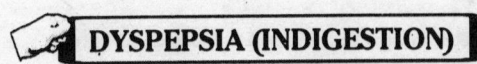

DYSPEPSIA (INDIGESTION)

Dyspepsia is any discomfort affecting the upper abdomen. It is synonymous with indigestion. Dyspepsia could be either a functional or organic disease.

Causes

It can be caused by a number of conditions, like ulcers, gall bladder diseases, pancreatitis, hepatitis and irritable bowel syndrome. It may also be due to rapid eating, inadequate chewing, swallowing of air and sometimes emotional stress.

Symptoms

The symptoms exhibited are a heaviness and bloating or fullness, more so after the meals, flatulence, heart burn and acid regurgitation. Often there may be a feeling of nausea and vomiting.

Diet Therapy

If it is a functional cause or some form of emotional stress responsible for indigestion, then individual counselling is needed. One must observe the principle of a balanced diet and regular meals in a stress-free atmosphere. It has got to be relaxed eating and proper mastication (chewing) that could restore normalcy. Food should be adequate, well-cooked and not too spicy. It is best to eat smaller meals, but more frequently, say 6-8 times a day.

In case of organic causes, one need to undergo specific treatment for that particular symptom or disease that has occasioned dyspepsia. In many cases of nervous origin, dyspepsia disappears once the psychoneurotic cause is removed. If it is due to organic causes, soft diet low in fat may be beneficial.

Dr (Mrs) Usha Jain has rightly commented:

Healthy Stomach is a 'Healthy Body'!

Almost all the digestive tract diseases have dyspepsia as the basic cause of the ailment. And 70% of all the diseases have their origin in the gastrointestinal tract.

According to Naturopathy, the major causes of dyspepsia are:

1. Irregular food habits
2. Heavy, late-night dinner
3. Very spicy foods
4. Beverages and Alcohol
5. Excessive physical or mental strain
6. Excessive use of medicines like aspirin, pain-killers, corticosteroids, non-steroidal anti-inflammatory drugs and other medicines taken on empty stomach.
7. Too much fried foods, sugars, sweets and starches.
8. Drinking excessive fluids in between the meals causes bloating of the stomach.
9. Irregular food habits also disturb the gastric secretions and kill the normal response to food.
10. Diseases like flatulence, abdominal pain and regurgitation of food into the food pipe—Reflux oesophagitis.

Precautions

1. Fasting on suitable liquids like tender coconut water, ashgourd water or cucumber/beet-root juice. These should be taken for 3-4 days.
2. Bland foods, cereals, fruits, vegetable salads and soup recommended.
3. Avoid fried foods and in-between-the-meal drinking of water.
4. Never over-eat. Always leave the dining table even when you still feel like eating bit more.
5. Avoid stale fruits and the left overs.
6. Thorough chewing of food is very important.
7. Swallow the food slowly when it is a liquid diet.
8. Follow the golden principle of diet therapy: *Avoid hurry, worry and curry* (hot), besides the usual anxiety.

Table 17.2 gives the special diet chart recommended by Dr (Mrs) Jain.

TABLE 17.2: DIET CHART FOR DYSPEPSIA

6.00 AM	Fasting on fruit and vegetable juice for 3 days -Tender coconut water sipped slowly in 10 minutes for 3-4 days. -Juice fasting is recommended for 40 days, if one can manage.	
7.00 AM	Carrot/ beet-root Juice taken with honey and lemon juice	1 cup
9.00 AM	Overnight soaked figs Munakka (Dried Currants) Almonds	2, 5 5
	Drink the soak water also	
	Fresh seasonal fruit juice like papaya, apples, spota, pears or guava	250 g
	Cold milk with honey	1 cup
11.00 AM	Tender coconut water	1 glass
12.00 Noon	Baked seasonal vegetables like bitter-gourd, tori, teenda and parwal	250 g
	Fortified chapattis	2-4 (25% wheat bran)
	Curd raita	
	Coconut chutney	
4.00 PM	Fresh seasonal fruit juice like papaya, custard apple, sapota	1 glass
7.00 PM	Seasonal vegetable soup	1 cup
	Vegetable dalia (porridge) eaten with curd raita and coconut chutney	2 cups
9.00 PM	Tea made with bran (1 tsp bran boiled in a cup of water, strain and mix with 2 tsp milk and 1 tsp honey).	1 cup

Source: Dr (Mrs) Usha Jain, Delhi.

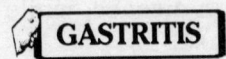 **GASTRITIS**

Gastritis is the painful inflammation of the gastric mucosa. There will be symptoms of anorexia, nausea, vomiting and epigastric pain.

Acute Gastritis

Acute gastritis usually follows repeated medication with aspirin, which causes irritation to gastric mucosa. Alcohol, irritant foods, radiation therapy and bacterial infections can also cause gastritis.

Chronic Gastritis

Chronic gastritis is associated with aging, peptic ulcers and conditions that cause chronic reflux of basic fluids from duodenum into stomach. A patient may also suffer from pernicious anemia.

Symptoms

The symptoms are mild and long-drawn. Chronic gastritis may lead to atrophy of the gastric mucosa, achlorhydria and loss of intrinsic factor resulting in vitamin B_{12} and iron malabsorption.

Diet Therapy

The conventional treatment includes using antacids, anti-secretory agents and antibiotics.

Diet therapy herein includes withholding the food for 1-2 days and then start with liquids. Later on, a bland diet is recommended.

In acute gastritis, withholding food for 24 hours will permit rest to the stomach. It should be followed by clear fluids the next day, before a full liquid or soft diet is resumed.

Avoid highly seasoned foods and those causing acidity.

In chronic gastritis, a liberal bland diet is advised.

Besides, vitamin B_{12} is given by injection to bypass the need for absorption.

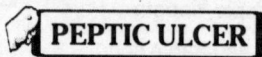

PEPTIC ULCER

It is one of the most common diseases that affects about 10% of the global population. It can occur at any age, although the middle adulthood shows the highest incidence of this disease.

Gastric and duodenal ulcers, along with complications of perforations occur more often in men than women. Peptic ulcers may occur with other diseases or with injuries like burns.

Peptic ulcer in itself is a benign disease, while gastric ulcers are more prone to develop into a malignant disease.

Symptoms

Basic symptoms of peptic ulcer are increased gastric tone and painful hunger contractions whenever the stomach is empty. This gnawing or piercing pain is usually relieved on eating. Sometimes, haemorrhage or bleeding is the first sign of these ulcers. Nutritional deficiencies are evident in low level of plasma proteins, anemia and loss of weight. Occasionally, there may be perforations and carcinoma, which would need surgical intervention.

Treatment

Anticholinergic drugs help reduce the acid secretions in stomach. Antacids buffer the excess acid present. Antihistaminic drugs act as antagonists to block histamine-stimulated gastric acid secretions.

Rest, both physical and mental rest helps in healing. Yoga is another new tool to effect perfect relaxation of mind and body.

Diet Therapy

One of the main consideration in peptic ulcer treatment is to avoid mechanical, chemical and thermal irritation. Hence, bland diet and restriction on dietary fibre are prescribed. The diet therapy is divided into four stages, depending upon the severity of the condition.

Stage One

This is the acute stage marked with lot of pain. Milk, on account of the buffering action of m ilk proteins, affords great relief. Fluids help neutralize the acids in the system. Milk, alongwith cream, up to 100 g/hour is advised. All leafy vegetables, fruits with skin and whole grain cereals are to be restricted. As the pain subsides, small doses of soft diet like pudding, custard and soft cooked eggs plus tender cooked fruits and vegetables may be resumed. As the condition improves, the quantity and variety of these soft foods may be increased.

Stage Two

Herein, milk or milk products are the main items. Six to eight feedings in a day are recommended. One must avoid green leafy vegetables and fruits, oilseeds and gas-forming vegetables like cabbage and cauliflower. Thermal irritation must be avoided by not using very hot or very cold foods. Avoid all hot or iced beverages and frozen desserts. To avoid chemical irritation, cut down on tea, coffee, gravies and spiced foods.

Stage Three

The diet regime in stage two should be liberalised and six feedings a day should suffice.

Stage Four

The amount of food each time remains the same, as in stage three. Gradually, once can resume well cooked foods, whole wheat flour and mashed pulses.

Foods Recommended

Weak tea and coffee
Refined cereals, bread and rice
Butter, esp. emulsified fat
Canned or cooked fruits

Lean tender meat
Cooked mashed pulses
Vegetables such as Potatoes, brinjals, lady finger and gourds

Avoid

- Alcohol and cola drinks
- Hot tea and coffee
- Whole grain cereal bread/chapattis
- Fried foods
- Spiced foods
- Raw fruits
- Pulses, dehusked
- Chocolates, sweets and nuts
- Vegetables like cabbage, cauliflower and peas

Table 17.3 and 17.4 gives the diet charts for different stages of peptic ulcers.

TABLE 17.3: SAMPLE MENU FOR PEPTIC ULCER (ACUTE PAIN PHASE)

7.00 AM	Milk with complan	1 glass
9.00 AM	Porridge with corn flakes	¾ cup
	Milk with sugar	1 cup
12.00 Noon	Cottage cheese	
	Mashed potato or noodles with cheese	
	Chapattis/bread	3-4
	Banana/stewed apple with custard	
	(*Minced meat/roast chicken for non-veg.*)	
3.00 PM	Milk	1 cup
	Biscuits	2
5.00 PM	Custard	1 cup
	Bread with butter	1-2 slices
8.00 PM	Sweet curd	1 cup
	Baked potato/mixed vegetables	1 bowl
	Chapattis	3-4
	Chinagrass jelly	1 cup
	Milk	1 glass
	(*Minced chicken/lamb stew for non-veg.*)	
10.00 PM	Milk	1 glass

Source: Dr. F. P. Antia. *Clinical Diagnostics and Nutrition*. Oxford University Press.

INFLAMMATORY BOWEL DISEASE (I.B.D.)

The term Inflammatory Bowel Disease is used to cover two diseases which have similar clinical and pathological features. These are:

(a) Ulcerative Colitis

(b) Crohn's Disease

The following tabulation marks out the distinctive points of these diseases which are usually marked by chronic bloody diarrhoea.

	Crohn's Disease	*Ulcerative Colitis*
1. Location	Anywhere in the bowel Diseased areas alternate with healthy tissues	Occurs in large intestine Usually starts in rectum and spreads upwards
2. Lesions	Involves all layers of intestinal wall	Confined to mucosal and sub-mucosal layers
3. Complications	Fistula —Obstruction —Stricture	Toxic Megacolon fistula Increased risk of colon cancer

There is a general weight loss, malnutrition syndrome, skin lesions and arthritic joint involvement. There is a severe loss of water and electrolyte leading to dehydration, fever and anemia in ulcerative colitis.

Diet Therapy

Nutritional support is an essential part of medical management of IBD. There are two objectives of diet therapy:

(a) Supporting the tissue healing process,

(b) Avoiding nutritional deficiency

Emphasis of treatment is to restore optimal nutrient intake. The main focus is on proteins and energy, minerals and vitamins, besides the texture of the food. The diet must supply about 100 g proteins/day, which is needed both for synthesis and healing. Regarding high energy, 2,500-3,000 kcal/day are needed to recoupe the losses caused by diarrhoea and the consequent weight loss. This would also help overcome the negative nitrogen balance and spare the proteins for tissue building. Extra vitamins needed for healing and increased protein and energy metabolism should be provided. These are thiamin, riboflavin, niacin and ascorbic acid. Trace elements like zinc are needed alongwith vitamin E.

One of the important points about food is to avoid residue that may cause irritation of the mucosa. Hence, it has got to be a very low-residue diet for IBD patients. Rekha Sharma (AIIMS) recommends the bland soft diet given in Table 17.4. The general guidelines for IBD treatment are given in Table 17.5.

TABLE 17.4: BLAND SOFT DIET FOR ULCERATIVE COLITIS

7.00 AM	Light tea	1 cup
9.00 AM	Tea/coffee	1 cup
	White bread or suji porridge with soy milk or suji upma	1 cup
	Cheese or egg white	2
	Butter or jam	1 tsp
11.00 AM	Buttermilk or light tea	1 cup
	Biscuits	2-3
1.00 PM	Soup	1 cup
	Dehusked pulses	1 cup
	Rice	1 cup or
	Chapattis (refined flour)	2-3
	Soft strained vegetables such as Potato, lauki, teenda, sitaphal	1 bowl
	Cheese or soft chicken or fish	
	Curd from soy milk	1 cup
	Banana or steamed fruit	1
4.00 PM	Tea	1 cup
	Sandwich	1 or
	Biscuits	2 or
	Egg white	2
7.00 PM	Dinner same as lunch	

Source: Rekha Sharma: *Diet Management*. Pub. Churchill Livingstone.

TABLE 17.5: GUIDELINES FOR NUTRITIONAL THERAPY IN IBD

Severity of disease	Nutritional treatment	Nutritional recommendations
1. Mild IBD	Limit foods that are irritating and/or are poorly absorbed	Decrease fibre intake esp. seeds, nuts, fruit peals, broccoli, dried beans. Limit food high on fat
2. Moderate IBD	Correct nutritional deficiencies Increase calorie intake	Increase energy intake to 300-500 kcal/day. Increase protein intake to 1.5-3 g/day. Supplement with multivitamin and minerals about 100-150 % of RDA
3. Moderate to severe incidence	Bowel rest	Use elemental enteral formulae orally or via feeding tube If total obstruction or fistula cannot be bypassed by feeding tube, then use parenteral nutrition

Adapted from Davis, J R and Shererk, K. *Applied Nutrition and Diet Therapy*.

Dr. Anita has given a special menu for Crohn's disease, as shown in Table 17.6.

TABLE 17.6: A SAMPLE MENU FOR CROHN'S DISEASE

8.00 AM	Quaker's oats	¾ cup
	Toast with honey	1
	Milk with sugar	1 glass
	(*Eggs 2-half-boiled or poached for Non-veg.*)	
12.00 Noon	Curd	1 cup
	Baked potato + mashed pumpkin	1 bowl
	Rice with dal water	1 bowl
	Chapattis	3-4
	Apple	
	(*Mutton soft-cooked for Non-veg.*)	
4.00 PM	Tea with cucumber sandwich	
7.00 PM	Buttermilk	1 cup
	Mashed potato/stewed vegetables	1 bowl
	Rice with dal water	1 bowl
	Chapattis	3-4
	Chinagrass jelly	
	Apple juice	1 glass
	Curds	1 cup
	(*Roast leg of chicken or baked fish for Non-veg.*)	

Source: Dr. F. P. Antia: *Clinical Dietetics and Nutrition*, Oxford University Press.

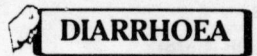

DIARRHOEA

One of the most common gastrointestinal disorder is diarrhoea which assumes serious form of dehydration. If not checked in time, it causes heavy mortality, more so in the infants. The infants' relatively high body water content and considerably larger area of intestinal mucosa, in comparison to the body surface area, causes a morbid evacuation of the bowels, the passage of watery stools increases in frequency. It may vary from 5 to 10 motions per day to one every few minutes. This severe condition may accompany various infections and diseases of the GI tract, such as ulcerative colitis and gastroenteritis.

The water (+ electrolytes) evacuation originates from small intestine. Normally, there will be about 10 litres of water in small intestine, mainly the secretions from stomach, liver, pancreas and the intestine itself. All this bulk, if not absorbed, is pushed down into large intestine (colon), which have a very limited capacity.

TABLE 17.7: DIET CHART FOR PEPTIC ULCER (REMISSION STAGE)

7.00 AM	Tea/coffee with biscuits	
9.00 AM	Porridge	1 cup
	Milk with sugar	1 cup
	Toast with butter	1
	Banana	1
	(*Scrambled egg for Non-veg.*)	
11.00 AM	Milk/Buttermilk	1 cup
	Biscuit	1-2
1.00 PM	Curd	1 cup
	Mashed Potato and carrot or vegetable casserole	
	Dal (pulses)	1 cup
	Rice + dal/Chapattis	3-4
	(*Roast chicken or tuna noodles casserole for Non-veg.*)	
4.00 PM	Fresh figs	
	Tea	1 cup
	Bread with butter	
7.00 PM	Buttermilk	1 cup
	Boiled potato/pumpkin or tendli with coconut	1 bowl
	Dal (pulses)	1 cup
	Chapattis	3-4
	Jelly/ice cream or Carrot halwa	
	(*Roast mutton/boiled fish/beef and onion stew for Non-veg.*)	
9.00 PM	Milk	1 glass
	Biscuits	2
	Bread with Butter	1-2

Source: Dr. F. P. Antia: *Clinical Diagnostics and Nutrition*. Oxford University Press.

In the normal course, colon receives about 500 ml of the undigested food mass from small intestine daily. Out of this, about 150 g is formed into feces and excreted out. And the feces comprise of 70% water. But this normal water loss is relatively a very small amount compared to the big drain involved in diarrhoea. It is this small water-holding capacity of the colon that creates a frequent urge to evacuate in diarrhoea.

Causes

Functional diarrhoea occurs due to many causes, the plain one being over-eating or eating something disagreeable or not easily digestible. It may also be caused by infections, nervous irritability, partially digested carbohydrates causing fermentation or excessive use of laxatives. Besides, some bacteria or parasites (worms) and toxins too cause diarrhoea. Occasionally, allergy to specific foods like milk, wheat, fish and eggs and stress causes diarrhoea. Lactose intolerance is another common cause in the infants.

Symptoms

Acute Diarrhoea

It is characterised by sudden and frequent bowel movements and excessive loss of water. There may be cramps, abdominal pain, vomiting and weakness caused by nutritional imbalance. Acute diarrhoea often accompanies conditions like gastroenteritis or ulcerative colitis.

Chronic Diarrhoea

It occurs when the condition persists for a fortnight or longer. Herein, the passage of food through small intestine is too rapid to allow any absorption. As such, it results in severe nutritional deficiencies.

Dehydration or excessive fluid and electrolyte loss is indeed a very serious condition that follows diarrhoea in the small infants. Its intensity, owing to the frequency and rapidity of stools, can often cause death. Dehydration is characterised by severe thirst, drying up of the mouth, loss of skin elasticity and reduced urinary excretion.

Treatment

The easiest and most effective treatment is the Oral Rehydration Therapy (ORT), which powders are easily available or reconstituted at home. ORT is a cheap fluid and electrolyte replacement mechanism that can save life.

The World Health Organisation recommends the following ORT formulas:

ORT Formula

Sodium chloride	3.5 g
Calcium bicarbonate	2.5 g
Potassium chloride	1.5 g
Glucose	20.0 g
Water	1.0 lit.

Other homely ORT mixtures are:

(A)	Glucose	20 g
	or	
	Sugar	40 g
	Boiled, cooled water	1 lit.
(B)	Rice Powder	20 g (2 heaped tsp)
	Water	1 lit.
	Boil for 5 minutes and then administer.	

ORT has to be started at the earliest onset of symptoms. Later on, when the condition has stabilized, buttermilk, coconut water or rice water can be given, to be followed by soft foods like cooked rice, mashed potatoes, curds and arrow-root powder. However, breast feeding of the infant must never be interrupted. Juice of fruits like orange, pomegranate, barley water with milk and sugar can be given. Carrot soup is an adequate recharger, replenishing sodium, potassium calcium, sulphur and magnesium. Bananas, which contain pectin, permit the growth of beneficial bacteria. Curds overcome harmful microflora and garlic kills parasites. Drugs like pectin and kaolin provide a mechanical binding effect, but do not help in cases of severe diarrhoea in the infants.

Since children with diarrhoea can soon develop 'Protein-Energy Malnutrition', hence the diet given to such children should be easily digestible and nutritionally balanced.

Following steps would ensure speedier recovery:

1. Breast milk be resumed as soon as soon as possible, not later than four hours of initiating the ORT.

2. Sufficient amount of ORs, rice kanji/sooji kanji, salted buttermilk, tender coconut water, light tea decoction, melon juice, sago + whey water, lime juice and sherbet should be given at frequent intervals.

3. Prefer a diet comprising of fresh softly cooked bananas or apple, soft cooked rice, sago gruel, rice gruel.

4. Ensure foods of high energy density, say a minimum of 60 kcal/kg.

5. For achieving higher energy inputs, one may add small quantity of fats and oils.

   Supplementary measures, ORT

   Starch-based ORs.
   Rice-based ORs.
   Sorghum-based ORs.
   Sweet potato water and wheat ORs.

Other ORs based on special solutes that may be used are:

   Glucose and glycine glucose polymers and amino acids
   Hydrolysed maltodextrin L-alanine glucose ORs.

Other home remedies include peeled banana or apple, cultured or soured milk, turmeric powder and garlic. In chronic diarrhoea cases, a soft protein-rich diet with vitamins and minerals should gradually be introduced, with larger amounts of fluids and milk.

A sample diet for chronic diarrhoea is given in Table 17.8.

Diet Therapy

Attempt must be made for the patient to take interest in his food, rather than his trying to avoid it. The diet must be protein-rich, such as tender meats and chicken, well-cooked fish and soft-boiled eggs. Spices must be altogether avoided. Milk should be taken liberally. To begin with, it has to be a low-fibre diet, which can later on graduate to moderate fibre diet. One must avoid raw vegetables and fruits which cause irritation. Vitamins and special iron and mineral supplementation helps restore the general tone and vigor of the body.

TABLE 17.8: DIET CHART FOR CHRONIC DIARRHOAEA

7.00 AM	Tea/coffee	1 cup
9.00 AM	Tea/coffee	1 cup
	Toast with butter	1
	Banana or peeled apple	1
1.00 PM	Curd	1 cup
	Dudhi (lauki) curry	1 cup
	Dal (pulses)	1 cup
	Rice	1 cup
	Chapattis	3-4
4.00 PM	Coconut water or orange juice	1 glass
	Suji upma	½ cup
7.00 PM	Curd	1 cup
	Red pumpkin curry	1 bowl
	Tendli with coconut	1 bowl
	Moong dal khichdi	1 bowl
	Chapattis	1-2
	Rice	½ cup

Source: S. Joshi. *Nutrition and Dietetics*. 1992, Tata McGraw Hill.

Avoid

- Whole milk
- Whole grains
- Whole pulses
- Fried mutton/foods
- Vegetable with seeds or skin
- Fruits with seeds
- Raw vegetables
- Spices and pickles

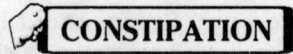 CONSTIPATION

Constipation is a disease of modern civilization, which, in turn, has become a cause for most of the other common ailments like rheumatism, arthritis, high blood pressure, appendicitis, cataract and cancers.

In constipation, the stools harden, causing considerable difficulty in bowel movement and leading to a very difficult and infrequent evacuation. It also causes, in severe cases, damage of the anal passage, which may occasionally lead to bleeding. In some people, the normal bowel movements are lethargic, consequently the stools are passed once in two or three days, a phenomenon that is very common in the West.

Constipation, which describes the symptoms of unsatisfactory defection, may be classified as follows:

1. Chronic Idiopathic Constipation for which the no cause has been found and it has been present for some time.
2. Irritable Bowel Syndrome, a functional syndrome in which constipation is one of the cardinal symptoms.
3. Colonic Inertia Constipation has no organic cause, but delayed transit through the ascending system.
4. Slow Transit Constipation, as in No.3, but delayed transit through colon and rectum.
5. Hindgut Dysfunction, chronic idiopathic constipation with delayed transit through the left colon and rectum.
6. Functional Outlet Obstruction has no organic cause, but delayed transit through the rectum.

Causes

Constipation may be caused by faulty dietary habits, irregular eating hours, poor muscle tone in the aged or those suffering from organic diseases like diverticulosis, intestinal spasm and excessive use of sedatives and opiates. Habitually prolonged use of laxatives/cathartics also leads to constipation. The modern man's fixation with pizzas and fast foods and the eventual lack of dietary fibre is another common cause of constipation.

Symptoms

The symptoms are lack of appetite, coated tongue, foul breath, giddiness and occasional headache, depression, nausea, pimples on the face and dark rings under the eyes. There may be diarrhoea alternating with constipation. Other symptoms are varicose veins, acidity and heart burn, constant fullness of tummy, insomnia and occasionally pain in the lumber region.

Diet Therapy

Maintain regularity in eating, rest and exercise and elimination time - all these restore the normal bowel movement. Laxatives may be occasionally used, but the ultimate treatment is diet.

Herein, the main emphasis is on the greater intake of dietary fibre through greater consumption of green leafy vegetables, fruits, bran, whole grain cereals and pulses. Increased fibre in the diet positively helps in two ways by:

(a) Augmenting the volume of stools,
(b) Decreasing the colonic transit time, thus speeding evacuation.

The effectiveness of indigestible residues (fibre) is not due primarily to the mechanical stimulus of distension, but rather to the chemical stimuli that arise from the destruction of hemicelluloses and celluloses by the intestinal bacterial flora. One of these stimulating product is fatty acids having low volatility.

TABLE 17.9: DIET CHART FOR CONSTIPATION

7.00 AM	Plain fresh water	1 glass
	Tea	1 cup
9.00 AM	Stewed figs	4 or
	Apricots	2 or
	Prunes	10
	Corn flakes with milk and sugar toast with honey	1
	Banana	
	(*Eggs 2-scrambled or ham and eggs for Non-veg.*)	
1.00 PM	Tomato soup cream of asparagus soup	1 bowl
	Buttermilk	1 glass
	Green salad—Radish, lettuce, tomato, carrot and beetroot	1 bowl served with dressing
	Pumpkin cooked or mixed vegetables	1 bowl
	Rice with dal/curry	1 bowl
	Chapattis	3-4
	Grapes	
	(*Stewed fish with lemon and mint dressing with boiled French beans for Non-veg.*)	
4.00 PM	Tea/Coffee	1 cup
	Bread slices	2
	Banana	1
7.00 PM	Cream of spinach soup or mixed vegetables soup	1 bowl
	Dal	1 bowl
	French Beans with boiled potato or onion	1 bowl
	Fried lady finger	½ bowl
	Chapattis	3-4
	Pumpkin jam or jelly	
	The patient must be made to drink 8-10 glasses of water every day	

Source: Dr. F. P. Antia: *Clinical Dietetics and Nutrition*, 1982, Oxford University Press.

It is better to introduce the extra fibre in the diet in a graduated manner so that the GI tract can easily adapt to fibre-related changes in bacterial proliferation, gas production and transit time. Avoid the use of refined cereals like white flour and maida etc. Fatty acids in the food like butter, cream, oils and bacon help stimulate the mucosal movements and so should be used more liberally. Liquid and high-fluid foods help, as also soups and a large amount of electrolyte and water.

Nutritionist, both of the West and the Orient, recommend water as the best fluid, followed by vegetable/fruit juice, milk, broth and beverages. Table 17.9 gives the sample menu of diet for constipation.

Since high fibre diet is the main recommendation, Table 17.10 spells out the foodstuffs that should be preferred and others which must be excluded in the diet of patients suffering from chronic constipation.

TABLE 17.10: HIGH FIBRE (ROUGHAGE) FOODS FOR CHRONIC CONSTIPATION

Type of foods	Foods included	Foods excluded
Beverages	All kinds including milk	None
Cereals	Whole wheat/bran bread	White bread
	Whole wheat porridge	Suji
	Oat meal	Refined flour chapattis
	Whole wheat chapattis	Sago, arrow-root
Legumes	All dals with husk	Dehusked dals
Meat Group	Meat/fish/chicken to be taken with green leafy vegetable	None
Vegetables	Green leafy vegetables (GLV)	Root vegetables
	Beans, peas, cauliflower	
Fruits	Guava, papaya, pomegranate and seetaphal	Fruit juice
	Other fruits with seeds and skin	
Fats/Oils	Normal requirement as desired	

Source: Rekha Sharma: *Diet Management*. 1999, B. I. Churchill Livingstone.

DR. (MRS.) USHA JAIN

The Naturopths view constipation as a deviation from 'Natural' norms of life, hence a refreshingly different approach

Causes

1. Taking greasy non-vegetarian foods, refined wheat products and soft non-bulk forming foods.
2. Lack of enough liquids and fluids.
3. Psychological causes like worry and anxiety etc.
4. Lack of physical activity that affects motility of colon.
5. Using Western type toilets which does not exert pressure on the posteriors.
6. Failure to make a habit of early morning evacuation and a bit of aversion with evacuation habits.
7. Medication adopted to control other diseases like sedatives and others for nervous disorders.
8. Diseases of GI tract also lead to constipation, such as hyperacidity, bad teeth, tumour, sluggish liver, colitis; spastic conditions of intestines due to excessive reliance on laxatives; diseases of colon and rectum; diabetes, uterine diseases; abnormal conditions of lower spine and enlargement of prostate glands.

Regulation Guidelines

1. Generous use of fruits like papaya, grapes, figs, pears, mangoes, grapefruit, goose-berry, guavas and oranges
2. All dried fruits like figs, prunes, raisins, apricots and plums have laxative effect.
3. Green leafy vegetables and other raw vegetables like spinach, lettuce, cabbage and cauliflower, Brussels sprouts, celery, alfalfa, turnips, pumpkin, peas and beets and asparagus.
4. Whole wheat, whole grains and wheat flour (unrefined).
5. Fruits with peel to be preferred like apples, guavas, pears, sapota and grapes.
6. Use brown bread, vegetable-chapattis and vegetable-dalia (porridge).
7. Greater use of dietary fibre like wheat bran, oats flakes, China grass, GLV, agar agar and isabgol.
8. Generous intake of water and fluids like lemon juice, fruit and vegetable juice.
9. Take 2-3 cupfuls of 'Copper-vessel Water' or green sun-charged water soon after getting up in the morning and then take a stroll after that in order to stimulate the bowels.
10. Soak dry fruits like figs, dates, raisins, 'Munakka' in milk/plain water. Take these, as also the 'Soak Water' befor going to bed or early in the morning.
11. Always sit in a squatting position (the old oriental style) for defecation. This puts pressure on lower abdomen and stimulates bowel movements. Using the old style toilet system proves very helpful.

Organic Laxatives

The organic laxatives, even when used for longer periods in chronic constipation, do not produce any ill effects.

These organic laxatives are:

1. Take 2-3 tsp Isabgol in milk or water at bed time or early morning.
2. Use 2 tsp Gulkand (Rose leaves paste in honey, sun-charged for 40 days).
3. Take powdered 'Harar' (Myrobalans, *Terminalia chebula*) with water at night. Better soak in water overnight and take 1 tsp with a pinch of salt early morning.
4. Steep pulp of Amaltas in water overnight. Strain it and take it early morning.
5. Bael fruit (Aegle marmelos) is considered to be a very effective laxative.
6. Use of Linseed in chronic conditions is strongly recommended.
7. Use 1-2 tsp Castor oil in milk or lemon juice at night.

Nature Cure

The following steps prove very useful:

1. Cold friction bath daily in the morning is quite helpful.
2. Use mud-pack or abdominal compress. The latter can be packed in 'Tesu' flowers.
3. Clean bowels daily with regular use of enema for a few days.
4. Use alternate hot and cold hip bath before retiring at night.
5. Using 'Red Oil' for abdominal massage relieves constipation
6. Practise Yogasanas, these help strengthen the abdominal and pelvic muscles and stimulate the peristalsis. These asanas are:

- Bhujang
- Shalabh
- Yoga-mudra
- Dhenur
- Hal-asan
- Puschi-uttana.

Another Yoga exercise recommended very strongly is:

'Shankh Prakshalan Kriya'.

TABLE 17.11: DR. (Mrs.) JAIN'S DIET CHART FOR CONSTIPATION (ROUTINE TYPE)

6.00 AM	Copper-vessel water or green sun-charged water	2-3 glassfuls
7.00 AM	Lime water with honey	1 glass
9.00 AM	Overnight soaked figs	2
	Almonds	5
	Munakkas (Dried currants)	10
	Milk with honey	1 glass or
	Milk with molasses in water	
	Ripe Papaya	250 g
11.00 AM	Green sun-charged water	1 glass
12.00 Noon	Seasonal fruit juice or vegetable juice, viz., Spinach, tomato, carrot—all mixed	1 glass
1.00 PM	Seasonal green vegetable salad,	1 bowl
	with sprouts—Alfalafa, green grams, beans, etc.	1 tsp
	Vegetable-chapattis or fortified chapattis	2-4 (+Bran 25%)
	Green Gooseberry (Amla) chutney with coriander, mint, onion and garlic	
4.00 PM	Seasonal juicy fruits—Papaya, pears, guava, etc.	1 glass
6.00 PM	Green sun-charged water	1 glass
7.00 PM	Green vegetables soup, including green leafy vegetables	1 glass
	Vegetable-Dalia with sprouts	1 bowl
	Steam-cooked seasonal green vegetables	1 bowl
	Curd raita—cucumber, onion, tomato, spinach, etc.	
	Green gooseberry chutney(+)	
9.00 PM	Soaked figs	2 with
	Amla powder	1 tsp

However, constipation is often observed to become a chronic problem. Table 17.12 gives a special diet chart for such a condition.

TABLE 17.12: DR. (Mrs.) JAIN'S DIET CHART FOR CHRONIC CONSTIPATION

6.00 AM	Copper-vessel water or green sun-charged water	2-3 glassfuls
7.00 AM	Overnight soaked saunf (Fenugreek) with Munakkas	15 Drink Soak water
8.00 AM	Spinach or bitter gourd juice add honey, if not diabeteic	1 tsp
9.00 AM	Overnight soaked figs	2
	Amonds	5
	Munakkas (Dried Currants)	10
	Seasonal fruit salad—papaya, pears, sapota, guava	250 g
	Bran tea	1 cup
	(*Boil 1 tsp bran in a cup of milk*)	
11.00 AM	Green sun-charged water	1 glass
12.00 Noon	Seasonal vegetable salad	250 g
	Sprouts-Alfalafa, green grams, beans, etc.	1 tsp
	Vegetable-chapattis	3-4
	(Wheat flour made into dough with raw grated green vegetables, but without water) or Fortified chapattis (50% Bran)	
	Coconut chutney with coriander, mint, onion, garlic and curry leaves.	
4.00 PM	Seasonal juicy fruits—Orange, pine-apple, sweet orange, grapefruit	1 glass
	(*Grapefruit is a very good cleanser*)	
6.00 PM	Green sun-charged water	1 glass
7.00 PM	Dinner same as lunch	
9.00 PM	Triphala powder	1 Tsp
	Amla	1 tsp
	Soaked figs	2
	with Munakkas	10
	Eat figs and mix all others in water and drink	

CHERIE CALBOLM SUPPLEMENT

Suggested Juicing Recipes for Crohn's Disease

Calcium-Rich Cocktail

3 kale leaves
Small handful parsley
4-5 carrots, greens removed
½ apple, seeded

Bunch up kale and parsley, and push through hopper with carrots and apple.

Digestive Special

Handful spinach
4-5 carrots, greens removed

Bunch up spinach and push through hopper with carrots

Potasium Broth

Handful parsley
Handful spinach
4-5 carrots, greens removed
2 stalks celery

Bunch up parsley and spinach leaves, and push through hopper with carrots and celery

Chlorophyll Cocktail

3 Beet tops
Handful parsley
Handful spinach
4 carrots, greens removed
½ apple, seeded

Bunch up beet tops, parsley and spinach, and push through hopper with carrots and apple

Harvest Soup

2-3 garlic cloves
1 kale leaf
1 large tomato
2 stalks celery
1 collard leaf, chopped
1 tsp croutons

Roll garlic in kale leaf and push through hopper with tomato and celery. Place juice in saucepan, add chopped collards, and gently heat. Garnish with croutons.

Garlic Express

Handful parsley
1 garlic clove
4-5 carrots, greens removed
2 stalks celery

Bunch up parsley and push through hopper with garlic, carrots, and celery

Ginger Fizz

¼-inch slice ginger root
1 apple, seeded
Sparkling water

Push ginger through hopper with apple. Pour juice into ice-filled glass. Fill glass to top with sparkling water

Suggested Juicing Recipes for Colitis

Calcium-Rich Cocktail

3 kale leaves
Small handful parsley
4-5 carrots, greens removed
½ apple, seeded

Bunch up kale and parsley and push through hopper with carrots and apple

Iron-Rich Drink

3 beet tops
4-5 carrots, greens removed
½ green pepper
½ apple, seeded

Bunch up beet tops, and push through hopper with carrots, followed by green pepper and apple

Folic Acid Special

2 kale leaves
Small handful parsley
Small handful spinach
4-5 carrots, greens removed

Bunch up kale, parsley and spinach, and push through hopper with carrots

Vegetable Express

2 lettuce leaves
1 small wedge cabbage
4-5 carrots, greens removed
3 broccoli flowerets
½ apple, seeded

Bunch up lettuce leaves, and push through hopper with cabbage, carrots, broccoli, and apple

Carotene Cocktail

Handful parsley
Handful spinach
4-5 carrots, greens removed
½ apple, seeded

Bunch up parsley and spinach, and push through hopper with carrots and apple

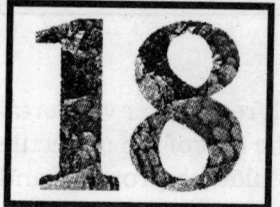

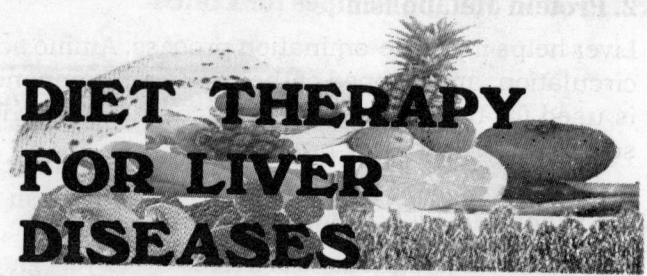

DIET THERAPY FOR LIVER DISEASES

LIVER—THE QUINTESSENTIAL WAREHOUSE

Liver is the largest gland of the body, accounting for nearly 3% of the bodyweight. More than the physical attributes, it is the one organ which performs a multitude of vital functions, of which over 500 functions have already been identified. Hence, it is called the 'Warehouse and Chemical Manufacturer' of the human body. These multiple functions may be grouped under five main heads:

1. Manufacture of vital substances, e.g. bile, prothrombin, firbrinogen, heparin and urea.

2. Regulation of body processes, e.g. detoxification, blood volume, reticuloendothelial activity and blood sugar level.

3. Metabolism of important nutrients like carbohydrates, proteins, fats, vitamins and minerals.

4. Storage of nutrients and other substances, e.g. glycogen, protein reserves, iron, copper, vitamins A, D, K and B complex.

5. Detoxification, e.g. alcohol, nicotine, and other toxic materials.

In view of its wider ramifications, all those concerned with the health (and nutrition) of the liver classify these group activities as listed below:

1. Detoxification Function

Liver helps degrade and detoxify materials like LSD, barbiturates, tranquilizers and hallucinogens. Detoxification is also involved in the esterification of cholesterol and conjugation and oxidation of steroids, besides the formation of bile pigments.

2. Protein Metabolism

Liver helps in the de-amination process. Amino acids, which reach liver via portal circulation, are stripped of their nitrogen component and the rest of the molecule is used for the production of glucose. It also synthesizes plasma proteins and serves as a reserve for proteins.

3. Carbohydrate Metabolism

One of the major functions of liver is to convert glucose into glycogen that provides energy reserves for the body. Excess carbohydrates are converted into fatty acids and neutral fat.

4. Lipid Metabolism

Production of fatty acids and triglycerides is another important function of liver. Further, cholesterol is synthesized by the liver and is eliminated in feces after its conversion to bile salts. Similarly, steroids are degraded in liver and excreted in the bile.

5. Vitamin and Mineral Metabolism

Carotenes are converted into vitamin A and stored in the liver. Other vitamins stored are vitamin D and vitamins of B group. It also stores important minerals like iron and copper.

6. Blood Formation

Liver is a major source of embryonic red blood cells and it is also involved in the production of blood platelets—thrombocytes.

7. Bile Formation

Bile is the main secretion of liver. It consists of bile pigments and bile salts, besides inorganic salts, proteins and cholesterol. The pigments: bilirubin and biliverdin are conjugated with glucuronic acid by the liver.

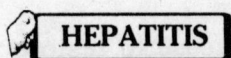 **HEPATITIS**

Hepatitis or inflammation of the liver is a common disease, of which the acute form is a self-limiting inflammatory condition. There are two types of hepatitis, viz., one is viral and the other is caused by drugs.

The Viral hepatitis results from viral infections, Virus A Hepatitis and Virus B Hepatitis. Herein, the infection is transmitted by fecal contamination of water or food or else parenterally by the use of contaminated syringes. Type B infection is a more severe disease.

Drug-induced hepatitis is caused mainly due to drug abuse, viz., alcohol, marijuana, hashish and heroine. Sometimes, it is also caused by hypersensitivity to sulfa drugs, penicillin and chloroform.

Symptoms

The injury to the liver cells in milder cases is reversible, but when it is a severe form, it causes extensive damage or necrosis of liver tissue, which in extreme cases, may lead to liver failure and death. The clinical symptoms are anorexia, nausea, vomiting, diarrhoea, fever, fatigue and loss of weight. Enlarged liver and spleen cause abdominal discomfort.

If hepatitis advances to a severe form, yellow bile pigments accumulate in the inflamed liver and spill into the blood, causing jaundice.

Jaundice, the major symptom of hepatitis, can have both nutritional and psychologic effects. Often malnutrition and impaired immuno-competence contribute to spontaneous infections and continuing liver disease. Jaundice initially occurs for 5 to 10 days, then deepens for 1-2 weeks and finally levels off and decreases with a convalescence period of 1-3 months.

Diet Therapy

Since exercise increases both the severity and duration of the disease, hence bed rest is the first step in treatment. The fluid intake must be increased to 300 -350 ml per day to avoid dehydration and also help improve appetite. However, optimum nutrition is the main therapy that helps in the speedy recovery of damaged liver cells and regaining the body tone and vigor.

The optimum diet calls for four-pronged strategy:

1. High Proteins

These are essential for liver cell regeneration. It also provides lipotropic agents like methionine and choline which help convert fats into lipoproteins and their removal from liver, thus preventing fatty infliteration. The diet must contain 75-100 g/day of high quality proteins.

2. High Carbohydrate

Diet should provide enough glucose to restore normal glycogen reserve and also meet the energy demands of the disease process. This glucose also spares the proteins for more important job of tissue regeneration. The diet must provide 300 - 400g of carbohydrate per day.

3. Moderate Fat

It will help make the food more palatable and attractive for anorexic patients. I could be milk, cream, butter, margarine and vegetable oils, say 100-150 g pe day.

4. High Energy

Normally 2500-3000 kcal are needed to meet the energy demands of tissue regeneration and to compensate for other losses from the disease.

The diet must be divided into 6-8 small meals and should be of liquid consistency to tempt the patient to eat something. As the condition improves, the texture of the food and frequency can be accordingly modified to make it more attractive. High protein beverages like protinules and protinex in milk should be given in between the meals.

One must avoid fried and high fat foods, nuts, chocolates and rich desserts, as also spiced foods. One must avoid root vegetables, tubers and fruits like banana, sapota and custard apple.

The Indian Council of Medical Research (ICMR)* has recommended the following sample diet in Table 18.1 for Indians. This diet provides:

Calories	1600 kcal
Proteins	65 g
Fat	40 g
Carbohydrates	245 g

TABLE 18.1: SAMPLE DIET FOR HEPATITIS (ICMR)

	Foodstuffs	Vegetarians (g)	Non-Vegetrians (g)
1.	Cereals	200	250
2.	Pulses	60	20
3.	Green leafy vegetables	200	200
4.	Other vegetables	200	200
5.	Fruits	200	200
6.	Milk	400 ml	200 ml
7.	Oils/Fat	20	20
8.	Poultry, without skin	—	100

While Dr. Antia's diet chart (Table 18.3) shows the diet regime for mild to medium jaundice cases, Table 18.2 gives a high carbohydrate diet for sub-acute state of hepatitis for the All India Institute of Medical Sciences (Delhi) patients, as advised by its Chief Dietician, Mrs. Rekha Sharma. This one provides:

Carbohydrates	350 g
Proteins	50 g
Fats	40 g

---

*ICMR recommendations for the Indians are equally applicable to most of the Third World Countries, unlike the irrationally rich diets of the West.

TABLE 18.2: HIGH CARBOHDYRATE DIET FOR HEPATITIS (SUB-ACUTE)

7.00 AM	Tea/coffee	1 cup
9.00 AM	Low fat milk (3%)	200 ml (1 glass)
	Bread with Jam—1 tsp	2 slices
	Fruit	1 medium
11.00 AM	Fruit Juice/Lemon with sugar or buttermilk	1 glass
1.00 PM	Rice or chapattis	75 g (3-4)
	Dal	100 g
	Potato	25 g (1 bowl)
	Curd	25 g (1 bowl)
	Sago kheer in milk	1 bowl with 1 g sugar
	Cooking fat	1 tsp
	Fruit	1 medium
4.00 PM	Tea with sugar	1 cup
	Arrow root biscuits	2
7.00 PM	Dinner same as Lunch	

Rekha Sharma: *Diet Management*, Churchill Livingstone, 1999.

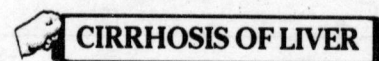 **CIRRHOSIS OF LIVER**

Cirrhosis of Liver is a chronic progressive disease of the liver in which the fibrous connective tissue replaces the functioning liver cells. Some forms result from biliary obstruction or liver necrosis, else from viral hepatitis and alcoholism. Alcohol and its metabolic products disturb liver metabolism and damage liver cells directly.

The clinical symptoms include nausea, vomiting, anorexia. Distension and abdominal pain. There is a low serum albumin level and edema due to protein deficiency. There is ascites and anemia from gastrointestinal bleeding and iron deficiency. The impaired circulation with increasing venous pressure may lead to oesophageal varices (*i.e.* enlarged veins), which may lead to fatal hemorrhage.

Figure 18.1 depicts the progression of pathology that eventually leads to the cirrhosis of liver.

Treatment

One of the main objective of treatment is to control blood ammonia levels. Antibiotics are used to limit the growth of intestinal bacteria and laxatives help speed up intestinal transit time. Oral antidiabetic agents are used to control hyperglycemia. Interferon and ribavirin are used to improve immune response in cirrhosis caused by viral hepatitis.

TABLE 18.3: SAMPLE MENU FOR JAUNDICE (MiLD TO MODERATE) OR VIRAL HEPATITIS

9.00 AM	Puffed rice	1 cup
	Skimmed Milk with 1 tsp sugar/ honey	1 cup
	Bread with butter/jam	2 slices
	Tea/coffee	1 cup
	Fruit	1 medium
	(*Half boiled eggs, 2 for Non-veg.*)	
11.00 AM	Fruit Juice/Sugarcane juice	1 glass
1.0 PM	Split Pea soup	1 bowl
	Rice	2 tsp
	Chapattis	3-4
	Thin dal	1 cup
	Cooked Pumpkin	½ cup
	Curd	25 g (1 bowl)
	Butter	1 tsp
	Mango/banana	1
	(*Roast mutton/baked chicken with tomato sauce for Non-veg.*)	
4.00 PM	Tea/Coffee	1 cup
	Biscuits/cake	
7.00 PM	Buttermilk	1 cup
	Boiled Potato	1
	Cooked cauliflower or mushroom, stuffed with egg plant	1 bowl
	Toast or khakhra	4
	Butter	2 tsp
	Grapes/stewed apricots	
	(*Meat or fish for Non-veg.*)	
9.00 PM	Skimmed milk	1 cup

Dr. F. P. Antia: *Clinical Dietetics and Nutrition*, Oxford University Press, 1982.

Diet Therapy

Diet Therapy is aimed at correcting the fluid and electrolyte imbalance and providing nutritional support for hepatic repairs. It should be started at the earliest before the disease gets advanced.

In infectious hepatitis, a high protein, high carbohydrate diet is recommended. But the protein level has to be controlled, if hepatic coma is suspected. About 35-50 g protein/day is adequate, but it could be increased to 80-100 g/day in cases of severe under-nutrition. However, the fat content should be kept low, less than 10 g/day. The calories should be provided in adequate amount about

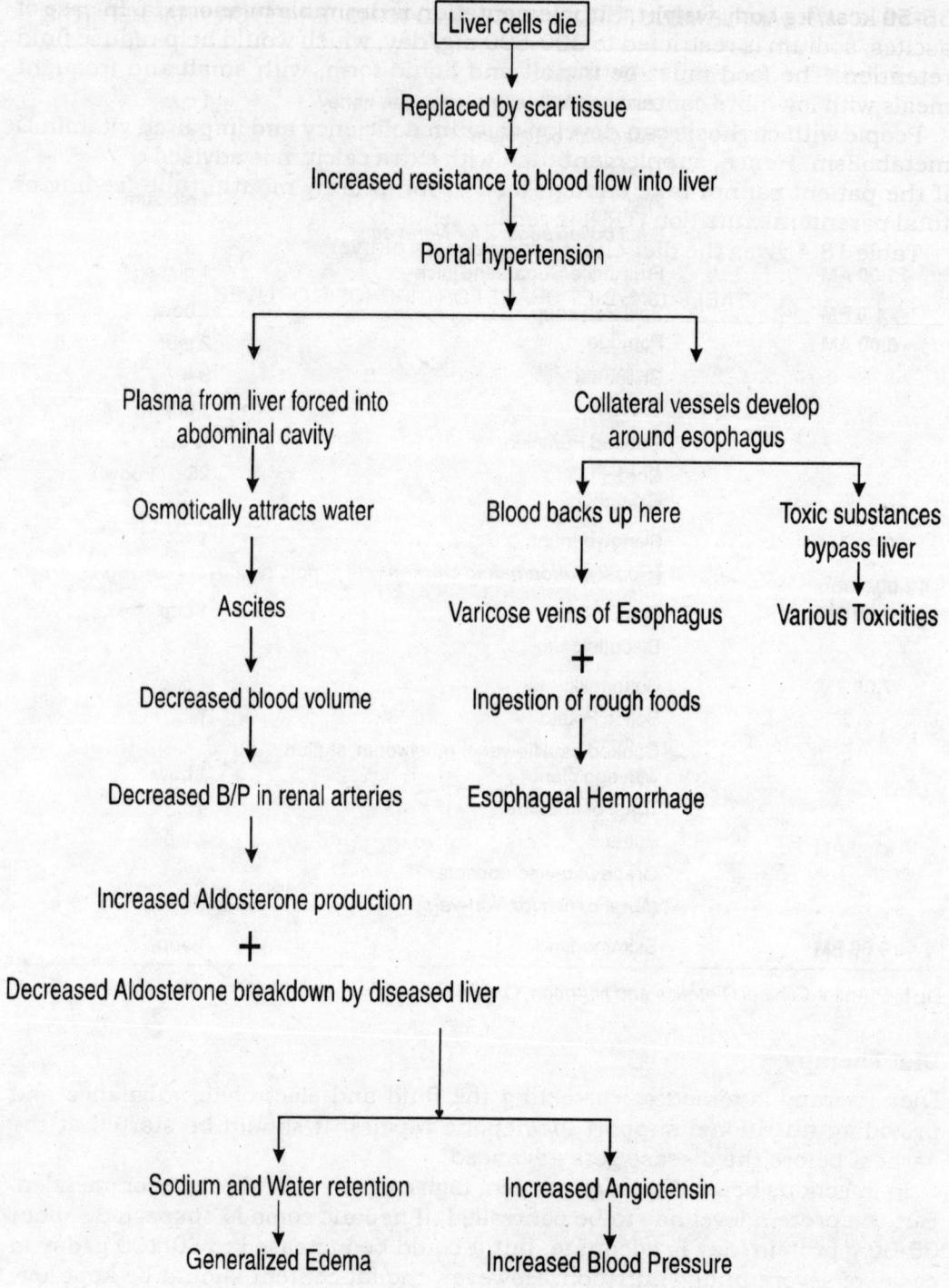

Fig. 18.1: Progression of Cirrhosis of the Liver

35-50 kcal/kg body weight. Supplementation is desirable in anorexia. In case of ascites, sodium is restricted to 300-500 mg/day, which would help reduce fluid retention. The food must be in soft and liquid form, with small and frequent meals with low-fibre content

People with cirrhosis can develop calcium deficiency and impaired vitamin D metabolism. Hence, supplementation with extra calcium is advised.

If the patient cannot take enough food or formula by mouth, tube feeding or total parenteral nutrition (TPN) is recommended.

Table 18.4 gives the diet chart for cirrhosis of liver.

TABLE 18.4: DIET CHART FOR CIRRHOSIS OF LIVER

8.00 AM	Porridge	¾ cup
	Skimmed Milk with sugar	1 cup
	Bread with Butter	2 slices
	Cottage Cheese	1 tbsp
	Tea/coffee	1 cup
	Orange	1
10.00 AM	Skimmed Milk	1 cup
12.00 Noon	Beet root/Russian salad	1 bowl
	Rice	2 tbsp
	Chapattis	3-4
	Thin dal	1 cup
	Cooked Brinjals	2-3 cups
	Skimmed Milk curd	
	Orange/sweet lime	1
	(*Stewed, grilled or smoked fish for Non-veg.*)	
4.00 PM	Tea/coffee	1 cup
	Almonds	8 or
	Groundnut	20
7.00 PM	Skimmed Milk	1 cup
	Boiled potato	1
	Vegetable lasagne with	3 tbsp
	Cottage Cheese or	
	Cooked Spinach	1 bowl
	Dal	1 cup
	Chapattis	4
	(*Roast chicken or baked chicken and noodle casserole for Non-veg*)	
9.00 PM	Skimmed Milk with	1 cup
	Skim Milk powder	2 tbsp

Source: Dr. F. P. Antia: *Clinical Dietetics and Nutrition.*

TABLE 18.5: DR. (MRS.) USHA JAIN'S DIET CHART FOR JAUNDICE

7.00 AM	Lemon squash with honey	1
7.30 AM	Amla powder with water/honey	1 tsp
9.00 AM	Butter milk (of toned milk)	1 glass
	Papaya/seasonal fruits	
11.00 AM	Tender Coconut water or ashgourd juice	1 glass
1.00 PM	Boiled seasonal vegetables	1 bowl
	Dry fortified Chapattis	2-4 (+25% Bran)
	Green vegetable salad	1 bowl
	Buttermilk	1 glass
4.00 PM	Orange juice or Sugarcane juice with ginger and lemon or sweet lime	1 glass
7.00 PM	Vegetable soup	1 glass
	Vegetable porridge	2 tsp
	Curd (toned milk)	1 bowl
	Amla chutney with mint, coriander, onion and garlic, all eaten with green salad	
9.00 PM	Amla powder with honey	1 tsp
	Soaked figs	2

Avoid

- Fats
- Fried Foods
- Spices
- Meat/Fish
- Maida
- Refined Cereal products
- Tea/coffee
- Alcohol
- Beverages

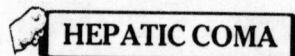 **HEPATIC COMA**

Hepatic coma is a syndrome of advanced liver disease. It is a neurologic disorder indicating extensive liver damage. It is characterised by varying degrees of consciousness, stupor and lethargy. Other symptoms include some personality changes, trembling of hands, loss of memory, hyperventilation and convulsions.

Due to entrance of ammonia into the cerebral circulation, it leads to many neurological disturbances. There is an imbalance of fluids and electrolytes. There will be signs of restlessness, mental confusion, delirium, drowsiness and hyper-irritability.

There is a very foul odor in the breath. Eventually, the patient relapses into coma, alongwith convulsions and death may occur.

Diet Therapy

The first and foremost step is to restrict proteins to the barest minimum level, say, 20-30 g/day. But it should be rich in calories (1500-2000 kcal/day) to prevent tissue breakdown. Glucose 300-400 g/day is recommended.

When the condition stabilizes, about 50 g high value proteins are advised, but the fluid intake should be restricted to 1000-1500 ml/day. Vitamin B complex and vitamin C supplementation is necessary. Attention must be paid to any deteriorating electrolyte imbalance, which should be corrected at once, lest it leads to some neurological problems. Supplementation with branched chain amino acids (BCAAs) helps improve the nitrogen balance in the system, although it does not improve the neurologic symptoms.

Table 18.6 gives the hourly diet chart for this disease.

TABLE 18.6: SAMPLE MENU FOR HEPATIC COMA

6.00 AM	Orange/sweet lime juice	150 ml with sugar 4 tsp
8.00 AM	Sugarcane juice	150 ml with glucose 2 tsp
10.00 AM	Rice or rava suji (porridge)	150 ml with sugar 3 tsp
12.00 Noon	Mashed banana with barley water	150 ml with sugar 2 tsp
2.00 PM	Tomato juice	150 ml with sugar 3 tsp
4.00 PM	Fruit juice	150 ml with sugar 2 tsp
6.00 PM	Vegetable soup (pureed and sieved)	150 ml with sugar 2 tsp
8.00 PM	Rice or suji porridge	150 ml with sugar 3 tsp
10.00 PM	Barley water	150 ml with sugar/honey 2 tsp

Source: S. Joshi. *Nutrition and Dietetics.*

N.B. Small meals frequently at 2-hour interval should be given if the patient is not in coma. If he is in a coma, it should be given by intra-gastric route.

HEPATIC FAILURE (Insufficiency)

This liver disorder occurs in severe hepatic diseases, when the liver function diminishes to 30% or less.

Heptic failure is characterised by a tendency to hemorrhage. Herein, prothrombin and fibrinogen levels are decreased and blood clotting is delayed. Due to accumulation of ammonia in blood, it leads to hepatic encephalopathy and hepatic coma, resulting eventually in death.

Treatment

Two drugs used for controlling ammonia levels are lactulose and neomycin. Vitamin K is advised to stop bleeding.

Diet Therapy

Protein levels should be kept at1.0-1.2 g/kg desirable body weight (DBW). This helps achieve a positive nitrogen balance. This protein level should be restricted to 0.7-0.8 g/ kg DBW in case of encephalopathy, but should never exceed 50 g/ day. If there is no improvement, then reduce the protein level by 10 g every 3rd or 4th day, till it comes down to 0.5 g/kg DBW.

Fluid intake-output balance is to be carefully controlled. Adequate calorie level must be maintained to avoid tissue catabolism. Usually, 2000 Kcal are needed per day. Sufficient carbohydrates are essentially a primary energy source. Branched chain amino acids (BCAAs) like Hepatamine are very helpful in maintaining adequate nitrogen balance and reduce the incidence of encephalopathy. These could be given as enteral feeding or through total parenteral nutrition therapy.

DISEASES OF GALL BLADDER AND PANCREAS

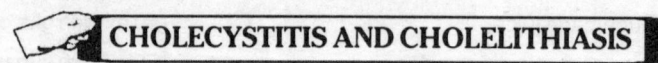 **CHOLECYSTITIS AND CHOLELITHIASIS**

Cholesyctitis is the inflammation of gall bladder which usually results from a low grade chronic infection.

In the normal course, cholesterol, bile's main ingredient, is kept in solution by other bile ingredients. However, when the gall bladder mucosa is inflamed or infected, its absorptive powers get affected. Under such conditions, cholesterol may precipitate, forming gall stones, composed solely of pure cholesterol. This condition is called 'Cholelithiasis' Excessive use of fat over a long period predisposes a man to gall stone formation, because of the constant stimulus to produce more cholesterol as a necessary ingredient to metabolise fat.

The symptom in both the conditions is severe abdominal pain. The patient gets the feeling of distension and fullness after eating, all the more so with fatty acids.

Treatment

Surgical removal of gall bladder, Cholecystectomy, is usually advised. Obese patients need to loose weight before the surgery. For small stones, ultrasound therapy and specific medication substitute for surgery.

Diet Therapy

1. Fat

Since fat is the principle cause of contraction of the diseased organ and the pain thereof, hence fat in the diet should be restricted to 20-30 g/day. Later on, depending upon his tolerance, it may be increased to 50-60 g/day. The fat control also helps control weight in obesity. This fat should not form more than 25-30% of the total kilocalories. For low-fat diet, one may refer Chapter 16.

2. *Kilocalories*

A low-fat diet advised above, helps in reducing weight and thus it helps in overall improvement in the condition.

3. *Cholesterol and Gas Formers*

Restriction on dietary cholesterol and vegetables like cabbage or legumes with high fibre (reported to be gas-forming) may be restricted.

The following diet regime in Table 18.7 is recommended for gall bladder diseases.

TABLE 18.7: DIET CHART FOR GALL BLADDER DISEASES

8.00 AM	Porridge	1 cup
	Skimmed Milk with sugar	1 cup
	Bread with Guava jam	2 slices
	Cottage Cheese	1 tbsp
	Tea/Coffee	1 cup
	Banana	1
12.00 Noon	Mixed vegetable soup or	1 bowl
	Rice	2 tbsp
	Chapattis	3-4
	Thin dal	½ cup
	Cooked Carrots with Pumpkin	1 bowl
	Skimmed milk curd	
	Papaya	1
	(*Minced Meat with boiled Potato and French Beans for Non-veg.*)	
4.00 PM	Tea/coffee	1 cup
	Biscuits	
7.00 PM	Vegetable Soup	3 tbsp or
	Cottage Cheese	
	Baked Potato/Caulifower	1 bowl
	Thin dal	1/2 cup
	Chapattis	4
	Buttermilk	1 glass
	Sago pudding/Apple pie	
	(*Meat/chicken grilled for Non-veg.*)	

Source: Dr. F. P. Antia: *Clinical Nutrition and Dietetics.*

PANCREATITIS

Acute inflammation of the pancreas is caused by the digestion of the pancreas tissue by its own enzymes, specially trypsin. Sometimes, gallbladder disease may cause a gall stone to enter the common bile duct and obstruct the flow from pancreas or cause a reflux of these secretions and bile into the pancreatic duct. This activates the powerful pancreatic enzymes within the gland. This does damage the tissue and causes pain. Sometimes, pancreatitis may be due to some infections or mumps. Normally, mild or moderate forms of this condition may subside completely.

Treatment

Treatment consists of intravenous feeding and replacement therapy of fluid and electrolytes, blood transfusion and medication with antibiotics. Gastric suction may be helpful.

Dietary Therapy

Nutritional support through parenteral feeding is helpful, because oral feeding could lead to entry of food into the intestine, which stimulates gastric secretion. With improvement in condition, a light diet can be given. However, coffee and alcohol must be avoided, since they stimulate pancreatic secretion.

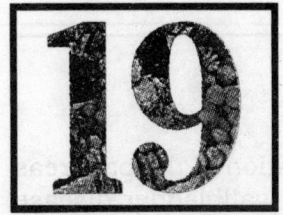

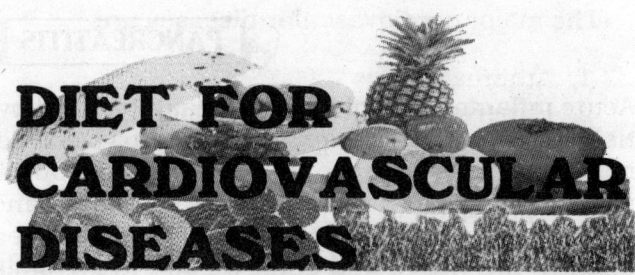

19

DIET FOR CARDIOVASCULAR DISEASES

THE CARDIOVASCULAR SYSTEM

The main function of the cardiovascular system is to supply the much-needed oxygen and nutrients to all the body cells. Any interruption in this crucial supply system for a few minutes invites death.

Of the four chambers of the heart, those on the right side receive the low-oxygen (de-oxygenated) blood from the body through the large vein: Vena Cava. It is then transported to the lungs, wherein carbon dioxide is exchanged for oxygen. Oxygenated (purified) blood is returned to the left side of the heart. It is then pumped into the rest of the body through the major artery: Aorta. There are valves in the heart which prevent the blood from flowing backwards. The enormity of the task performed by the heart muscles, through pulsation, can be gauged from the fact that these contract and relaxe 72 times every one single minute, i.e. over 100,000 times a day. And the body's 'Pace-maker' that coordinates the heart beat is the sino-arterial node, a specialised tissue in the right atrium.

The blood vessels serve as the freeway system of the body. The arteries carrying pure blood branch into smaller and still smaller arterioles and finally culminate into filament-like capillaries. It is these capillary-beds which provide the 'Exchange Station' between the arteries and the veins. These capillaries are so narrow that the red blood cells pass through them in a single file. Here, oxygen and nutrients are transferred from the blood to the tissues and in return, carbon dioxide plus other cellular wastes are absorbed by the blood. This widespread intricate web of capillaries, arteries and veins mean that by the end of the cycle, blood would have travelled through thousands of miles (some reports put it at 60,000 miles), of interconnecting blood vessels in order to furnish clean blood to all the body tissue. It is not the blood passing through the chambers that provides nourishment to the heart muscles. That job is done by the coronary arteries. And it is these coronary arteries which are the main target, nay the victims of the heart disease.

The major cardiovascular diseases are

1. Atherosclerosis
2. Hypertension (Increased Blood Pressure)
3. Ischaemic Heart Disease
4. Angina Pectoris
5. Cardiac Infarction.

Diabetes, high blood pressure and hyperlipidaemia are the common disease which are metabolically co-related with the incidence of CVD

The magnitude of this problem is shown by the fact that today, half of all the deaths in the west are attributed to the CVD. In USA alone, an estimated 3400 persons suffer a heart attack every day, i.e. more than two heart attacks every minute. Nearly 2 million adults continue to suffer from rheumatic or congestive heart disease. The American Heart Association estimates the total cost of CVD at $ 98 billion in medical bills and production losses in mid 1998. And this deadly syndrome is catching up everywhere in the developing countries.

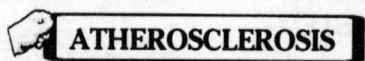 **ATHEROSCLEROSIS**

Underlying Disease Process

Atherosclerosis is the main disease of the Cardiovascular System. It is characterised by gradual deposition of fat that results in narrowing of the lumen of blood vessels, thus obstructing the flow of blood. The typical lesions are raised fibrous 'plaques' on the interior surface, 'Intima' of the blood vessels, which contain fatty materials like lipoproteins, the carrier of blood cholesterol. Even an unaided eye can detect these crystals in the softened cheesy debris of advanced lesions. This degeneration may allow a blood clot, 'Embolus' to develop and cut off the blood flow in the affected artery. And if this artery happens to be a major one like the coronary artery, then a heart attack occurs.

Deprived of oxygen and nutrients, the cells die in this condition called 'Ischaemia'. The localised tissue is called the 'Infarct' and when it affects the coronary artery supplying to the cardiac muscles: Myocardium, the disease is called Myocardial Infarction.

Of late, the research in the CVD has pinpointed three major causes for these plaques, the basic root of atherosclerosis and the main culprit for most of the cardiovascular diseases, viz. injury to the blood vessels and formation of clots (thrombosis), genetic factors and lipid (cholesterol) disorders.

Contrary to the popularly-held belief, atherosclerosis is not a sudden development. Rather, it is a slow onging process, developing at the rate of 1-2% from childhood in the form of 'Fatty streaks' in the artery walls. It is only in the advancing years, 40-50 onwards that it tends to assume serious proportion and restricts blood supply.

The arteries affected most are the aorta, coronary arteries and those supplying to the brain and kidneys. When one or more coronary artery is affected, it is called Coronary Artery disease (CAD). A blocked coronary artery results in a heart attack, the first warning signal of which is Angina pectoris or the pain in the chest.

Among the causes of atherosclerosis are damage to the artery wall by carbon monoxide in cigarette smoke, virus infections and hypertension. The damaged cell fragments stimulate the growth of arterial muscle which release 'Thromboxane'. It is the latter which causes the artery to constrict which sets in a chain reaction of accumulation of fat in the artery wall. Of the various contributory factors of atherosclerosis, cholesterol and lipoproteins are the major causes of this disease.

Cholesterol

Atherosclerosis is closely associated with blood fat levels. As this fat level specially cholesterol rises, so does the risk of the disease. The Framingham Study (1970s) found that as blood cholesterol levels rose from 150 mg % to 260 mg %, the risk of heart disease escalated three-fold. On the other hand in countries like Asia, where the cholesterol level is low, there is very little incidence of heart diseases. The Lipid research Clinics in USA have shown that for every 1% decline in blood cholesterol, a person reduces the chances of developing heart disease by 2%.

Lipoproteins

To transport cholesterol and other fats within the body, the blood packages them into different water soluble bubbles, called Lipoproteins. These are complexes of fat (lipids) and proteins that travel in the blood. Depending upon the density of fat and proteins, the lipoproteins are of four types:

1. **Chylomicron** are large globules composed primarily of triglycerides (TGs) and choletserol carried to the liver and other tissues.
2. **Very Low-density Lipoproteins (VLDLs)** are intermediate lipoproteins produced in the liver that carry TGs. These are mainly fats produced in the body.
3. **Low-density Lipoproteins (LDLs)** are high in cholesterol, but contain few TGs. The proportion of protein herein is much larger than VLDLs and chylomicrons. They are the main transporters of cholesterol from liver to the tissues and are produced from the VLDLs.
4. **High-density Lipoproteins (HDLs)** contain some TGs and some cholesterol, but they have large amount of proteins and phospholipids. They transport cholesterol from tissues to the liver.

In case there is too much cholesterol carried in the LDLs, a person's risk for heart disease is greater. But in the HDLs, the risk factor is very low. Increased concentration of certain cholesterol-carrying lipoproteins in the plasma are closely related to an increased risk of heart disease. But they can also be helpful in evaluating the effect of dietary changes and the consequent effectiveness of diet therapy. The three terms used in this measurememt of lipids are

1. **Hyperlipidaemia** is the condition which shows increased level of blood lipids.

2. **Hypercholesterolemia** is an increased level of cholesterol in the blood.

3. **Hypertriglycridaemia** is an increased serum triglyceride level.

In contrast, the term Hyperproteinaemia refers to the levels of different types of lipoproteins like VLDL, HDL etc. A man above 55 should not have more than 220 mg/100 ml serum cholesterol and the triglycerides should not exceed 150 mg per 100 ml.

Atherosclerosis and the heart disease are often called 'Silent Diseases'. They go on advancing unnoticed, till severe pain, angina pectoris develops. For those people with total cholesterol above 150 mg% and a high ratio of total cholesterol to HDL-cholesterol show greater incidence of disease, but then dietary control helps in a big way—to be dealt with later.

MYOCARDIAL INFARCTION

Acute Myocardial Infarction is the most common cause of death in the West. Myocardial Infarction results from prolonged myocardial ischaemia, with necrosis of myocytes due to interruption of blood supply to an area of the heart. The most common cause is occlusive thrombus superimposed on a ruptured or ulcerative atheromatous plaque.

Smoking, hypertension and hypercholesterolaemia are the main risk factors for the formation of atherosclerotic plaques. And sheer stress causes rupture of these plaques.

Infarction usually affects the left ventricle and intraventricular septum, though the right ventricle may be affected occasionally. Cardiogenic shock, due to systolic or diastolic dysfunction, is the common form of death.

Treatment

The treatment consists of administration of apirin and thrombolytic therapy with Streptokinase, Anistreplase and Rt-PA. Intravenous β-blockers are strongly recommended for patients without contraindications, who do not receive thrombolytic therapy. Angioplasty is used in cases of acute myiocardial infarction.

Dietary Therapy

The dietary therapy recommended for myocardial infarction, as also for congestive heart failure, is shown in Table 19.1.

TABLE 19.1: DIET CHART FOR MYOCARDIAL INFARCTION

7.00 AM	Light tea	1 cup
9.00 AM	Light tea	1 cup
	Bread slice	1 or
	Porridge	½ cup
	Egg white	1
	Low-fat milk	1 cup
11.00 AM	Fruit juice	1 cup
1.00 PM	Clear soup	1 cup
	Khichdi	1 cup or
	Bread slices	2
	Curd	1 cup
	Custard	½ cup or
	Jelly	1 bowl
4.00 PM	Tea	1 cup
	Biscuits	2
7.00 PM	Clear soup	1 cup
	Sandwich or khichdi or soft rice	1 cup
	Soft pureed vegetables or mashed potato	1 cup
	Cooking oil	5 g
9.00 PM	Low-fat milk	1 cup

Source: Rekha Sharma. *Diet Management*. Churchill Livingstone.

This diet contains:

Proteins	38 g
Fat	25 g
Carbohybdrates	135 g
Calories	1000 Kcal

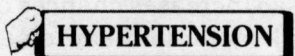 **HYPERTENSION**

Hypertension or blood pressure is the blood's force against the artery walls, as it is pumped out from the heart. In the normal course, blood pressure varies during the day; it increases with excitement, anxiety or physical activity. After the event is over, it returns to normal. However, when it remains elevated for considerable time, it is called Hypertension or High Blood Pressure. Technically, it refers to sustained increase in diastolic pressure, systolic pressure or both. When the heart contracts, it is called the 'Systolic Pressure', it is usually the larger number on the top in a reading (*i.e.* 120/80). Diastolic pressure is the lower figure when the heart relaxes. The normal blood pressure for different age groups is shown in Table 19.2. This range of blood pressure is as follows:

Normal Blood Pressure	120/80 or less
Borderline Hypertension	140-160/90 or less
Hypertension	160/95 or more

TABLE 19.2: NORMAL BLOOD PRESSURE

Age years	Systolic Range			Diastolic Range		
	Min.	*Av.*	*Max.*	*Min.*	*Av.*	*Max.*
15-19	105	117	120	73	77	81
20-24	108	120	132	75	79	83
25-29	109	121	133	76	80	84
30-34	110	122	134	77	81	85
35-39	111	123	135	78	82	86
40-44	112	125	137	79	83	87
45-49	115	127	139	80	84	88
50-54	116	129	142	81	85	89
55-59	118	131	144	82	86	90
60-64	121	134	147	83	87	91

It is reported that in USA, one in every four persons suffers from hypertension. High blood pressure results from an imbalance between the cardiac output and the peripheral resistance. The following factors, individually or in concert, lead to such an imbalance:

1. Heredity
2. Mental tension
3. Excessive intake of table salt
4. Obesity and excessive weight
5. Sedentary life
6. Smoking and alcohol.

Amongst the known causes, these are atherosclerosis, tumour on renal gland or kidney malfunction. Stress also increases chances of premature heart disease. Hypertension is the primary risk factor for heart disease and stroke. It is called the '*Silent Killer*', because of no outward physical sign of high blood pressure.

The health hazards that have their origin in high blood pressure are:

1. Atherosclerosis
2. Heart failure
3. Arterial inflammation
4. Aneurysms of aorta
5. Renal troubles
6. Reduced life expectancy.

The best defence against this condition is prevention and treatment of the existing hypertension. But in more than moderate hypertension, it calls for effective treatment. Dietary factors contribute a great deal in prevention of hypertension. These factors include maintenance of bodyweight and proper levels of essential minerals like sodium, chloride, calcium, magnesium, cadmium, dietary fibre and alcohol.

Yoga

Since too much cholesterol carried in the LDLs is the main culprit in promoting the incidence of heart diseases, the recent report of the AIIMS, New Delhi about the Yoga combating Cholesterol in the Times of India dt. 19-11-2002 conclusively proves the healing impact of Yoga.

According to Dr. Bijlani, Head of Physiology Deptt, AIIMS, where this study was conducted, the major gains accruing after the Yogasanas were:

1. Decrease in the average blood glucose from 120 to 107.
2. Decrease in Total Cholesterol from 195 to 185.
3. The Low density lipoproteins (LDLs) went down from 120 to 110.
4. The Very Low density lipoproteins (VLDLs) went down from 30 to 25..

On the other hand, the 'Good Cholesterol', viz. High-Density Lipoproteins (HDLs) were found to have gone up marginally from 40 to 41, after the patients had done the Yogasanas.

Once again, Yoga has claimed the merit when it comes to treating the cardiovascular diseases.

Yoga Exercises have proved extremely beneficial to patients of high blood pressure. 'Shavasana' has yielded the best results over 4-8 or 12 weeks.Other yoga asansas found very useful are

Padmasana
Vajrasanas
Yogamudra
Matsyana
Matsyendrasana.

For hypertension (high blood pressure), Table 19.3 gives the sample diet containing low sodium level. Also see special supplements for Cherie Calbom's recommendations for hypertension.

TREATMENT FOR CARDIOVASCULAR DISEASES

Medication is a very helpful measure in treating CVD and a wide array of drugs are available, as under:

1. Vasodilators: are the drugs that help increase the vessel's diameter, thus permitting greater flow of blood in the coronary arteries.

2. Beta Blockers help by relaxing the heart muscle and control blood pressure.
3. Digoxin protects the ventricles from the effects of arterial fibrillation.
4. Atropine is helpful by increasing the rate of heart beats in conditions like bradycardia.
5. Diuretics are used in case of heart failure. They help reduce the volume of blood in circulation and also reduce the level of sodium.

TABLE 19.3: SAMPLE MENU FOR HIGH BLOOD PRESSURE (LOW SODIUM DIET)

7.00 AM	Tea/coffee with sugar	1 cup
9.00 AM	Grape fruit juice	1 cup
	Porridge with cream and sugar	1 cup
	Puffed rice with milk	½ cup
	Toast with butter	2
	Sweet lime	
12.00 Noon	Vegetable soup with sour lime	1 cup
	Baked potato	1
	Cauliflower/cluster beans	1 cup
	Chapattis	3-4
	Banana	1
	(*Mutton chop for non-veg.*)	
4.00 PM	Tea with sugar	1 cup
	Bread with jam	2
	Unsalted cashewnuts	8 or
	Groundnuts	20
7.00 PM	Buttermilk	1 cup
	Cooked brinjals	1 cup
	Tomato and potato pie	1 bowl
	Rice with dal	1 cup
	Chapattis	3-4
	(*Roast chicken/veal casserole with boiled potato for non-veg.*)	

Source: Dr. F. P. Antia: *Clinical Diagnostics and Nutrition, Oxford University Press*, 1982.

DIET THERAPY FOR CVD

Notwithstanding a host of latest medicines available in the field, the best form of treatment that has long-lasting effect is the Diet Therapy. Indeed, the Diet Therapy ought to precede the drug therapy. This point is borne by the special dietary recommendations made in Table 19.4 by the WHO that go a long way to prevent heart diseases.

Besides the weight control (reduction in the obese patients), dietary fat regulation helps bring down cholesterol levels which is another major plank in both prophylactic and curative treatment. And many of these salts and minerals help regulate the blood pressure (hypertension). As such, calorie balance, fats and carbohydrates, plus proper control and maintenance of salt balance are the principle planks of the diet therapy in dealing with the Cardiovascular diseases.

1. Ideal Body Weight

There is a direct relationship between body weight and hypertension, and consequently other heart diseases. It is recommended that calorie intake be reduced by about 1000 kcal, which would help the patient return to normal body weight. A bed-ridden patient should not have more than 1000-1200 kcal/day.

TABLE 19.4: DIETARY RECOMMENDATIONS FOR CVD PREVENTION (WHO)

	Food ingredients	Higher limit	Lower limit
1.	Total energy from fats (%)	30	15
	—From SFA	10	0
	—From PUFA	7	3
2.	Cholesterol level	< 300 mg	0
3.	Total energy from proteins (%)	15	10
4.	Total energy from carbohydrates (%)	75	55
5.	Total dietary fibre (g/day)	40	27
6.	Non-starch polysachharides (NSP) (g/day)	24	16
7.	Free sugar (g/day)	10	0
8.	Fruits and vegetables (g/day)	—	400
9.	Pulses, nuts and seeds (g/day)	—	30
10.	Salt (g/day)	6	—

Greater the body weight, greater the work load on the heart and hence greater the incidence of CVD, a common phenomenon in the High-diet, Higher-weight West. Obesity is the net effect of dietary imbalance between energy intake and expenditure. Obesity may be caused by genetic, psychogenic, metabolic or hereditary factors. In the developing countries, the 'Desirable Body Mass Index (BMI)' should be within the range of 18.5 and 20. The BMI of more than 23 is closely linked to common heart disease.

When the weight is lost, the volume of blood declines, thus altering the hormones related to blood pressure, which eventually goes down. If the ideal weight is maintained, then many cases of mild to moderate hypertension can be tackled without resorting to medicines. This fact means avoiding many undesirable side-effects of hypertensive drugs.

Regular exercise is another very helpful step. Both exercise and weight loss can help reduce blood pressure by normalising other body processes.

2. Dietary Fat

A high-fat diet increases the incidence of blood pressure. Avoid the use of saturated fats through meats etc. Instead, one should shift to vegetable oils and such foods which have only polyunsaturated fatty acids (PUFA). These PUFA or the essential fatty acids are the building blocks for prostaglandins, the hormone-like substances in the blood, which regulate blood pressure by dilating blood vessels and excreting greater amount of sodium and water.

Omega-3 fatty acids, viz., Eicosapentaenoic acid (EPA) and other Docosahexaenoic acid (DHA) in sea-foods have been found very useful. They alter platelet activity and reduce platelet aggregation, thus lowering the risk of coronary thrombosis. They decrease the risk of VLDL and significantly increase anti-inflammatory effect.

Vegetarian diets of whole grain bread and cereals are low-fat diets and hence decrease the risk of hypertension. Herein, the high fibre intake and potassium content help in bringing down blood pressure to normal. If the fat content of diet is reduced to 25% or less, salt is restricted and the ideal body weight maintained, it could help eliminate hypertension by 85%, without using any medicine.

Amongst the vegetable oils, safflower (Kardi) oil gets the top ranking as an anti-hypertensive agent, followed by corn oil, soyabean oil and sesame oil. Safflower oil, becasue of the high linoleic acid content, offers considerable benefits, while coconut oil and palm oil, which contain high saturated fats, are to be avoided.

Essential fatty acids like linolenic acid (ALNA-n_3) and linoleic acid (LA-n_6) should be incorporated into the diet, as they help effectively lower the cholesterol level of the blood.

The percentage of LA-n_6 in safflolwer, soyabean, sunflower oils, corn and cottonseeds is more than 50% of the total fatty acids, while in rice bran, coconut oil, ghee and vanaspati, it ranges from 20-40%. An ideal ratio of LA/ALNA should be 5-10, hence soyabean is specially recommended. Else, mustard oil in combination with groundnut or sesame (til) oil may be used. PUFA level can be increased by incorporating 100 g fish oil in the diet.

Table 19.5 shows the quality of fats in the vegetable oils.

Another very important plank of dietary therapy is to avoid, as much as possible, the cholesterol intake through foods like eggs, meats, butter and cream etc.

3. Carbohydrates

Amongst the starches and carbohydrates, sugars, glucose, sucrose and fructose, if taken in excess, cause 'Hyperlipidaemia'. Instead, the complex carbohydrates like whole grain flour and legumes should be consumed, as also fresh fruits and raw vegetables which offer greater dietary fibre. Greater the consumption of these complex carbohydrates, greater the capability of the system to resist the onset of any CVD. Other foods like garlic help reduce substantially the blood cholesterol levels in the body.

TABLE 19.5: QUALITY OF FATS IN VEGETABLE OILS

	Oil	PUFA/SFA	LA/ALNA (n_6/n_3)	Preferred Medium
1.	Soybean oil	High	Ideal	Best source
2.	Mustard oil	Ideal	Low	
3.	Coconut oil	Low	Ideal	
4.	Palm oil	Low	Ideal	
5.	Ghee	Low	Ideal	
6.	Vanaspati	Low	Ideal	
7.	Safflower oil	High	Very high	
8.	Sunflower oil	High	Very high	
9.	Groundnut oil	Ideal	High	GN + Mustard oil
10.	Rice Bran oil	Ideal	Fair	
11.	Sesame (Til) oil	Fair	High	Til + Mustard oil

4. Minerals

(a) Sodium

High salt diet increases blood pressure, besides constricting the arterial walls. The desired levels of sodium is 500 mg/day, which dose is obtained through normal diet, but in the USA, the consumption of sodium goes upto 5000 mg with all the harmful consequences.

Chloride, the other component of salt, is also linked to hypertension. The kidney produces an enzyme, Renin, which regulates the level of water and sodium. Chloride discourages the secretion of renin enzyme and thus it could lead to higher blood pressure.

(b) Potassium

A diet high in potassium, like fruits and vegetables, protects against hypertension. An increased potassium intake helps lower the systolic and diastolic blood pressure.

Following tabulation gives different categories of potassium-containing fruits and vegetables in common use:

Group A:	High potassium vegetables	High potassium fruits/juices
	Artichokes	Apricots
	Beans, lentils	Avocados
	Broccoli	Bananas
	Brussels sprouts	Cantaloupes
	Carrots, raw	Dates
	French fries	Figs
	Greens	Honeydew melons
	Lima beans	Mangoes
	Parsnips	Nectarines
	Potato, baked	Orange,—Juice
	Pumpkin	Papayas
	Spinach	Prunes
	Sweet potato	Raisins
	Tomato	Rhubarb
	Winter squash (butternut)	Water melon
	Tomato juice	Apricot nectar
		Prune juice

Group B:	Low-potassium vegetables	Low-potassium fruits/juices
	Asparagus	Apple, apple juice
	Beets	Applesauce
	Cabbage	Blueberries
	Carrots, cooked	Cherries
	Cauliflower	Cranberries—Juice
	Celery	Fruit Cocktail
	Corn	Grapefruit—Juice
	Cucumber	Grapes—Juice
	Eggplant	Lemons
	Green beans	Limes
	Green peppers	Peaches, fresh
	Kale	Pears, fresh—Nectar
	Lettuce	Pineapple—Juice
	Okra	Plums
	Onions	Raspberries
	Potato, presoaked	Strawberries
	Radish	Tangerines
	Wax beans	
	Zucchini	

(c) Calcium

When diets are supplemented with 1000 mg calcium/day, it lowers the diastolic pressure in mild to moderate cases of hypertension. Blood pressure also declines when calcium is added to high-sodium diet.

(d) Magnesium

Magnesium deficiency is related to an increase in blood pressure. Use of magnesium-rich foods like nuts, dried beans and peas, and sea-foods is recommended to lower the blood pressure.

(e) Cadmium

Cadmium is reported to increase the risk of hypertension. Smokers inhale a very large amount of cadmium from cigarettes.

Similarly, consumption of alcohol in large quantity leads to higher blood pressure.

As such, diets with moderate intake of calories, carbohydrates and modified fats (PUFA), but having abundance of proteins and low sodium are specially recommended in CVD. Vitamins and mineral supplementation is not necessary when large quantity of fruits and vegetables are being taken in diet.

Prudent Diet

Prudent Diet can play a very significant role in minimising the incidence and magnitude of cardiovascular diseases.

The American Heart Association recommends Prudent diet, as shown in Table 19.6. Of late, even these recommended figures have been revised, as indicated in Table 19.7, for high blood lipid levels.

TABLE 19.6: PRUDENT DIET NORMS IN USA

		Prudent diet	Usual American diet
1.	Total kilocalories	Sufficient to maintain ideal body wt.	Often very excessive
2.	Cholesterol (mg/day)	300	600-800
3.	Total fats—as % of kcal	30-35	40-45
	(a) Saturated fatty acids	Max.10	15-20
	(b) MUFA	15	15-20
	(c) PUFA	10	5-6
	(d) P/S ratio—(c/a)	1–1.5 = 1	0.3 = 1
4.	Carbohydrates—as % of kcal	50-55	40-45
	(a) Simple sugars	10	15-20
	(b) Complex carbohydrates	30-35	20-25
5.	Proteins—as % of kcal	12-20	12-15
6.	Sodium—m eq	130	200-250

Low-Sodium Diet

A low-sodium diet, recommended for high blood pressure and cardiac diseases, is also indicated in conditions like nephritis and toxaemia of pregnancy.

Depending upon the patient's condition, it may be:

(a) Mild restriction, about 2-3 g sodium/day
(b) Moderate restriction, about 1-2 g sodium/day
(c) Severe restriction i.e. less than 1 g sodium/day

The salt equivalent (units) are:

One teaspoon salt = 1500-2000 mg sodium
One m Eq = 23 mg sodium.

One must avoid use of extra salt on the dining table.
Restrict animal foods, as they are rich in sodium.
Restrict vegetables high in sodium like beet root, spinach, carrots and celery.
Avoid baking soda (sodium bicarbonate) in preparing foods, vegetables and pulses, field beans, amaranth and knol khol.

Since a low-sodium diet is bland and unappetising, salt-substitutes like Sodium-free calcium gluconate and moderate herbs and spices can be used for seasoning. One must avoid using chilli powder, since it contains added salt.

Sodium Depletion

There is a risk of sodium depletion, especially in hot weather when lot of sodium is lost through sweat. This can also happen in case of vomiting, diarrhoea, surgery and renal damage.

The symptoms of sodium depletion can be seen in the form of general weakness, abdominal cramps, oliguria, azotaemia and some acid-base imbalance.

The following tabulation shows the sodium level of different foodstuffs.

Low Sodium	Moderate Sodium	High in Sodium
Chapattis	Maize	Bread
Fruits	Puffed rice flakes	Biscuits, cakes
Cabbage	Corn flakes	Butter
Cauliflower	Leafy vegetables	Pasteries
Tomatoes	Carrots	Processed cheese
Peas	Radish	Meat extracts
Onions	Milk, curds	Pickles
Nuts	Lean meats	Sausages
Sugar, honey	Fish	Foods (+ baking soda)
Oil/cream	Poultry	Salted snacks

GUIDELINES FOR CVD DIET

1. Better use skim milk; avoid butter, cream and milk products.
2. Prefer white meats (chicken) over red meats (pork, mutton, beef).
3. Avoid all fried foods. Prefer oven or 'Tandoor'-baked items.
4. Heavy Indian sweets like barfi and cakes/puddings be avoided.
5. Restrict cholesterol content of diet to 250-350 mg/day.
6. Roasting in aluminum foil-wrapped foods is recommended.

Avoid

- Milk products such as cream, barfi, processed cheese, ice creams, puddings
- Animal fats, viz., butter, ghee, bacon fat; also lard, coconut and palm oils
- Fatty meats, organ meats like kidney, liver, brain
- Oily fishes like sardines: shell-fish like prawns and lobsters
- Oily or fried foods
- Nuts, dried fruits and oilseeds like groundnuts
- Salted foods like papads, chutneys and foods canned in brine
- Bakery products, dough nuts, pasteries
- Sausages and oil-based dressing

TABLE 19.7: REVISED NORMS FOR PRUDENT DIET

		Step One	Step Two
1.	Total fat, as % of kcal	< 30	< 30
	(a) Saturated fatty acids	< 10	< 7
	(b) MUFA	10-15	10-15
	(c) PUFA	10	10
2.	Carbohydrates, as % of kcal	50-60	50-60
3.	Proteins	15-20	15-20
4.	Cholesterol (mg/day)	< 300	200

Foods-Restricted Usage

1. Cereals—wheat, rice, sorghum (jowar), etc.
2. Pulses and lentils
3. Lean meats, fish, egg white and sausages
4. Vegetable oils
5. Sugar and jaggery
6. Common table salt
7. Root vegetables—potatoes, sweet potatoes, beet root, yam and pink radish
8. Noodles, spaghetti, bread
9. Milk without cream, cow's milk.

Foods – Unrestricted Usage

1. Green leafy vegetables, preferably raw vegetables
2. Garlic and onion
3. Tamarind, sour lime and vinegar for seasoning
4. Thin buttermilk, skim milk
5. Spices in moderate amounts
6. Coconut water
7. Clear soups

Table 19.8 gives an overview of different foods and beverages for a healthy heart.

TABLE 19.8: FOOD CHART FOR A HEALTHY HEART

Foods	Prefer	Limit (reduce)	Avoid
Cereals	Wheat, rice, ragi, bjara, maize, jawar	Foods prepared with maida like white bread and biscuit	Cakes, pastries, naan roti, roomali roti, noodles.
Pulses	Whole and sprouted and dals	—	—
Vegetables	Green leafy vegetables and other vegetables	Roots and tubers	Fried vegetables, banana chips, canned vegetables
Fruits	Fresh fruits		Dried fruits, canned fruits in syrup
Dairy products	Low fat milk, butermilk, skimmd milk	Full-cream milk, milk powders	Cheese, butter, khoa, condensed milk, cream
Eggs	Egg white	—	Egg yolk
Animal foods	Fish	Chicken	Prawns, shrimps, all types of meat
Fat	More than one type of vegetable oil	Total fat intake	Oily dishes, butter, ghee coconut oil, vanaspati, deep-fried foods
Sugar and Sugar products	Jaggery	Sugar in any home-made beverages	Sweets like chocolates, ice creams
Nuts and Oilseeds		All nuts and oilseeds	
Beverages	Fresh fruit juice (without sugar), light tea	Coffee, cola, soft drinks	Alcohol
Salt	Foods in natural state	Too much salt in preparations	Pickles, papads, sauces, salt biscuits, fried crispies

The Indian Council of Medical Research (ICMR) has recommended a special diet with low-cholesterol and reduced saturated fats, as shown in Table 19.9. These foods can help lower the plasma cholesterol levels.

TABLE 19.9: SPECIAL DIET FOR HEART PATIENTS (ICMR)

Foodstuffs	Amount (g)
Cereals	300
Pulses	50
Green leafy vegetables	50
Other vegetables	100
Roots and tubers	100
Fruits	100
Skimmed milk	400 ml
Sugar	30
Oil/fat	30

This ICMR diet will provide:

Calories	2400 kcal
Proteins	70 g
Fats	55 g
Carbohdyrates	400 g

Diet Regimes

Since the incidence and magnitude of the cardiovascular diseases are very much varied, hereunder we present a series of diet regimes/charts from different practising dieticians in India. The diseases covered in this concluding part of the Diet therapy for CVD are:

1. Ischaemic heart disease
2. High blood pressure-low cholesterol diet
3. Congestive hearty failure

Besides, we present the special diet chart recommended by the pre-eminent naturopath and practising dietician of Delhi, Dr (Mrs) Usha Jain.

TABLE 19.10: DIET CHART FOR ISCHAEMIC HEART DISEASE

7.00 AM	Tea with milk 50 ml	1 cup
9.00 AM	Porridge or	1 cup
	Bread slice	1
	Egg white	1
	Milk with sugar	1 cup
1.00 PM	Curd	1 cup
	Green leafy vegetable	1 bowl (200 g)
	Dal (pulses)	1 bowl
	Cheese	25 g
	Chapattis	2
	Cooking fat	5 g
4.00 PM	Tea with milk 50 ml	1 cup
	Biscuits	2-3
7.00 PM	Green leafy vegetables	1 bowl (200 g)
	Dal (pulses)	1 bowl (125 g)
	Chapattis	3
	Rice	75 g
	Cooking Fat	5 g
9.00 PM	Milk	1 glass

Source: Rekha Sharma: *Diet Management*.

This diet provides:

Calories	1400 kcal
Proteins	60 g
Fats	40 g
Carbohydrates	200 g

TABLE 19.11: DIET CHART FOR HIGH BLOOD PRESSURE
(LOW CHOLESTEROL, HIGH HDL DIET)

Time	Item	Quantity
7.00 AM	Tea/Coffee with sugar	1 cup
9.00 AM	Low fat milk	1 cup
	Whole wheat porridge	1 cup (50 g) or
	Whole wheat bread	1 slice or
	Oats	50 g
	Cheese	25 g or
	Egg white	1
1.00 PM	Curd (low fat milk)	1 bowl
	Green leafy vegetable	1 bowl (125 g)
	Dal (whole pulses)	1 bowl
	Fortified chapattis	3-4 (+ 25% Bengal gram)
	Cooking oil	5 g
	Fruits	200 g
4.00 PM	Soya upma	50 g or
	Sprouts	1 tsp
	Tea	1 cup
7.00 PM	Green leafy vegetables	125 g
	Rice khichdi with	
	Whole bengal gram	50 g
	Chapattis	4
	Cooking oil	5 g
	Sugar	20 g

Source: Rekha Sharma. *Ibid.*

This diet provides:

Calories	1500 kcal
Proteins	64 g
Fat	25 g
Carbohydrates	254 g

TABLE 19.12: DIET FOR CONGESTIVE HEART FAILURE

8.00 AM	Puffed rice	¾ cup
	Skim milk with sugar	1 cup
	Toast with jam	1
	(*Poached egg—one for non-veg.*)	
11.00 AM	Buttermilk	1 cup or
	Orange juice	½ cup
1.00 PM	Tomato/green bean soup	1 cup
	Cooked/steamed pumpkin	1 bowl
	Dal (pulses)	½ cup
	Rice	2 tsp
	Chapattis	2
	Banana	1
	(*Chicken soup/chicken broth roast turkey or minced meat— 2 slices for non-veg.*)	*2 tsp*
4.00 PM	Tea/coffee	1 cup
	Biscuits	2
5.30 PM	Sweet lime juice	1 cup
7.00 PM	Vegetable/leak soup with lemon juice	1 cup
	Cooked carrots or cluster guar beans	1 cup
	Curd (skim milk)	1 cup
	Chapattis	2
	Ice cream	½ cup
9.00 PM	Skimmed milk	1 cup

Source: Dr. F. P. Antia: *Clinical Diagnostics and Nutrition.*

This diet provides:

Calories	1500 kcal
Proteins	50 g
Fats	30 g
Carbohydrates	255 g

DR. (MRS) USHA JAIN SUPPLEMENT

TABLE 19.13: A REFERENCE DIET CHART FOR CARDIOVASCULAR DISEASES

7.00 AM	Crushed garlic with	3-5 cloves
	Honey with amla powder	1 tsp
	Fresh amla juice	1 tsp
7.30 AM	Lemon (1) honey sqash	
8.00 AM	Tender coconut water	1 glass
9.00 AM	Overnight soaked figs with	2
	Almonds	5
	Munakka (Dried Currants)	10
	(*Eat these together and drink 'soak water'*)	
	Seasonal fruit salad	125 g or more
	Buttermilk	1 glass
11.00 AM	Seasonal fruit juice or vegetable juice— ashgourd, cucumber, bottlegourd	1 glass
	(*Ashgourd juice is highly recommended for CVD*)	
1.00 PM	Seasonal green vegetable salad	125 g
	Sprouts—alfalfa, moong (green grams)	2 tbsp
	Cooked/steamed vegetables	1 bowl
	(*Add spinach if constipated*)	
	Chapattis	3-4
	Amla chutney (+ coriander, mint, onion, garlic)	
	Curd raita (+ cucumber, spinach, mint, bottlegourd)	
3.00 PM	Tender coconut water	1 cup
5.00 PM	Seasonal juicy fruits	1 bowl
7.00 PM	Dinner as lunch or vegetable soup	1 cup
	Vegetable porridge	1 bowl
	Green vegetable salad	1 bowl
	Chutney and raita (above)	
9.00 PM	Soaked figs 2 with amla powder	1 tsp

DR (MRS) USHA JAIN'S GUIDELINES

Avoid

- Sugar
- Salt
- Fried foods
- Saturated fats
- Meats
- Pickles
- Spices
- Canned foods
- Tea/coffee
- Beverages
- Alcohol
- Smoking

For Obese Patients

Juice fasting for 3 days—ashgourd juice or tender coconut water given every 3 hours, to be sipped very slowly in 10 minutes. Reduce the quantity and add green salad or fruit salad one at a time.

For Ischaemia Patients

Beet/carrot juice 1 cup and amla juice 1 tsp with honey 1 tsp. Overnight soaked raisins 10 (drink 'soak water' also) with lemon-honey squash 1 glass.

For Heart Patients

Bed rest.
Beet/carrot juice with lemon-honey or amla juice, 1 tsp, to be taken every 3 hours. Apple puree, stewed apple with honey
Apple juice and amla juice for 3-7 days or carrot + orange juice
After 7 days, add cereal porridge + fruit salad + toned milk.

For Angina Pectoris (For pain)

Onion juice with crushed garlic and honey with
Lemon juice or ginger 1 tsp, morning and evening

CHERIE CALBOM SUPPLEMENT

Suggested Juicing Recipes for Atherosclerosis

Ginger Hopper

¼-inch slice ginger root
4-5 carrots, greens removed
½ apple, seeded

Push ginger through hopper with carrots and apple.

High-Calcium Drink

3 kale leaves
Small handful parsley
4-5 carrots, greens removed

Bunch up kale and parsley, and push through hopper with carrots.

Garden Salad Special

3 broccoli flowerets
1 garlic clove
4-5 carrots or 2 tomatoes
2 stalks celery
½ green pepper

Puch broccoli and garlic through hopper with carrots or tomatoes. Follow with celery and green pepper.

Potassium Broth

Handful parsley
Handful spinach
4-5 carrots, greens removed
2 stalks celery

Bunch up parsley and spinach leaves, and push through hopper with carrots and celery.

Suggested Juicing Recipes for Hypertension

Sweet Potassium Shake

¼ cantaloupe
1 banana

Juice cantaloupe. Place juice and banana in blender or food processor, and blend until smooth.

Sweet Calcium Shake

1 pint strawberries
6 oz. silken tofu

Juice strawberries. Place juice and tofu in blender or food processor, and blend untill smooth. Garnish with strawberry.

Sweet Magnesium Smoothie

1 pint blackberries
1 ripe banana
2 oz silken tofu
1 tsp Brewer's yeast

Juice berries. Place juice, banana, tofu, and yeast in blender or food processor, and blend untill smooth. Garnish with black-berries. Drink 1 hour before bedtime.

Calcium-Rich Cocktail

3 kale leaves
Small handful parsley
4-5 carrots, greens removed
½ apple, seeded

Bunch up kale and parsley. and push through hopper with carrots and apple.

Potassium Broth

Handful parsley
Handful spinach
4-5 carrots, greens removed
2 stalks celery

Bunch up parsley and spinach leaves, and push through hopper with carrots and celery.

Harvest Soup

2-3 garlic cloves
1 kale leaf
1 large tomato
2 stalks celery
1 collard leaf, chopped
1 tsp croutons

Roll garlic in kale leaf, and push through hopper with tomato and celery. Place juice in saucepan, add chopped collards, and gently heat. Garnish with croutons.

Garlic Express

Handful parsley
1 garlic clove
4-5 caroots, greens removed
2 stalks celery

Bunch up parsley and push through hopper with garlic, carrots, and celery.

Magnesium Drink

1 garlic clove
Small handful parsley
4-5 carrots, greens removed
2 stalks celery
Parsley sprig for garnish

Wrap garlic in parsley, and push through hopper with carrots and celery. Pour juice into glass, and garnish with sprig of parsley.

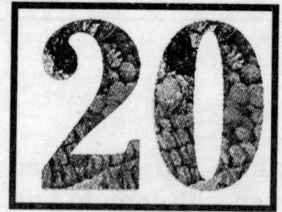

20 DIET AND DIABETES MELLITUS

Diabetes Mellitus is a metabolic disorder in which the ability to oxidize the primary fuel, glucose, is lost altogether. The glucose accumulates in the blood and is excreted in urine, thus causing excessive urination, thirst and hunger and multiple complications in the body systems.

Diabetes Mellitus is rather a group of diseases in which the hormone, insulin, is not manufactured by the β cells of the islets of Langerhans of Pancreas or is produced in very small amount and then not utilized by the body. Figure 1 shows the consequences of insulin deficiency and its wider ramifications. Diabetes Mellitus is classified into five types, as under:

Type I: IDDM, Insulin-dependent Diabetes Mellitus, which usually appears in the youth below 25 years of age. It is also called juvnile onset of Diabetes Mellitus. They are usually underweight and show no insulin response when fed large amounts of glucose. They are prone to ketosis, i.e. excess of ketone bodies in the blood that could lead to coma and death.

Type II: NDDM, Non-Insulin-dependent Diabetes Mellitus, which may be obese or non-obese type. It usually appears in middle age.

Type III: GDM, Gestational Diabetes Mellitus, which occurs during pregnancy and the blood glucose level returns to normal after delivery.

Type IV: SDM, Secondary Diabetes Mellitus, which includes other types of diabetes associated with pancreatic/hormonal disease, adverse drugs and genetic syndromes.

Type V: IGT, Impaired Glucose Tolerance, which shows abnormal plasma glucose levels, earlier called 'Borderline Diabetes'.

Table 20.1 compares the two types of diabetes.

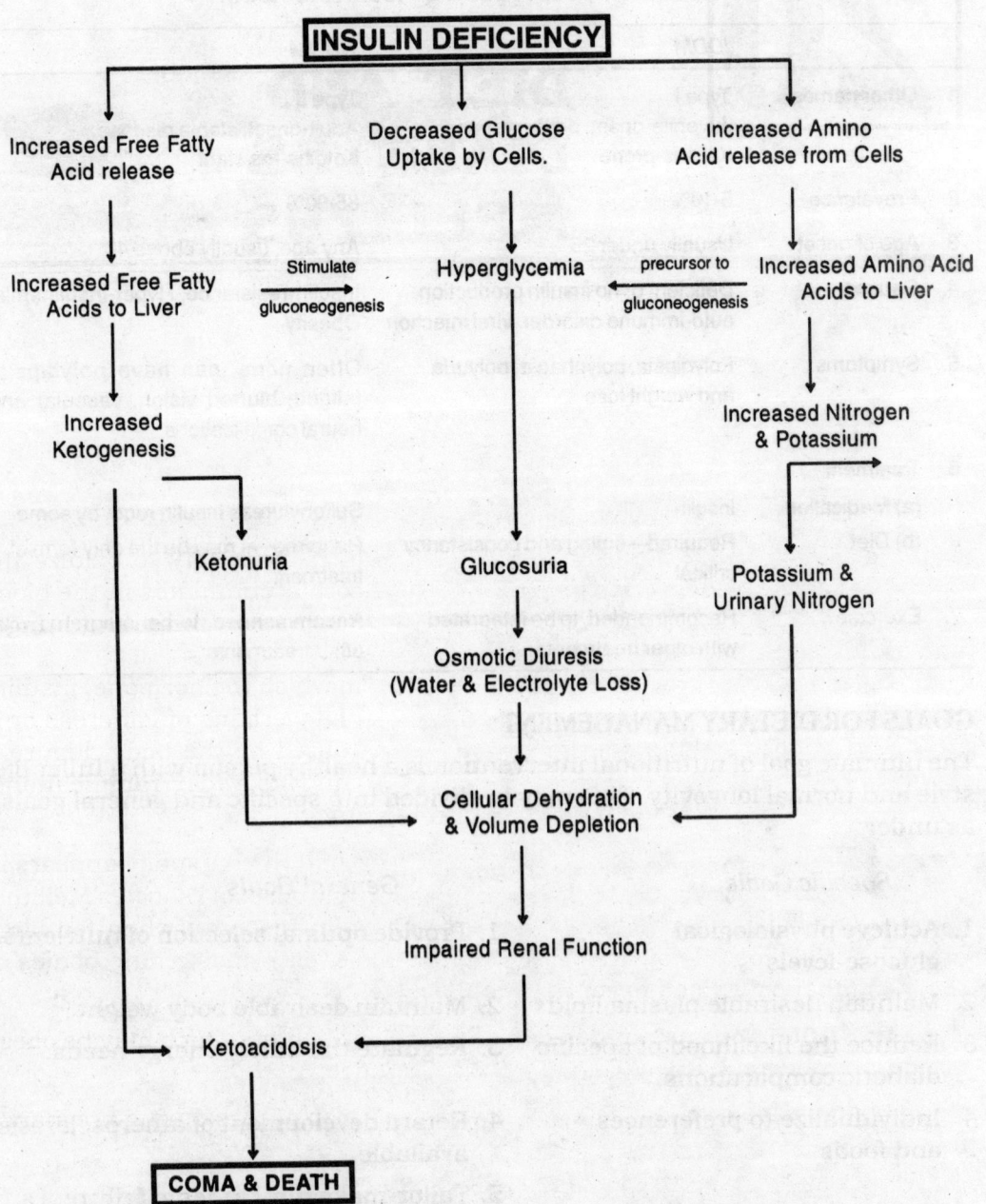

Fig. 20.1: Metabolic Consequences of Insulin Deficiency

Source: *Metabolic and Endocrine Physiology* Year Book, Chicago, 1973.

TABLE 20.1: COMPARISON OF IDDM AND NDDM

		IDDM	NDDM
1.	Other names	Type I Juvenile-onset, brittle disease, Ketosis-prone	Type II Adult-onset, stable disease, Ketosis-resistant
2.	Prevalence	5-10%	85-90%
3.	Age of onset	Usually under 25	Any age, usually above 40
4.	Causes	Deficient or no insulin production, auto-immune disorder, viral infection	Insulin-resistance, Hyper-insulinemia, Obesity
5.	Symptoms	Polydipsia, polyphagia, polyuria and weight loss	Often none, can have polydipsia, fatigue, blurred vision, vascular and neural complications
6.	Treatment		
	(a) Medication	Insulin	Sulfonylureas Insulin reqd. by some
	(b) Diet	Required—timing and consistency critical	Required—it may be the only form of treatment
7.	Exercise	Recommended, to be integrated with other treatments	Recommended, to be integrated with other treatments

GOALS FOR DIETARY MANAGEMENT

The ultimate goal of nutritional intervention is a healthy person with a fuller life style and normal longevity. This may be divided into specific and general goals, as under:

Specific Goals

1. Achieve physiological glucose levels
2. Maintain desirable plasma lipids
3. Reduce the likelihood of specific diabetic complications.
4. Individualize to preferences and foods

General Goals

1. Provide optimal selection of nutrients.
2. Maintain desirable body weight
3. Regulate the timely energy needs.
4. Retard development of atherosclerosis available.
5. Tailor-make diet for renal failure.
6. Address special requirements, as in pregnancy or lactation.

Table 20.2 compares various insulin preparations in USA and their timings of action.

TABLE 20.2: USUAL TIMINGS OF ACTION OF INSULIN PREPARATIONS (IN HOURS)

	Type	Onset	Peak	Maximun Duration
1.	Regular	0.5 - 1	2 - 3	4 - 6
2.	N P H	2 - 4	4 - 10	14 - 18
3.	Lente	3 - 4	4 - 12	16 - 20
4.	Ultra-lente	6 - 10	?	20 - 30

Source: Shils *et al. Nutrition in Health and Disease.*

DIABETES MELLITUS

Diabetes Mellitus has become a widespread disease, affecting one out of every 20 persons. Of these, 15% are IDDM and 85% NDDM type. Diabetes complications have now become the fifth-ranking cause of death in USA. It causes 50% of all the amputations of the lower extremities in adults, 25% of all kidney failures and is the leading cause of blindness in adults in USA. The economic impact of diabetes is estimated to be over $20 billion in America. Of the total 177 million diabetics in the world, India alone accounts for 33 million cases.

Causes

Diabetes strikes men and women, young as well as old. The most common factors causing diabetes are:

1. Heredity
2. Improper dietary habits
3. Inadequate physical exercise
4. Side effects of drugs.
5. Effect of hormones
6. Psychological factors
7. As a sequel to other diseases like pancreatitis and heart attacks.

Symptoms

The symptoms include elevated blood glucose (hyperglycemia), increased appetite (polyphagia), increased thirst (polydipsia) and increased urination (polyuria) and unplanned weight loss. The glucose loss through excretion, *i.e.* glycosuira may go up to 100 g per day. This excessive loss results in osmotic diuresis and so the increased volume of urine. These symptoms may persist for months together in the maturity-onset diabetes.

In juvenile-onset type, complications may set in if early treatment is not given. Fatty acid levels in blood and liver shoot up. The excessive fat metabolism results in increased acetone, aceto-acetic acid and β hydroxy butyric acid, which lead to ketosis, ketonemia and ketonuria. In advanced cases, the patient exudes acetone odor. Besides, there is extensive breakdown of proteins to provide energy to the body, which is obtained by de-amination of amino acids. In advanced cases, anorexia sets in, followed by nausea and vomiting. The excessive loss of water and electrolytes in urine results in dehydration and even death. This may occur due to combined effect of hyperglycemia, ketosis, acidaemia and dehydration. Occasionally, there may be blurring of vision, skin irritation and other infections. In women, skin irritation is specially noticed around vulva, owing to heavy concentration of glucose in urine.

Blood Glucose Level

In the normal course, fasting glucose concentration of the blood is 70-110 mg/100 ml. When this level goes up to 170 mg/100 ml, it shows the presence of sugar in urine. But in cases of severe diabetes, the glucose level may shoot up to 400 mg/100 ml.

Complications of Diabetes

These may be acute or chronic complications. In acute complications of diabetes, hypoglycemia or insulin shock occurs. It is characterized by nervousness, weakness, excessive sweating, nausea and vomiting and convulsions.

Diabetic acidosis and coma are the other complications which are accompanied by weakness, headache, anorexia and abdominal pain. The two types of coma are hypo-glycemic and hyperglycemic, as shown in Table 20.3.

TABLE 20.3: DIABETIC COMAS

Distinguishing Features	Hypoglycemic Coma	Hyperglycemic Coma
1. Onset	Very rapid, within minutes	Gradual, after several days
2. Cause	Inadequate food, excessive physical labour, excessive medication	Carelessness in treatment, Some infectious diseases
3. Symptoms		
Thirst	Absent	Present
Hunger	Extreme	Absent
Vomiting	Rare	Very common
Abdominal pain	Absent	Very common
Skin	Moist	Dry
Tremors	Common	Absent
Eyeballs	Normal	Soft
Pulse	Fast (or normal) and strong	Fast and feeble
Breathing	Normal or shallow, odorless	Deep, fast, laboured, with acetone smell
General Appearance	Pale and weak	Florid and hungry

The chronic complications of diabetes include cataract (retinopathy), impairment of renal functions (nephropathy) and damage to nerve fibres (neuropathy). It has been observed that diseases of small and large blood vessels occur more frequently in the diabetic patients. There is also a tendency to recurrent myocardial infarction with an increase in the incidence of congestive heart failure. There may be ulceration, sepsis of feet and in severe cases even gangrene that may necessitate amputation of the foot.

General Management of Diabetes

The fundamental principles of treating the diabetics are early detection and prevention of complications.

For diagnosis, a 75 g dose of glucose is used and 2 blood tests are taken—fasting and a 2-hour plasma glucose. In the latter, plasma glucose value of 200 mg/dL indicates diabetes. The normal level is 140 mg/dL. The values between 140 and 200 mg/dL are called Impaired Glucose Tolerance (IGT). The second test relates to glycohemoglobin. Higher the level of circulating glucose, higher the concentration of glycohemoglobin. The measurement of Hemoglobin Aic provides an effective tool for evaluating long term management of diabetes and its proper control.

The treatment objectives are five-fold:

1. Maintenance of optimal nutrition
2. To provide calories for reasonable body weight, normal growth and development.
3. To maintain glycemic control
4. To achieve optimal blood lipid levels.
5. Prevention of degenerative complications.

In the overall analysis, well-planned food habits and exercise, balanced with aggressive insulin therapy is the best prescription for treatment and control of diabetes.

Insulin Therapy

Hypoglycemic drugs can be given either as oral tablets or insulin injections. Oral tablets containing sulphonylureas are Tolbutamide and Chlorpropamide. These are helpful in majority of the cases of maturity-onset type. Insulin is used in emergency, this could be short-acting, medium-acting and long-acting insulin.

1. Short-acting Insulin like cystalline insulin and Semilente insulin cover a period of 4-6 hours and are taken before breakfast and dinner. The carbohydrate distribution in this regime is

Breakfast	2/5 of carbohydrates
Lunch	1/5 of carbohydrates
Dinner	2/5 of carbohydrates

2. Medium or Intermediate-acting Insulins are Isophane or Natural Protamine Hegedron (NPH), lente and globin. NPH is the most popular drug. Taken before breakfast, the peak action is reached in 8-10 hours and lasts for a total of 24 hours. The carbohydrate diet distribution is as under:

Breakfast	1/7 of carbohydrates
Lunch	2/7 of carbohydrates
Mid-afternoon	1/7 of carbohydrates
Dinner	2/7 of carbohydrates
Bed-time	1/7 of carbohydrates.

3. Long-acting Insulin or Protamine Zinc Insulin (PZI) and Ultralente Iletin Insulin. Their use is not so common, given alone or with regular insulin at breakfast. The carbohydrate distribution is 1/5th, 2/5th and 2/5th respectively, with an extra 20-40 g carbohydrates given at bed-time.

Occasionally two types of insulin may be mixed and given as one single injection.

Diet Therapy

Diet therapy is the main cornerstone of managing diabetes. It is a very individualistic regime, each patient being given the requisite amount of calories as his condition calls for the obese requiring a low-calorie diet as under:

Following guidelines could help determine the exact amount of the nutrients required by a patient:

1. Proteins

For most persons, it is calculated as 1.25 -1.5 g/kg body weight. This goes up to 2 g/kg when extra proteins are needed for replenishment; also for growing children, pregnant and lactating women.

3. Carbohydrates

A man needs 100 g carbohydrates/day to prevent ketosis and protein breakdown. And he can store 1800 kcal from carbohydrates as liver glycogen (i.e. 450 g CHO). A diabetic must consume complex carbohydrates like rice, wheat, jowar and ragi up to a maximum of 250 g/day.

Amylopectins are rapidly digested and amylose is slowly digested. Therefore, foods with higher proportion of amylose should be preferred, e.g.

Amylose content of Bengal gram	=	33%
Amylose content of wheat	=	25%
Amylose content of potato	=	23%.

3. Fats

Fats to the tune of ±10 g of the protein content of diet could be used. These should have 10% share of PUFA,. Cholesterol in the diet should be below 300 mg/day. This could be done by avoiding the fats of animal origin and greater use of vegetable oils.

TABLE 20.4: CALORIES FOR DESIRED BODY WEIGHT (DBW)-CALORIES/KG

Condition	Sedentary Worker/ aged	Moderate Worker	Heavy Worker
Normal	30	35	40
Obese	20-25	30	35
Underweight	35	40	40-50

4. *Fibre*

Dietary Fibre plays a major role in diabetes management. It has therapeutic value and may reduce the prevalence of the disease. The plus points of high fibre intake are:

(1) Results in slow digestion and absorption
(2) Decrease post-prandial plasma glucose
(3) Increases Tissue insulin sensitivity
(4) Stimulates glucose use
(5) Attenuates hepatic glucose output
(6) Decreases counter-regulatory hormone release, such as glucogen
(7) Lowers serum cholesterol
(8) Lowers fasting and post-prandial serum triglycerides
(9) May alternate hepatic cholesterol synthesis
(10) May increase satiety level between the meals.

5. *Sweeteners*

There is no need to restrict sucrose. Rather, it should be substituted as carbohydrates. Nutritive sweeteners like fructose, sugar alcohols (sorbitol, mannitol and xylitol) have significant advantage over sucrose. Non-nutritive sweeteners like acesulfame K, aspartame and sachharin are approved by the FDA and can be safely consumed from 20 g to 35 g per day.

A case of mild diabetes can be easily managed with a controlled, balanced diet. But in advanced cases, it must be supplemented with insulin therapy.

There are **3Rs** that should guide the care and management of diabetes patients, viz.

Regularity
Routine
Regulation.

Reduction of body weight results in better functioning of the β-cells and increased sensitivity. The total calorie requirement can be calculated according to the desirable body weight (DBW), as shown hereunder:

1. Diet Alone

Physical Details

Age	25 years,	Obese,	148 cm tall
Actual Body weight	52 kg	DBW	45 kg

1. Weight to be reduced: 52 – 45 kg = 7 kg

2. Total calories required: 25 × 45 = 1125 kcal

3. Protein requirement: 1.54 g/kg body weight, *i.e.* 68 g/day
   Calories through Proteins: 68 × 4 = 272 kcal

   Non-Protein Calories: Total calories – Protein share, *i.e.*
   $$1125 – 272 = 853 \text{ kcal.}$$

4. Calorie intake from carbohydrates – 50%, *i.e.* 426 kcal
   Amount of carbohydrate: 4 cal/g of carbohydrates
   $$= 426 ÷ 5 = 105 \text{ g carbohydrates/day}$$

5. Calorie intake from fat: 50% of non-protein calories and 9 cal/g of fat
   $$426 ÷ 9 = 47 \text{ g of fat}$$

6. Total requirement for 1125 kcal diet:

Proteins	68 g
Carbohydrates	105 g
Fat	47 g

This regulated diet must be adhered to till the desirable body weight is accomplished. In the second follow-up stage, the calorie intake is increased—
$$30 × 45 = 1350 \text{ kcal.}$$
And these carbohydrates must be proportionately divided into 1/5th, 2/5th and 2/5th for the three major meals of the day.

2. Diet and Oral Therapy

The diet with oral tablets should have moderate calories at breakfast, but higher calorie levels at lunch and dinner time. The recommendation is 1/5th , 2/5th and 2/5th respectively.

3. Diet with Insulin Injections

When supplemented with insulin injection, it permits more flexibility. Herein, it is the time of insulin injection which decides the diet pattern, as shown in Table 20.5.

TABLE 20.5: CARBOHYDRATE DISTRIBUTION WITH INSULIN

	Insulin	Breakfast	Lunch	Afternoon Snacks	Dinner	Bedtime
1.	Short-acting insulins	2/5	1/5	—	2/5	—
2.	Intermediate-acting insulins	1/7	2/7	1/7	2/7	1/7
3.	Long-acting insulins	1/5	2/5	—	2/5	CHO 20-40 g
4.	Regular insulin at breakfast	1/3	1/3	—	1/3	CHO 20-40 g

DIET GUIDELINES

1. Eat complex starches like wheat, jowar, bajra and ragi, in place of simple sugars like glucose, sucrose and fructose in items like honey, table sugar and fruit juices.

2. To fortify the protein contents, mix soya flour or gam flour with wheat flour for making chapattis.

3. Use whole grain pulses like bengal grams, green grams, soyabeans, instead of split and dehusked dals.

4. Use maximum of green leafy vegetables like cabbage, cauliflower, carrots, lettuce, tomatoes and onions as the main fillers in the diet. Prefer dietary fibre-rich foods and pulses, plus raw vegetables, instead of refined foodstuffs and cooked vegetables or peeled fruits. Potatoes, apples, sapota and pears with their skin are recommended.

6. Use minimum of fats. Better cook in non-stick pans.

Food Exchange System

The Food Exchange System for planning diabetic diet is based on the concept of food equivalents. It was developed jointly by the American Diabetic association and American Dietetic association. Six food groups are listed in this Exchange system, viz. starch/bread, meat, vegetables, fruits, milk and fats. In India, legumes and pulses are also included. Foods from one group may be freely exchanged with those of others.

A brief illustrative description of these six groups is given in Table 20.6.

A sample menu, using this Food Exchange lists is shown in Table 20.7. Let us say, we have to plan for a day's menu as under:

Energy	2200 kcal
Carbohydrates	275 g
Proteins (20%)	110 g
Fat (30%)	75 g

TABLE 20.6: FOOD EXCHANGE SYSTEM FOR DIABETES

	Food Group	Unit of Exchange	Carb. g	Prot. g	Fats g	kcal	Characteristic Items
1.	Milk	1 cup					
	Skimmed		12	8	—	90	Skimmmed or very low fat
	Low fat		12	8	5	120	
	Whole milk		12	8	8	150	
2.	Vegetables	½ cup	5	2	—	25	Medium CHO
3.	Fruits	Varies	15	—	—	60	Varies with CHO value
4.	Bread	Varies	15	3	—	80	Variety of bread, cereals,
			– 1				vegetables equ.
		slice					1 slice bread
5.	Meat						Protein foods
	Lean		—	7	3	55	Exchange unit equ.
	Medium fat		—	7	5	75	Protein value of 25 g
	Higher fat		—	7	8	100	Lean meat
5.	Fat	1 Tsp					Food fat items equ. to
	PUFA		—	—	5	45	1 tsp margarine/
	MUFA		—	—	5	45	olives/ avocados/
	Saturated ·		—	—	5	45	mayonnaise

Source: Sue R. Williams. *Nutrition and Diet Therapy.*

TABLE 20.7: DIET CHART FOR DIABETES

Breakfast	Medium shreded wheat cereal	
	Poached egg on whole grain toast	One
	Bran muffin	One
	Margarine	One tsp
	Low fat milk	One cup
	Sliced fresh peach	One
	Coffee/tea	
Lunch	Vegetable soup with wheat crackers	
	Tuna sandwich on whole wheat bread	
	Fresh pear	
Afternoon Snack	Crackers	10
	Peanut butter	2 tsp
	Orange	
Dinner	Pan-boiled well-trimmed pork chop	
	Brown rice	One cup
	Green beans	Half cup
	Green salad	
	Italian dressing	One tbsp
	Apple sauce	Half cup
	Bran muffin	One
Evening Snack	Popped Pop corn	Three cups
	Cheese	One oz
	Low-fat milk	One cup

Source: Sue R Williams, Ibid.

To amply illustrate the Food Exchange, another exercise for a 2000 kcal Diabetic diet is shown in Table 20.8, This has been recommended by Shils *et al.* in the book: *Modern Nutrition in Health and Disease* (8th Edition)

That apart, we give two more diet charts to suit different cases in the Indian conditions, say low calories and high calorie diets, as being prescribed in the All India Institute of Medical Sciences, New Delhi.

TABLE 20.8: WORKSHEET FOR DEVELOPING A 2000 FOOD EXCHANGE PLAN

Exchange	Serving	Energy kcal	Carbohydrate g	Proteins g	Fats g
Starch/bread	8	640	120	24	Trace
Meat and substitutes	3	165	—	21	9
Vegetables	7	175	35	14	—
Fruits	7	420	105	—	—
Milk	2	180	24	16	Trace
Fat	10	450	—	—	50
Total amount	—	2030	284	75	59
Target		2000	290	75	60

TABLE 20.9: DIABETIC DIET FOR 1200 KCAL

			Carbohydrate g	Proteins g	Fats g
7.00 AM	Tea (50 ml milk)	I cup	2	1	1
9.00 AM	Milk—200 ml	1 glass	9	6	6
	Porridge	50 g or			
	Bread slices	2	30	4	—
1.00 PM	Fort. chapattis	(3) -60 g	45	6	—
	Dal with husk	1 bowl	15	5	—
	Curd	125 g	6	4	3
	Green leafy vegetables	200 g	3	1	—
	Cooking fat	5 g	—	—	5
4.00 PM	Tea (50 ml milk)	1 cup	2	1	1
	Biscuits	3	15	2	—
7.00 PM	Fort. chapattis	(2) -40g	30	4	—
	Dal with husk	1 bowl	15	5	—
	Curd	125 g	6	4	3
	Green vegetables	200 g	3	1	—
	Cooking fat	5 g	—	—	5
9.00 PM	Milk	200 ml	9	6	6

This diet supplies:

Carbohdyrates	150 g
Protein	50 g
Fats	30 g
Total calories	1230

TABLE 20.10: DIET CHART FOR DIABETES-1800 KCAL

		Carbohydrate g	Proteins g	Fats g
7.00 AM	Tea (50 ml milk)	l cup	2	1	1
9.00 AM	Milk (200 ml)	1 glass	9	6	6
	Porridge	50 g or			
	Bread slices	230	4	—	
	Butter	10 g	—		8
	Cheese	25 g or			
	Egg	1	—	5	5
1.00 PM	Fort. chapattis	(4)-80 g	60	8	—
	Dal with husk	1 bowl	15	5	—
	Curd	125 g	6	4	3
	Green leafy vegetables	200g	3	1	—
	Cheese	25 g	—	4	3
	Cooking fat	10 g	—	—	10
	Fruit	100 g	10	—	—
4.00 PM	Tea (50 ml milk)	1 cup	2	1	1
	Biscuits	3	15	2	—
7.00 PM	Fort. chapattis	(5) - 100 g	75	10	—
	Dal with husk	1 bowl	15	5	—
	Curd	125 g	6	4	3
	Green vegetables	200 g	3	1	—
	Cooking Fat	5 g	—	—	5
9.00 PM	Milk	200 ml	9	6	6

This diet supplies:

Carbohydrates	249 g
Proteins	67 g
Fats	51 g
Calories	1800

Source: Rekha Sharma: *Diet Management*.

DIETARY PRECAUTIONS

Since diet plays a crucial role in the treatment and prevention of Diabetes mellitus, hereunder we give special regime of foods to be avoided or used in a restricted manner and the other foods which could be taken *ad libitum*.

Avoid

- Sugar and sugar Products
- Jams and jellies
- Fried foodstuffs
- Groundnut and coconut oil
- Butter, cream, margarine and ghee
- Fatty and organ meats
- Shell and oily fish
- Cakes, pastries and doughnuts
- Alcohol and soft drinks.

Following foodstuffs be used, in a restricted manner:

Cereals, viz., jowar, bajra, ragi, wheat and rice
Noodles, spaghetti and macroni
Root vegetables, viz., potato, yam, sweet potato and colocasia
Vegetable oils, viz., saffola, soya oils
Lean meats, fish and eggs
Pulses and fruits.

Ad lib. Consumption

Raw and green leafy vegetables
Cabbage, cauliflower,
Celery and brusells sprouts,
Thin buttermilk, skimmed milk
Clear soups
Spices, moderate amounts

EXERCISE

Regular physical activity helps in controlling diabetes. Long brisk walk, jogging exercises and swimming help maintain proper body weight and tone up the cardiovascular system, all the more so in IDDM cases. Others with NDDM need light exercise to control their blood glucose and lipid levels. In the long run, exercise improves body metabolism and also contributes to the well-being of the patients. It is reported to enhance the insulin action on the body tissues.

One has got to be vigilant in regulating the insulin dosage. If the pre-exercise level of blood glucose is too low, hypoglycemia can result during exercise. If it happens to be too high and there is deficiency of insulin, then the exercise may cause further increase in blood glucose and also ketosis. It is recommended that one should take supplementary snacks, especially carbohydrates before and during the exercise to help maintain blood glucose levels within normal range.

Summing up, regular exercise helps by:

1. Lowering the blood pressure, since high blood pressure increases the chronic problems associated with diabetes.
2. Reducing risk factor of atherosclerosis by lowering triglycerides and VLDLs, as also cholesterol and increasing HDLs.
3. Reversing the resistance to insulin.
4. Increasing the blood glucose lowering effect of injected insulin, thus requiring reduced dosage of insulin.
5. Increasing the sensitivity to insulin and improving glucose tolerance.
6. Improving glycogen control and also cardiovascular fitness.

Yoga

Yoga exercises play a very important role in controlling diabetes. The Indian Journal of Medical Sciences reported an experiment at the Jiwaji University, Gwalior. Diabetic soldiers, number 180 were made to perform Ujjayi and Bhastrika Pranayama for about 45 minutes every day for 3 months. Almost all the patients reported marked improvement in their condition. Other Yogasanas that proved greatly beneficial are:

Uddiyabandh

Trikonasana

Yogamudra

Paschitmottasana

Matsyasana

Dhanurasana

Konasana

Shavasana.

In Naturopathy, acupressure and magnet therapy have helped a great deal, more so by controlling high blood pressure and CVD.

DR (Mrs) USHA JAIN SPPLEMENT

TABLE 20.11: DIET CHART FOR DIABETES

7.00 AM	Green sun-charged water (else in copper vessel) with a clove of garlic	1 glass
8.00 AM	Bittergourd juice with lemon juice (Depending upon glucose level)	1 cup
9.00 AM	Seasonal green vegetable salad with sprouts, viz., Alfalfa, moong, Bengal gram methi (Red gram—moth is highly recommended)	125 g
	Buttermilk with 'jeera, roasted', methi powder (blood sugar level)	1 glass
12.00 Noon	Steamed seasonal vegetables, viz., Ash gourds and pumpkin, spinach, amaranth and green methi	125 g
	Vegetable chapattis + 2 tbsp diabetic atta (proteins) + jowar, bajra, barley + 1 tsp grated vegetables + wheat bran + almonds deoiled cake	3
	Green amla chutney with green turmeric and curry leaves	
3.00 PM	Tender coconut water + green ginger + ashgourd juice + carrots and amla juice, mixed	1 cup
5.00 PM	Juicy fruits, viz., grapefruit, kandhari pomegranate, sweet lime, kino, orange, malta, chokotra	1 glass
7.00 PM	Green vegetable soup	½ cup
	Steam-cooked barley/maize + vegetable porridge	125 g
	Eat with seasonal green salad + amla chutney and raita	
9.00 PM	Fruits, viz., papaya, pears, apples	

Obese Patients

Avoid cereals for 3 days.

Use mixed fruit and vegetable salad with butter milk for 3 days.

Methi seeds soaked overnight with 1 tsp curd, depending upon sugar level.

CHERIE CALBOM SUPPLEMENT

Suggested Juicing Recipes for Diabetes Mellitus

Digestive Special

Handful spinach
4-5 carrots, greens removed

Bunch up spinach and push through hopper with carrots

Potassium Broth

Handful parsley
Handful spinach
4-5 carrots, greens removed
2 stalks celery

Bunch up parsley and spinach leaves, and push through hopper with carrots and celery.

Chlorophyll Cocktail

3 beet tops
Handful parsley
Handful spinach
4 carrots, greens removed
½ apple, seeded

Bunch up beet tops, parsley, and spinach, and push through hopper with carrots and apple

Garden Salad Special

3 broccoli flowerets
1 garlic clove
4-5 carrots or 2 tomatoes
2 stalks celery
½ green pepper

Push broccoli and garlic through hopper with carrots or tomatoes. Follow with celery and green pepper.

Tomato Salad Express

Handful spinach
Handful parsley
2 tomatoes
½ green pepper
Dash tabasco sauce

Bunch up spinach and parsley, and push through hopper with tomatoes and green pepper. Add tabasco sauce

Garlic Express

Handful parsley
1 garlic clove
4-5 carrots, greens removed
2 stalks celery

Bunch up parsley and push through hopper with garlic, carrots, and celery

Calcium-Rich Cocktail

3 kale leaves
Small hundful parsley
4-5 carrots, greens removed
½ aple, seeded

Bunch up kale and parsley, and push through hopper with carrots and apple

Low-Sugar Pop

1 apple, seeded
¼ lime
Sparkling water

Juice apple and time. Pour juice into tall, ice-filled glass. Fill glass to top with sparkling water

Pancreas Tonic

3 lettuce leaves
4-5 carrots, greens removed
Handful green beans
2 Brussels sprouts

Bunch up lettuce leaves and push through hopper with carrots, green beans, and Brussels sprouts

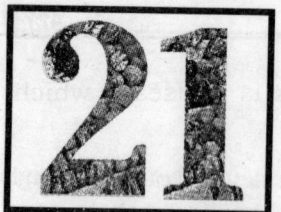

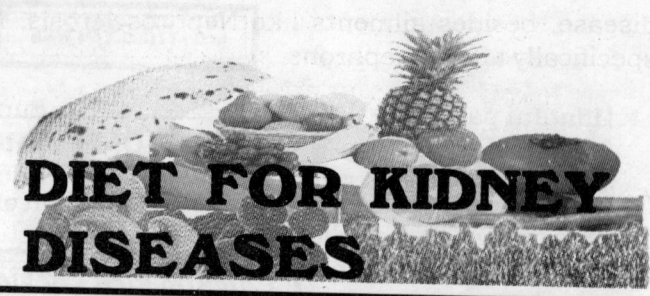

DIET FOR KIDNEY DISEASES

Kidneys are the body's filtering agents which help maintain the water balance, electrolyte level, the normal pH and osmotic pressure of the blood by flushing out all the metabolic byproducts, toxic substances and other unwanted material accumulated in the blood. The functional unit herein is Nephron, which consists of a glomerulus or tuft of capillaries surrounded by the Bowman's capsule. There are over a million nephrons in each kidney which filter more than 2500 pints of blood every day.

Each capsule is attached to a long-winding tubule through which passes the fluid from the blood contained in the glomerulus. Urine is produced in the nephrons and emptied in the pelivs of the kidney, from where it flows through the ureters into the urinary bladder. A normal pair of healthy kidneys filter about 130-150 litres fluid every day, out of which about 15 litres is eliminated as urine from the body. This volume goes down to 0.5 litres following water deprivation and increased to 20.0 litres folowing ingestion of very large quantities of water. This goes to show the immense reabsorption capacity of the kidneys.

Nephrons, as such, perform four basic functions, viz.

1. Filter most constituents from entering the blood, save red blood cells and plasma proteins.
2. Reabsorb the needed substances, as the filterate continues along the winding tubules.
3. Secrete additional ions to maintain acid-base balance.
4. Excrete unwanted material in the concentrated urine.

Kidney troubles are the fourth largest health problem and in USA alone, it kills 60,000 persons every year. The diseases of kidneys usually involve the nephrons, glomerulus and the tubules. Kidney stones or urinary calculi is another disease, besides ailments like Nephrosclerosis. Nephritis is a disease which specifically affects nephrons.

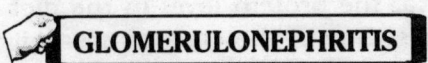
GLOMERULONEPHRITIS

Glomerulonephritis is primarily an inflammation of glomeruli. It may be acute or chronic and generally follows streptococcal infections of respiratory tract, such as tonsillitis, sinusitis, influenza and pneumonia. It is more common in children than in the case of adults.

Symptoms

These are characterized by haematuria and protinuria, i.e. blood and albumin in urine, along with some nitrogen retention. Often, there is oedema, hypertension, shortness of breath and water retention along with circulatory congestion. Renal insufficiency leads to oliguria or anuria, i.e. reduction in urine or no urine, which marks the onset of acute renal failure. There will be swelling around the ankles, puffiness around the eyes, nausea and vomiting. Chronic Glomerulonephritis is marked by frequent urinatioin and nocturia. Sometimes, nephrotic syndrome develops, as seen by the symptoms of massive oedema and protinuria.

Diet Therapy

A: *Acute Glomerulonephritis*

The recovery process may take a few weeks or even months. Diet management is done through fluid balance and by maintaining proper protein and energy balance.

Fluid Balance

Maintain proper fluid balance by adjusting the intake of fluids to match the fluid output. In case of oliguria, the patient must be given 500-700 ml fluid per day.

Proteins

The amount of protein is restricted in case of renal failure or oliguria, when the blood urea nitrogen is elevated. It should not exceed 40 g proteins per day. But albuminuria and proteinemia conditions demand larger intake of proteins. These proteins should be of higher biologic value like eggs, fish, and meat etc. The protein level may be gradually increased over the next 10-15 days.

Energy

The main treatment centres on bed rest, when he needs lesser calorie intake, otherwise the RDA must be maintained. In case the protein intake has to be reduced, then non-protein calorie diet like butter, margarine, vegetable oils, jellies, sugar and low-protein desserts are recommended, as also soft drinks.

B: *Chronic Glomerulonephritis*
Proteins

In the case of proteinuria, the protein level in the diet must be increased to compensate for the losses. But in the case of urea nitrogen retention in the blood, the protein level should be lowered to 40g or less per day. The proteins must be of higher biologic value.

Carbohydrates and Fats

These must be provided in liberal measure in order to save the catabolism of tissue proteins. This would also prevent starvation ketosis.

Sodium

It is restricted to 500-1000 mg/day in case of oedema and oliguria. Otherwise, the sodium intake is maintained between 2000 and 3000 mg/day. One must monitor and avoid sodium depletion in case of large excretion of urine. The latter may result in weakness, nausea and shock.

Potassium intoxication may occur in severe oliguria. This would call for dialysis, hence potassium level should also be monitored.

Tables 21.1, 21.2, 21.3 and 21.4 give the food exchange lists and the diet chart for acute and chronic glomerulonephritis.

TABLE 21.1: FOOD EXCHANGE LIST FOR ACUTE/CHRONIC GLOMERULONEPHRITIS

	No. of Exchanges	Proteins g	Sodium mg	Calories kcal
Milk	2	10	30	200
Legumes and pulses	2	12	30	200
Meat/fish	½	5	–	50
Green leafy vegetables	2	–	20	–
Other green vegetables	2	–	20	100
Fruits	2	–	20	100
Cereals	9	18	225	900
Sugar	25 g	–	–	100
Fats	2 g	–	–	200
Total		**45**	**345**	**1850**

Sodium-restricted in case of edema.
If no edema, sodium intake can be increased to 2000-3000 mg.
(1 tsp contains 1500-2000 mg sodium)

TABLE 21.2: JOSHI'S SAMPLE DIET CHART FOR GLOMERULONEPHRITIS–I

7.00 AM	Tea	1 cup
9.00 AM	Bread	2 slices
	Egg	1
	Small orange	1
	Tea	1 cup
1.00 PM	Chapattis	1
	Vegetables	¾ cup
	Rice	1 cup (medium)
	Curd	½ cup
4.00 PM	Tea	1 cup
	Rice poha	¾ cup
	Banana	½
7.00 PM	Chapattis	1
	Vegetables	¾ cup
	Rice	1 cup
	Pulses	1 cup (medium)
	Curd	½ cup

TABLE 21.3: Dr ANTIA'S DIET FOR GLOMERULONEPHRITIS–II

7.00 AM	Tea/coffee	1 cup
9.00 AM	Toast	2
	Butter	2 tsp
	Jam	1 tsp
	Tea/coffee	1 cup
11.00 AM	Milk with sugar	1 cup or
	Milk shake	1 glass
1.00 PM	Boiled potatoes with	
	Butter	2 tsp
	Rice (taken with milk)	4 tbsp
	Chapattis	2
	Caramel puddings	
4.00 PM	Tea	1 cup
	Biscuits	3
	with Butter	1 tsp
7.00 PM	Boiled Pumpkin	1 bowl
	Chapattis	2 or
	Bread	1 slice
	with Butter	2 tsp
	Chocolate cake with cream	1 tsp

Dr Antia insists that there shold be no salt in cooking, else on dining table. Further he advises that the vegetables double-boiled and drained off.

This diet offers:

Proteins	30 g
Carbohydrates	255 g
Fats	63 g
Calories	1700 kcal

TABLE 21.4: DR. (Mrs.) JAIN'S DIET CHART FOR NEPHRITIS

7.00 AM	Green Sun-charged water	1 glass
	Crushed Garlic	1 clove
	Kulthi (pulses) soaked in water	1 tbsp
8.00 AM	Silky hair on Corn cob's decoction	1 tbsp
	(Helps remove accretions in kidneys)	
9.00 AM	Corn (baby) Cob soup	1 glass
	Seasonal fruit/vegetable salad	1 bowl
12.00 Noon	Corn Cob soup	1 glass
	Green vegetable salad	1 bowl
	Fortified Chapattis	3-4
	Gooseberry (amla) chutney	
4.00 PM	Seasonal fruit juice—Papaya, sapota, pomegranate, citrus fruits	1 glass
7.00 PM	Corn dalia (porridge)	2 cups
	Green vegetable salad	1 bowl
	Kulthi (pulses) soak water	1 cup
9.00 PM	Seasonal fresh fruit	1 bowl
	Soaked Figs	2
	Kulthi (pulses) soak water	1 cup

N.B. Kulthi is a special pulse crop growing in the high altitude areas and is reputed to have proved very efficacious in treating Renal diseases.

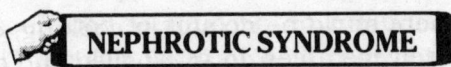

NEPHROTIC SYNDROME

Also called Nephrosis, it is a disease usually of small children that may be caused by glomerulonephritis, other infections, reactions and drugs. There is a massive loss of proteins in urine. The blood levels of plasma proteins goes down but cholesterol shows marked increase. Protein loss may range from 3-16 g/day in the adults. In children, this loss goes up to 50 mg/kg body weight. There will be accumulation of body fluids, as seen by the swelling of eyelids and legs. This syndrome is normally reversed by corticosteroids or immuno-suppressive drugs.

Diet Therapy

The aim of Diet Therapy is to minimise oedema, control urinary albumin losses and retard progression of renal diseases and prevent protein malnutrition.

Proteins

The daily intake of proteins is increased to 100-200 g. The proteins must be of high biologic value. High protein supplements, especially those with low sodium concentration are recommended.

Calories

Sufficient calorie intake must be ensured, say 50-60 kcal/kg body weight.

Sodium

Low sodium diet is recommended in case of oedema. A dose of 500 mg sodium will suffice.

As such, the nutritionists recommend a high protein, high carbohydrate diet with low sodium. Tables 21.5 and 21.6 give the diet carts for Nephrotic syndrome.

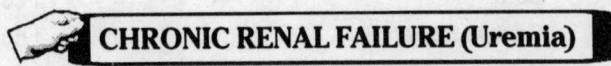

CHRONIC RENAL FAILURE (Uremia)

Uremia is the excessive retention of urinary constituents in the blood. It is the toxic condition of terminal manifestation of renal failure. The condition of renal insufficiency may become chronic with progressive degenerative changes in renal tissue and a marked depression of all the renal functions. The principal cause of uremia are chronic glomerulonephritis, nephrosclerosis and chronic pyelonephritis.

In the early stages, kidneys lose their ability to excrete concentrated urine when fluid intake is very low. But when excess fluid is taken, it results in much diluted urine not being excreted. Due to the presence of large amounts of nitrogenous wastes, it is unable to maintain a constant blood pH of 7.4. In advanced cases, since the excretion of all the wastes of potassium, nitrogen and phosphates is not possible, it leads to their greater concentration in blood. Accumulation of sodium and water leads to oedema. This gets further aggravated by a decrease in serum albumin on account of both loss in urine and poor intake of diet. In children, it may lead to renal rickets. The terminal stage of renal failure is marked by convulsions, vomiting and diarrhoea and finally it leads to coma.

TABLE 21.5: DIET CHART FOR NEPHROTIC SYNDROME–I

8.00 AM	Cornflakes	1-2 cups
	Dalia with Skimmed Milk and sugar	1 cup
	Cottage Cheese	2 tbsp
	Toast	1
	Tea/Coffee	1 cup
	(Eggs poached/omlette—2 for Non-veg.)	
10.00 AM	Skimmed Milk fortified	1 cup
	with skimmed milk powder	2 tbsp
	Banana	1
1.00 PM	Buttermilk	1 cup
	Green vegetable salad	1 bowl
	Cooked Brinjals	1 bowl
	Rice	2 tbsp
	Dal	1 cup
	Chapattis	4
	Groundnut	15
	(Minced meat 4 tbsp for Non-veg.)	
4.00 PM	Tea/Coffee	1 cup
7.00 PM	Cottage Cheese	3 tbsp
	Curd	1 cup
	Cooked Spinach	1 cup
	Dal	1 cup
	Chapattis/Khakhra	2
	(Roasted chicken leg for Non-veg.)	
9.00 PM	Skimmed milk fortified	1 cup
	with skimmed milk powder	2 tbsp

Source: Dr. F. P. Antia, *ibid.*

This diet provides:

Proteins	110 g
Carbohydrates	252 g
Fats	72 g
Energy	2100 kcal

TABLE 21.6: DIET CHART FOR NEPHROTIC SYNDROME–II

7.00 AM	Tea	1 cup
9.00 AM	Ragi porridge	1 cup (Finger Millets)
	Banana	1 small
	Egg	1
1.00 PM	Chapattis	2
	Vegetables	¾ cup
	Rice	1 cup
	Pulses	1 cup
	Curd	1 cup
4.00 PM	Tea	1 cup
	Suji Upma	¾ cup
7.00 PM	Chapattis	2
	Vegetables	¾ cup
	Rice	1 cup
	Pulses	1 cup
	Curd	1 cup
9.00 PM	Milk with Casilan	1 glass

Source: Joshi, S A, *ibid*.

N.B. Vegetables and fruits containing sodium less than 10 mg % should be used.

Symptoms

Chronic renal failure is characterised by symptoms of anemia, loss of weight, hyper-tension and osteodystrophy, accompanied by pain in the bones and joints. In advanced cases, increased capillary fragility leads to gastrointestinal bleeding. Nervous system involvement brings muscular twitching, burning sensation in the extremities. Cheyne-stroke respiration, marked by irregular, cyclic type breathing, indicates acidosis. There may be ulceration of the mouth and foetid breath. The body resistance to infection severely goes down. Uremia calls for frequent haemodialysis every few hours, say thrice a week.

Diet Therapy

Following imperatives be kept in mind while planning the diet for cases of renal failure:

1. Provide enough calories,
2. Regulate the protein levels of diet,
3. Ensure sufficient intake of fluids, besides sodium and potassium,
4. Supplement the diet with calcium, iron, minerals, vitamins B complex and vitamin

However, the phosphates must be restricted.

Energy

The calorie intake must be sufficient to avoid undue tissue loss and acid protein replenishment, say between 2000 and 3000 kcal/day. Sago diet is especially recommended. Rice porridge is also recommended, besides ice cream and soft sweet products like rasgullas and gulab jamuns.

Proteins

High biologic proteins, 1 g/kg body weight, are mandatory with haemodialysis. Those not on dialysis should be given only 0.6 g proteins/kg body weight. Non-protein calories should come from fats, sugars, fruits and vegetables, besides low-protein supplements.

Carbohydrates and Fats

Carbohydrates should account for 60% of the total calories. Cholesterol must be restricted up to 300 mg/day. For fats, PUFA is recommended, the PUFA-saturated fat ratio should be 1 : 1.

Sodium and Potassium

Sodium must be restricted in oedema, hypertension and congestive heart failure, say 1-2 g/day. Potassium intake for dialysis patients is 2500 mg/day, while for those not on dialysis need to be given 1500-200 mg potassium. Since animal proteins are rich in potassium, their intake should be constantly monitored. Other minerals like phosphorus should be restricted to 600-750 mg/day. Calcium supplementation of 1.5-2.0 g/day and vitamin D 30,000-40,000 IU is recommended twice a week. This would prevent hyperthyroidism.

Fluids

Water balance must be strictly monitored to avoid dehydration or water intoxication. Normally, 400-600 ml fluid is recommended per day. But the dialysis patients need 1000 ml. As such, these patients on dialysis gain weight, one pound/day, owing to water retention. However, this excess weight is taken care of by dialysis. Table 21.7 gives the RDA for acute renal failure.

TABLE 21.7: RECOMMENDED DIETARY ALLOWANCE FOR ACUTE RENAL FAILURE

Nutrient	Amount
Protein	0.6-0.8 g/kg body weight
Energy	45-55 kcal/kg body weight
Potassium	30-50 m Eq/day
Sodium	20-40 m Eq/day
Fluid	Replace output from the previous day plus 500 ml
Phosphorus	Limited as needed

Tables 21.8 and 21.9 give the diet charts for renal failure.

TABLE 21.8: FOOD EXCHANGE LISTS FOR CHRONIC RENAL FAILURE

(Prot. 30-40 g, Sod. 500 mg, Calories 2000)

		No.of Exchanges	Proteins (g)	Sodium (mg)	Calories (kcal)
1.	Milk	1	5	20	100
2.	Legumes and Pulses	1	6	10	100
3.	Meat/Fish	1/2	5	–	50
4.	Green Leafy Vegetables	2	–	35	–
5.	Green Vegetables	3	–	20	150
6.	Fruits	2	–	20	100
7.	Cereals	8	16	20	800
8.	Sugar	50 g	–	–	200
9.	Fats	4G	–	–	400
	Total		**32**	**125**	**1900**

TABLE 21.9: DIET CHART FOR RENAL FAILURE

7.00 AM	Tea	1 cup
9.00 AM	Potato paratha	1
	Banana	1
	Tea	1 cup
1.00 PM	Chapattis	2
	Spinach curry	1 cup
	Pulses	1 cup (medium thick)
	Rice	½ cup
4.00 PM	Tea	1 cup
	Suji upma	¾ cup
7.00 PM	Chapattis	1
	Cabbage curry	1cup
	Egg curry	1 cup
	Rice	1 cup
	Orange/sweet lime	1

Source: Joshi, S A, *ibid.*

N.B. All preparations should be made with minimum salt.

No extra salt should be served on the dining table.

PORTABLE DIALYSIS

The CADP, continuous ambulatory portable dialysis, is a home dialysis process that introduces dialysis directly into the peritoneal cavity, where it can be exchanged for fluids that contain metabolic waste products. The patients on CADP need special nutrition support and care, as follows:

1. Protein intake is increased to 1.2-1.5 g/kg body weight.
2. Phosphorus level is limited to 1200 mg/day, by restricting the use of phosphorus-rich foods like nuts and legumes to one serving a week and dairy products to half a cup and one egg everyday.
3. Potassium intake must be increased by eating lots of fruits and vegetables.
4. Liberal intake of fluids will help prevent dehydration.
5. Avoid fats and sweets to control triglycerides and HDL levels.
6. Maintain lean body weight by including the calories by dialysis into total meal plan.
7. Concerted efforts should be made to encourage the patients to eat more.

Table 21.10 gives the diet chart for the renal patients on dialysis.
Concluding this chapter on kidney diseases, we give five special diets from all over the globe.

1. Low Purine Diet for Renal Calculi

Breakfast	Lunch	Dinner
Fruit	Egg/cheese dish	Egg/cheese dish
Refined cereal/egg	Cooked vegetable/ Green salad	Cream of vegetable soup, if desired
White toast	White bread	Starch (potato/substitute)
Butter 1 tsp	Potato	Cooked vegetables
Sugar	Fruit/simple dessert	Butter 1 tsp
Coffee	Milk	Green salad
Milk, if desired		Fruit/simple dessert, Milk

2. Low Methionine Diet for Renal Calculi (Cystine Stones)

Breakfast		Lunch		Dinner	
Fruit juice	1 cup	Soup	1 cup	Meat	56 g
Fruits	100 g (1/2 cup)	Sandwich	1	Starchy	100 g
Toast	1 slice	Fruits	200g (1 cup)	Vegetables	(1/2 cup)
Butter	1 tsp	Soy milk	240 ml	Green salad	1 serving
Jelly	2 tsp	Sugar	1 tsp	Bread	1 slice
Sugar	1 tbsp	Cream	1 tbsp	Dessert	1 serving
Beverage		Beverage		Cream	1 tbsp
				Butter	1 tsp
				Sugar	1 tsp
				Beverage	

Diets Nos. 1 and 2 from S R William's: *Essentials of Nutrition and Diet Therapy*, Pub. Mosby.

TABLE 21.10: DIET CHART FOR RENAL PATIENTS ON DIALYSIS (50 G PROTEINS)

			Carbo-hydrates g	Prot-eins g	Fats g	Sodium mg	Potass-ium mg	Phosph-orus mg
7.00 AM	Tea with sugar	1 cup	12	1	1	4	30	20
9.00 AM	Bread	2 slices	30	4	–	25	20	–
	Milk	1 cup	9	6	6	32	240	200
	Butter unsalted	25 g	–	–	20	–	–	–
	Egg	1	–	5	5	65	48	110
	Arrowroot biscuits	4	20	–	–	1	6	–
1.00 PM	Chapattis fortified with arrow root powder							
	(50g : 55g)	4	58	3	–	5	84	10
	Rice	25 g	19	–	2	18	–	–
	Curd	125 g	6	3	3	40	150	110
	Vegetables	125 g	3	1	–	20	150	20
	Sago khichdi	50 g	43	–	–	–	–	–
	Fruit	100 g	9	1	–	15	84	20
	Cheese	25 g	–	4	3	60	29	35
	Cooking oil	10 g	–	–	10	–	–	–
4.00 PM	Tea	1 cup	12	1	1	4	30	20
	Sago vada	2 cups	43	–	10	–	–	–
7.00 PM	Chapattis	4	58	3	–	5	84	10
	Rice	25 g	19	–	2	18	–	–
	Curd	125 g	6	3	3	40	150	110
	Vegetables	125 g	3	1	–	20	150	20
	Dehusked pulses	25 g	15	5	–	6	120	40
	Cooking oil	10 g	–	–	10	–	–	–
9.00 PM	Milk	1 cup	9	6	6	32	240	200

Source: Rekha Sharma: *Diet Management.*

This diet contains:

Carbohydrates	374 g
Proteins	50 g
Fats	80 g
Sodium	665 mg
Potassium	1633 mg
Phosphorus	905 mg
Calories	2400 kcal

3. Low Calcium Diet (200 mg Ca)

Breakfast		Lunch		Dinner	
Fresh Orange juice	100 ml	Cooked Beef steak	100 g	Cooked Lamb chop	90 g
White Bread toast	1	Potatoes	100 g	Potatoes	100 g
Butter	15 g	Tomatoes	100 g	Frozen green Peas	80 g
Rice krispies	15 g	Bread	25 g	Bread	25 g
Cream (20% butter fat)	35 g	Butter	15 g	Butter	15 g
Sugar	7 g	Honey	20 g	Jam	15 g
Coffee/Tea/distilled water		Apple sauce	20 g	Peach sauce	20g
		Coffee/Tea/distilled water		Coffee/Tea/distilled water	

This diet chart provides total calcium—198.68 mg, *i.e.*

Breakfast	81.22 mg
Lunch	56.57 mg
Dinner	60.59 mg

4. Low Phosphorus Diet (Phosphorus 1 g and Proteins 40 g)

Breakfast	Lunch	Dinner
Fruit Juice	Meat 56 g	Meat 56 g
Refined Cereal	Potato	Potato
Egg	Cooked vegetables	Cooked vegetables
White Toast	Green salad	Green salad
Butter	White Bread	White Bread
Milk ½ cup	Butter	Butter
Tea/Coffee	Milk ½ cup	Dessert
	Tea/Coffee	Tea/Coffee

5. Acid-Ash Diet

Breakfast	Lunch	Dinner
Grape Fruit	Creamed chicken	Broth
Wheatna	Steamed Rice	Roast Beef gravy
Scrambled Egg	Green Beans	Buttered Noodles
Toast	Stewed Prunes	Sliced Tomato
Butter	Bread	Mayonnaise
Plain jam	Butter	Vanilla Ice cream
Sugar	Milk	Bread
Cream		Butter
Tea/Coffee		

N.B. Diet charts nos. 3-5 from Mitchell. *Nutrition in Health and Disease*, J. B. Lippincot Co. New York, 1976.

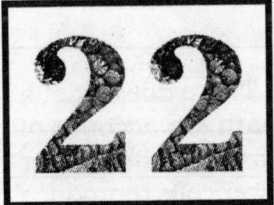

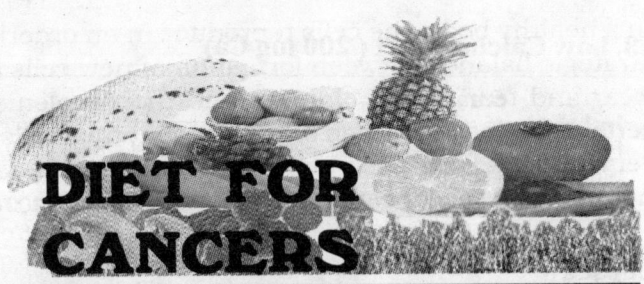

DIET FOR CANCERS

Earlier, when asked what they feared most, the Americans would say 'Cancer'. This dreaded disease is now causing the same spell in developing countries like India and China.

Cancer is the unrestrained growth and spread of the abnormal cells in the body. These malignant cells invade the surrounding healthy tissues. By metastasis, the cancer cells spread through blood and lymph systems, consequently forming new cancerous growths in other parts of the body. Usually, the bland term, 'Cancer' is used to describe the disease, since it manifests in a multiplicity of forms, as under:

1. Lung Cancer
2. Colo-rectal Cancer
3. Breast Cancer
4. Prostate Cancer
5. Liver Cancer
6. Leukemia and Lymphoma
7. Female Reproductive System Cancer
8. Urinary Tract Cancer
9. Brain Cancer
10. Gastrointestinal and Pancreatic Cancer.

From the public health angle, cancer is a very serious health hazard. It is the second largest killer, next to heart disease, accounting for about 20% of the total deaths in USA every year.

CANCER CELLS

In a healthy body, the cells reproduce in an orderly manner. There does exist a strategic balance between formation of new cells and the death, on account of wear and tear, of the old cells and their replenishment. Normal cells, under certain contingencies, can convert to abnormal cells. These cancer cells reproduce very fast. They are solely concerned with growth, rather than function, while the normal cells are concerned mainly with function, rather than growth.

Causes

There are multiple causes that produce cancer, though the exact cause(s) is not definitely established. However, the contributing factors or the predisposing causes are fairly well-known. These causes are:

1. Genetical factors
2. Environmental factors
3. Occupational hazards
4. Personal habits, like alcohol and smoking
5. Dietary factors-both deficiencies and excesses.
6. Stress.

Eminent Oncologist, Dr. Charles B. Simone has categorically listed the 'risk factors' for cancer as shown in Table 22.1.

TABLE 22.1: CANCER RISK FACTORS

Risk factor	Associated human cancer
1. Nutritional factors 　High-fat, low fiber	Breast, colon, rectum, prostate, stomach, mouth, pharynx, esophagus, pancreas, liver, ovary, endometrium, thyroid, kidney, bladder
Iodine deficiency	Thyroid, breast
Aflatoxin (fungus product)	Liver
2. Obesity	Breast, endometrium, colon
3. Tobacco use 　Smoking, chewing, snuffing	Lung, larynx, mouth, pharynx, head and neck, esophagus, pancreas, bladder, kidney, breast
Passive inhalation	Lung, cervix, breast, oral
4. Alcohol	Mouth, pharynx, esophagus, gastrointestine, pancreas, liver, head and neck, larynx, bladder
5. Age greater than 55	Many organ sites
6. Immune system malfunction	Lymphoma, carcinoma

7. High blood pressure	Breast, colon
8. Environment	Leukemia, lung, skin, other sites
9. Sedentary lifestyle	Breast, colon, other sites
10. Stress	Implicated in multiple sites
11. Hormonal	
Late/never pregnant	Breast
Fibrocystic breast disease	Breast
DES(diethylstibestrol)	Breast, vagina, cervix, endometrium, testicle
Conjugated estrogens	Breast, liver
Androgens (17-methyl position)	Liver
Undescended testicles (especially after age 6)	Testicle
12. Sexual-Social	
Female promiscuity	Uterine cervix
Poor male hygiene	Penis
Male homosexuality (Promiscuity)	Kaposi's sarcoma, anus, tongue
13. Radiation	
X rays, etc. (ionizing)	Skin, breast, myelongenous leukemia, thyroid, bone
Sunlight (UV) excessive in fair-skinned people who burn easily	Skin
14. Pesticides	Lung, prostate, liver, skin
15. Occupational	
Petroleum, tar, soot	Lung, skin, scrotum
Boot and shoe manufacture and repair	Nasal sinus
Furniture and cabinet making industry	Nasal sinus
Rubber industry	Lung, bladder, leukemia, stomach
Chemists	Brain, lymphoma, leukemia, pancreas
Foundry workers	Lung
Painters	Leukemia
Printing workers	Lung, mouth, pharynx
Textile workers	Nasal sinus

Table 22.2 shows the initial linkages between diet and cancer.

The underlying cause of this malignant disease is the fundamental loss of control over normal cell reproduction. Several inter-related causes contribute to the degeneration of cells, viz. mutations, carcinogens, radiation, oncogenic viruses and stress factors.

TABLE 22.2: DIETARY FACTORS AND CANCER

Contributing Factors	Preventive Factors
High fat intake	High fibre intake
Alcohol	Vegetables
Nitrites, Nitrites and Nitrosamines	Vitamin A and Carotenoids
Fungus toxins (Aflatoxins)	Vitamin C
Cooking	Vitamin E
Sachharine cyclamates	Selenium

The mutant genes may be inherited, although environmental factors like pollution also play important role in cancer development. Chemical carcinogens (hydrocarbons) also interfere with the cell structure and functions. Smoking, pesticide residues, air and water pollutants, food additives and occupational hazards, all these lead to cell degeneration. Radiation damage from X-rays, reactive materials and toxic wastes lead to chromosome breakage that pave the way to development of carcinoma. The oncogenic or tumour-producing viruses that interfere with the function of regulatory genes have already been identified in the animals. Psychic disturbances and trauma are the physiologic events triggered by stress and thus convert anxiety into malignancy.

There are two stages in the development of cancer.

1. An Initiation Phase
2. A Promotion Phase

In the initiation phase, the normal body cells get exposed to cancer-causing substances, called the mutagens or carcinogens. These adversely affect the cell metabolism, which then get transformed into abnormal cells. During the second phase of promotion, the abnormal cells multiply and proliferate very fast. In the normal course, the latter phase may last for years and the cancerous growth may remain undetected for 10-20 years or more. The affected body organs must be exposed to certain conditions during both the initiation and promotion phases for the cancer to develop. There are found many substances in the food that promote cancer. The food additives: Nitrosamines, used to preserve meat, are initiators of cancer, while alcohol does not initiate but promotes the growth of pre-existing cancer cells. But diet can also be preventive, like the low-fat, high-fibre diet, which also happens to be rich in vitamins A and C, besides trace elements.

Table 22.3 shows the cancer initiators and promoters.

Nutritional deficiencies, as well as dietary excesses, significantly contribute to cancer development. A diet low in fact and alcohol, but high in dietary fibre, vitamins A and C and mineral selenium inhibit the initiators and discourage promotion of several types of cancers. On the other hand, higher intake of fats contribute to greater incidence of breast and colon cancers. Meat intake also contributes to colon cancer. Excessive usage of alcohol, as also smoking, are associated with cancer of the mouth, pharynx larynx, throat and lungs. Similarly, prolonged use of tobacco (chewing) contributes to oral cancer.

TABLE 22.3: COMMON DIETARY INITIATORS AND PROMOTERS OF CANCER

	Initiators	Promoters
1.	Nitrosamines	Sachharine
2.	Benzo (a) pyrenes in barbecued meats	Excess dairy fat
3.	Pesticides (malathion, parathion, kepone, DDT)	Citrus oil
4.	Aflatoxin	12-0-tetradecanoyl-phorbol-13-acetate
5.	Polychlorinated biphenyl (PCB)	High temperatures (43-45 degree centigrade)
6.	Polyvinylchloride (PVC)	Alcohol
7.	Heavy Metals—lead, mercury, arsenic compounds	Surface active agents—Sodium lauryl sulfate
8.	Tannic acid	Some herbs Streptomyces.

Broadly speaking, there are two types of cancer tumours, viz.

(a) Sarcoma arising out of connective tissue,
(b) Carcinoma arising out from epithelial cells.

Both these types are malignant cancers.

The National Academy of Sciences (NAS), USA has categorically stated that 'Cancer of most sites is influenced by dietary patterns'. As such, it is no exaggeration that there is so much a man can do to prevent the initiation and promotion of cancers.

Cancer Therapy

There are 3 main planks of cancer therapy, viz.

1. Surgery
2. Radiotherapy
3. Chemotherapy

Surgery

Early diagnosis of operable tumours often leads to successful surgical treatment of a large number of cancers. However, optimum nutritional status, before taking up surgical intervention, and maximal nutritional support in the post-operative stages are fundamental to speedier recovery.

Radiation

Radiation in cancer treatment has developed around controlled use of X-rays with two types of tumours:

(a) Those responding to therapy with a dose level that is tolerable to the health of normal tissues,

(b) Those which can be targetted without causing damage to the overlaying vital organ tissues.

Radiation is done by using X-ray, radiation isotopes (Co-60) and atomic particles derived from radioactive materials.

Chemotherapy

A large number of anti-neoplastic drugs are now available for treating cancer tumours. These chemotherapeutic agents may be divided into six categories, viz.

1. Alkaloids
2. Alkylating agents
3. Antibiotics
4. Antimeta bolites
5. Enzymes
6. Hormones

These chemotherapeutic agents may be used in two ways:

(a) Combined when a combination of drugs are used in a coordinated manner,

(b) Adjuvant therapy, when it is used in conjunction with other treatments, such as surgery or radiotherapy to increase the cure rate.

Problems Related to Cancer Treatment

The cancer therapy, be it surgery, radiation, chemotherapy or immunotherapy, is known to have many side-effects which further complicate the condition. Table 22.4 categorically lists the side effects of surgical intervention.

However, the severity of chemotherapy manifests in many toxic effects like bone-marrow effects (anemia and bleeding), gastrointestinal effects (nausea, vomiting, stomatitis, ulcers and anorexia) and hair follicle effects (alopecia or baldness). The systemic reaction in advanced cases may lead to cachexia. Often, there is the imbalance of decreased intake and increased demand, resulting in negative nitrogen balance, which is an indication of body tissue wasting. The gastrointestinal surgery can cause 'dumping' problem.

TABLE 22.4: NUTRITION SIDE EFFECTS OF CANCER SURGERY

	Site of Surgery	Side Effects Noticed
1.	Head and neck	Impaired chewing and swallowing
2.	Esophagectomy	Diarrhoea, steatorrhea and esophageal stenosis
3.	Vagotomy	Gastric stasis, diarrhoea, fat malabsorption
4.	Gastrectomy	Dumping syndrome, hypoglycemia, mal-absorption, possible deficiency of iron, calcium, vitamin B_{12} and fat soluble vitamins
5.	Pancreatectomy	Diabetes Mellitus; possibly malabsorption of fats, proteins, fat soluble vitamins and minerals
6.	Small Bowels	Malabsorption of nutrients
7.	Ileostomy	Sodium and water losses, vitamin B_{12}, fat malabsorption; bile salt diarrhoea

Source: Charuhas P. M. *Topics in Clinical Nutrition*, 1993, Aspen Pub.

Diet Therapy

Cancer is the one disease that is amenable to a whole host of foodstuffs that prevent or retard progress of cancer in the human body. Dr. Simone has given a very exhaustive list of three *'Natural Food Protectors'*, as shown in Table 22.5.

The basic principles of diet therapy in cancer are two-fold:

1. To meet the increased metabolic demands of the disease and also to prevent catabolism as far as possible,
2. To alleviate the symptoms of disease and its treatment through adaptation of food and the feeding process.

Two important principles involved herein are a personal nutritional assessment and vigorous nutrition-support therapy. It is indeed very difficult to replenish a nutritionally-depleted patient than to maintain a good nutritional status in a patient from the outset. As such, it calls for a detailed personal history in order to determine a patient's individual needs, tolerance and preferences. The vigorous diet care often makes all the difference in success rate of medical therapy. Hence, the nutritional needs may be determined on the basis of energy, proteins, vitamins and minerals, also fluid requirements.

1. Energy

Greater energy demands are placed on the cancer patients. There must be more than enough carbohydrates in order to spare proteins for the vital tissue synthesis. An adult patient with good nutritional status requires about 2,000 kcal/day for maintenance needs. But a more malnourished patient would call for 3,000-4,000 kcal/day.

TABLE 22.5: NATURAL FOOD PROTECTORS

Protector	Food Source	Protective Action
Carotene	Carrots, sweet potatoes, yams, pumpkins, squash, kale, broccoli cantaloupe	Neutralizes free radicals and singlet oxygen radicals; enhances immune system; reverses pre-cancer conditions; high intake associated with low cancer rate
Indoles	Cabbage family: cabbage, broccoli, cauliflower, mustard green, etc.	Destroys estrogen, known to initiate new cancers, especially breast cancer
Isoflavones	Legumes: beans, peas, peanuts	Inhibits estrogen receptor; destroys cancer gene enzymes; inhibits estrogen
Lignans	Flax seed, walnuts, fatty fish	Inhibits estrogen action; inhibits prosta-glandins, hormones that cause cancer spread
Polyacetylene	Parsley	Inhibits prostaglandins; destroys benzo-pyrene—a potent carcinogen
Protease Inhibitors	Soybeans	Destroys enzymes that can cause cancer to spread
Quinones	Rosemary	Inhibits carcinogens or co-carcinogens
Sterols	Cucumbers	Decreases chotesterol
Sulfur	Garlic	Inhibits carcinogens, inhibits cancer spread, decreases cholesterol
Terpenes	Citrus fruit	Increases enzymes to break down carci-nogens; decreases cholesterol
Triterpenoids	Licorice	Inhibits estrogens, prostaglandins; slows down rapidly dividing cells, like cancer cells

2. *Proteins*

Efficient protein use promotes tissue building, prevents catabolism and helps make up tissue deficits. For maintenance purpose, a protein level of 80-100 g/day is recommended. It could go up to 100-200 g proteins/day in malnourished cases.

3. *Vitamins and Minerals*

Key vitamins and minerals control protein and energy metabolism through their multiple roles in cell enzyme systems, as also in structural development and tissue integrity. Table 22.6 shows the role of important vitamins and minerals in relation to cancer prevention.

TABLE 22.6: ROLE OF VITAMINS AND MINERALS IN CANCER PREVENTION

Action	(a) Cancer Risk Reduction (b) Deficiency Cancer	Rich Foods	Special Observations
Vitamin A (a) Retinol (b) β Carotene Inhibits initiation and promotion phase, 1. Inhibits growth of abnormal cells 2. Alters immune fnctions, improves body's defences 3. Strengthens cell membranes 4. Alters cell production	Cancer of mouth, larynx, oesophagus, breast, cervix. bladder, lungs, colon, stomach, prostate **(Nos. 1-3)** (b) Cancer rate highest in low vitamin A patients **(Nos. 4-5)**	(a) Animal foods-milk, eggs, liver, meat. (b) dark green and orange vegetables–carrots, broccoli, winter squash, sweet potato, pumpkin, spinach, pears, apricots, cantaloupes, water melons plus cheese and non-fat milk	Necessary for growth of epithelial tisues. Epithelial cancers account for half of all the cancers Lung cancer rates lower in smokers with high fruits and vegetable usage RDA—4,000-5,000 IU for night blindness; Cancers 10,000-25,000 IU
Vitamin C 1. Inhibits nitrites conversion in stomach, **(Nos. 3, 3a)** 2. Improves cell resistance to damage. **(No. 11)** 3. Enhances Immunity 4. Strengthens body's defences against damage by oxidation	(a) Cancer of Stomach throat and Bladder. **(Nos. 6-10)**	Vegetables, fruits—citrus, strawberry, broccoli, Cantaloupe, potatoes, asparagus;	
Vitamin D Controls basic cell functions	Cancer of breast and colon **(Nos. 12, 13)**	Yeast, fish liver oils Fortified milk, Sunlight on skin	Inadequate synthesis of vitamin D involved in colon cancer
Vitamin E 1. Tocopherols antioxidant. 2. Inhibits conversion of Nitrites **(No. 14)** 3. Assists Selenium, inhibits cancer growth **(No. 3)**	Cancer of stomach; Non-malignant cancer of breast **(No. 14)**	Whole grains, Wheat oil. nuts and beans: germ Vegetable oils–soyabean oil, corn of, safflower oil	Vitamin E content: of oils declines when they are refined/bleached

Folic Acid	1. Maintains genetic code of cells. 2. Regulates Cell division and growth 3. Converts damaged cells to normal cells **(No. 15)**		Dark green leafy vegetables—spinach, lettuce, broccoli, legumes, bets, orange, cantaloupe, liver	Easily lost on over-cooking or improper storage and processing
Vitamin B$_6$	1. Strengthens body's immune system 2. Protects against initiation of cancer **(No. 16)**		Whole grain bread/cereals, lean meat. Chick, fish soyabeans, driedbeans, peanuts, walnuts, bananas, cabbage, cauliflower, potato	Lost during cooking and canning or refining or grains
Iron	Helps proper functioning of immune system	(b) Deficiency risk of stomach **(No. 14)**	Liver, meat eggs, whole grains, green leafy vegetables, nuts, legumes	RDA 18 mg
Selenium	1. Antioxidant 2. Stimulates immunity **(No. 19)** 3. Strengthens defences 4. Detoxifies cancer-causing Cd and Hg. **(No. 18)**	(b) Cancer of GI tract, lungs, breast and lymph systems	Cereals grown in selenium-rich soils; leanmeat, sea-food. Organic supplements like Seleno-methionine and Seleno-cystein have effect on inhibition of cancer	People with very low selenium levels have twice the risk of cancer than those with high selenium.
Zinc	1. Regulation of genetic code within the cells 2. Maintain healthy immune system. **(No. 3)** 3. Helps in healing of tissues	(b) Deficiency can lead to prostate cancer **(No. 20)**	Whole grain bread/cereals; Low fat milk, lean meats, Sea-foods, oysters, liver, eggs, cheese, milk	

N.B. This comprehensive tabulation was compiled from diverse sources in the National Medical Library, Delhi. The bold numbers in the parenthesis provide reference to the special bibliography given at the end of this chapter.

Dr. Charles B Simone strongly recommends a combination of vitamins and minerals as food supplements as shown in Table 22.7. He also recommends taking as a food supplement the calcium formula shown in Table 22.8.

TABLE 22.7: SUPPLEMENTATION PROGRAM

Nutrient	Adult		Children (Age 1-4)	
	Amount	% U.S. RDA*	Amount	% U.S. RDA
Beta-Carotene	20 mg	***	1 mg	***
Vitamin A (Palmitate)	5,000 IU	1,000	834 IU	33
Vitamin D (Ergocalciferol)	400 IU	100	400 IU	100
Vitamin E (di-tocopherol)	400 IU	1,333	15 IU	150
Vitamin C (Ascorbic acid)	350 mg	580	60 mg	150
Folic acid	400 mcg	100	200 mcg	100
Vitamin B_1 (Thiamine)	10 mg	667	1.1 mg	157
Vitamin B_2 (Riboflavin)	10 mg	588	1.2 mg	150
Niacinamide	40 mg	220	9 mg	100
Vitamin B_6 (Pyridoxine)	10 mg	500	1.12 mg	100
Vitamin B_{12} (Cyanobalamin)	18 mcg	300	4.5 mcg	150
Biotin	150 mcg	50	25 mcg	20
Pantothenic acid (de-calcium pantothenate)	20 mg	200	5 mg	100
Iodine	150 mcg	100	70 mcg	100
Copper (Cupric oxide)	3 mg	150	1.25 mg	125
Zinc (Zinc gluconate)	15 mg	100	10 mg	125
Potassium	30 mg	#	2 mg	#
Selenium (organic)	200 mcg	**	20 mcg	**
Chromium (organic)	125 mcg	**	20 mcg	**
Manganese (Gluconate)	2.5 mg	**	1 mg	**
Molybdenum	50 mcg	**	25 mcg	**
Inositol	10 mg	#	0	N/A
Para aminobenzoic acid	10 mg	#	0	N/A
Bioflavonoids	10 mg	#	10 mcg	#
Choline (Choline bitartrate)	10 mg	#	5 mg	#
L-Cysteine	20	#	0	N/A
L-Arginine	5 mg	#	0	N/A
Histidine	N/A	N/A	10 mg	**
Leucine	N/A	N/A	10 mg	**
Isoleucine	N/A	N/A	10 mg	**
Lysine	N/A	N/A	10 mg	**
Threonine	N/A	N/A	10 mg	**

\# No nutritional requirement established.
* Percentage US RDA for Adults and Children.

TABLE 22.8: CALCIUM FORMULA

Nutrient	Dosage	% U.S. RDA*
Calcium (Calcium carbonate)	500 mg	50
Magnesium (Magnesium oxide)	140 mg	36
Silicon	2 mg	#
Boron	2 mg	#
L-Theronine	2 mg	#
L-Lysine	2 mg	#

*Percentage U.S. Recommended Dietary Allowance (U.S. RDA) for adults and children 4 or more years.
No U.S. RDA established.

4. *Fluids*

Cancer patients must ensure adequate fluid intake for two reasons:

1. To replace gastrointestinal losses or losses through infections and fevers.
2. To help the kidneys dispose off the metabolic breakdown products from the destroyed cells and from the toxic drugs used in treatment.

This could call for 2-3 litres fluids to be supplied daily.

Table 22.9 gives the important foods which have cancer-preventive properties. Later on, Table 22.10 categorically lists major phytochemicals which have proven anti-cancer properties. It also shows the food sources of these phytochemicals. Thus, one finds a huge cornucopia of organic resources to fight cancer, without having to resort to the cumbersome, liability-ridden conventional cancer therapy.

TABLE 22.9: CANCER-PREVENTIVE FOODSTUFFS

High	Garlic, Cabbage, Liquorice, Soyabeans, Ginger; Carrots, Celery, Parsnips
Medium	Onions, Tea, Turmeric, Orange, Lemon, Grapefruit, Whole Wheat, Flax, Brown Rice, Tomato, Eggplant, Pepper, Broccoli, Cauliflower, Brussels Sprouts
Moderate	Oats, Barley, Potato, Sage, Mint, Cucumber, Rosemary, Thyme, Chives, Cantaloupe, Berries

(Adapted from Cancer-preventive Foods and Ingredients by Caragay in Food Tech. April, 1992)

TABLE 22.10: PHYTOCHEMICALS, BIOLOGICAL ACTIVITIES AND FOOD SOURCES

Group	Examples	Main Food Sources	Activities/Functions
Non-starch Polysachharides			
Fibre and Related Compounds	Soluble-Pectins and gums	Fruits (apples, citrus) Oats, Soyabean, algae	Lowers serum cholestrol
	Insoluble Celluloses	Cereals (wheat, rye) Vegetables	Prevents cancers, alleviates constipation
	Resistant/retrograde starch	High-amylose starches, processed starches, whole grains, seeds	Prevents colon cancer
Phytates		Cereals, grains, soyabeans	Binds minerals, prevents colon cancer
	Oligosachharides	Chicory, soyabeans, artichokes, onion	Modify gut microflora, cancer prevention
Flavonoids	Flavonols, Quercetin, Kaempferol	Vegetables (onion, tomatoes), wine, tea	Antioxidants
	Flavonones, Tangertin, Naringenin, Hesperitin	Citrus fruits	Cancer prevention, Imune modulation
Tea Polyphenols	Catechins, Epicatechins	Green tea	Antioxidant
Derived Tannins	Theoflavins, Thearubigens,	Black tea, red wine, roasted coffee	
Isoflavonoids	Daidzein, Genistein	Soyabean products	Anti-oestrogenic, prevents cancer
Lignans	Secoisolariciresinol,	Rye bran, berries, nuts	Antioxidant, anti-oestrogenic
Glycosinolates	Glucobrassicin, Indoles	Cabbage, broccoli, mustard, watercess	Phase II induction
Phenols	Ethyl phenol, Gallic acid, Tannins	Raspberry, black tea, strawberries	Antioxidants
Monoterpenes	D-Limonene, Perillyl alcohol	Citrus fruits, herbs, cherries	Phase I and II induction, Anti-tumour activity
Phytosterols	Campesterol, Stigmasterol	Veg. oils (soyabean, sunflower oil)	Lowers serum cholestrol
Organo-sulphides (Allium compounds)	Diallyl sulphide, S-allylcysteine	Garlic, onion, leeks	Phase II induction, cancer prevention

Nutritional Management

The spectrum of special nutritional management includes four mechanisms or forms of feeding the patient, two enteral forms and two parenteral forms. However, the age-old dictum of diet management, *i.e.*

'If the Gut works, use it.'

must be capitalized upon to the maximum possible extent.

Enteral Feeding

For cancer patients, an oral diet with supplementation is the most effective form of nutritional support. Based on the personal history, adjustments must be made in the texture, temperature of the foodstuffs and the choice thereof, depending upon tolerance and preference levels.

In case of sore mouth and stomatitis which pose difficulties in eating, foods with high liquid content or gravy are recommended. Lactose intolerance, as a result of chemotherapy, calls for nutrient supplement formula with a non-milk protein base. Many such commercial supplements are now available in the market.

Tube Feeding

Tube feeding is advised when the patient is unable to eat or swallow anything. The route of entry may vary from the traditional naso-gastric tube to alternate surgical placements of esophagostomy, gastrostomy and jejunostomy tubes. Patients can also be fed by pump-monitored slow drip during the night, which literally frees him from the cumbersome tube being used during the day.

Parenteral Feeding

In case the gastro-intestinal system cannot be used, then parenteral feeding is resorted to. It could be in two forms:

1. Peripheral Parenteral Nutrition (PPN), used briefly to administer solutions of dextrose, amino acids, vitamins and minerals with intermittent fat emulsions.
2. Total Parenteral Nutrition (TPN) to meet greater nutritional support requirements stretched over a longer period of time through a larger central vein. Herein, one could feed more concentrated formulations.

The parenteral feeding, despite occasional doubts and reservations, has proved to be a significant means of turning metabolic status from catabolism to anabolism, thus saving a critical situation and avoiding the grave consequences of development of cancer cachexia.

Chemotherapy Complications

Many side effects or complications of chemotherapy and other drug therapies, which can otherwise aggravate the situation, can be avoided by suitable dietary modifications, as shown in Table 22.11.

TABLE 22.11: DIETARY INTERVENTION FOR DRUG THERAPY COMPLICATIONS

	Complications	Dietary Intervention
1.	Anorexia or Loss of Appetite	More frequent feeding with a varied menu; even a few bits/sips every hour can add up to sufficient calories and protein level in the system
2.	Sore mouth/Sore Throat	Soft foods like banana, pears, apricots, cottage cheese, mashed potatoes, scrambled eggs, pureed vegetables or pureed meats, liquids, milk shakes
		Mix foods with butter, gravy/sauces. Use anaesthetic lozenges/spray to benumb the mouth/throat to enable the patient to eat without difficulty
3.	Altered sense of taste/smell	Prepare foods that look and smell good
		Use flavour seasonings. Try tart foods as orange or lemonade. Seek advice about good mouth care
4.	Dry Mouth	Sucking sugar-free hard candy can help produce saliva
		Use soft pureed foods, also foods with sauces and gravies
		Sip water every few minutes to help in swallowing
5.	Nausea	Use anti-emetic drugs. Eat small amounts and slowly drink liquids throughout the day, Use curds, soft fruits and vegetables like stewed apples and bananas
		Drink beverages that are cooled and chilled
		Avoid eating for 1-2 hours before radiation or chemotherapy
6.	Vomiting	Use anti-emetic drugs. Avoid eating till vomiting under control
		Once vomiting is under control, try small amounts of clear liquids—1 tsp every ten minutes and gradually increase the amount finally to 2 tbsp every 30 minutes. Later on, give full liquid diet.
7.	Diarrhoea	Drink plenty of fluids. Eat small amounts throughout the day. Use foods rich in sodium and potassium like bananas, peach, apricot and boiled mashed potatoes. Try curd, porridge, grape juice, smooth peanut butter, white bread, coffee/cheese. Try clear liquid diet during the first 12 hours after diarrhoea
		Avoid very hot or very cold foods/drinks.
8.	Constipation	Plenty of fluids, 8-10 glasses/day
		Take a hot drink an hour before the normal stool time. Eat high fibre foods, fresh fruits and vegetables with skin. Add bran to chapattis/cereals. Take regular exercise
9.	Weight Gain	Try limiting the weight gain
		Use diuretics to get rid of extra fluids
10.	Tooth Decay	Rinse mouth after every meal
		Use soft tooth brush
		Consult dentist about special problems
11.	Lactose Intolerance	Use soyabean formulae and aged cheese and soya milk

TEN COMMANDMENTS FOR CANCER DIET

These are the diet patterns that help reduce considerably the risk of developing cancer.

1. Maintain an ideal body weight
2. Reduce the level of fats in the diet. It should be less than 30% of the total dietary calories.
3. Increase the intake of dietary fibre.
4. Increase the intake of vitamins A and C-rich foods.
5. Make the maximum consumption of cruciferous vegetables like cauliflower, cabbage and broccoli.
6. Restrict the use of salt-cured, smoked nitrite-cured foods.
7. Avoid all sorts of contaminated foods.
8. Restrict the use of alcohol to a moderate level.
9. Be careful to avoid foods that contain carcinogens and mutagens.
10. Feed in small amounts, but at more frequent intervals.

The consumption of low-fat, high-fibre diet throughout life might aid in prevention of cancers, cardiovascular diseases hypertension, obesity and diabetes. Incidentally, many of the foods that are full of vitamin A are also high in vitamin C. The following steps would help increase the daily intake of these two vitamins vital for cancer prevention.

1. Vegetable and fruit juice.
2. Salad should become a compulsory item of diet.
3. Even mid-meal snacks should be restricted to raw vegetables and fruits.
4. Serve only fruit for dessert.
5. Substitute sweet potato for white potato.
6. Top the cereals with fresh fruit.
7. Add chopped green chillies to the non-vegetarian diet.
8. Use tomato sauce to the exclusion of other sauce/pasta.
9. Dark green leafy vegetables must be incorporated into the daily menu.
10. Maximise the consumption of cruciferous vegetables.

Cruciferous vegetables like cabbage, cauliflower and broccoli contain both vitamins A and C, as also dietary fibre. Besides, they also contain indoles - a cancer-fighting substance.

Vitamin A comes in two forms:

(a) Retinol-supplied by foods of animal origin such as milk, meats, eggs and fish.

(b) β carotenes, found only in fresh fruits and vegetables. Dark orange carrots have more vitamin A (β carotenes) than pale, light colored carrots. Similarly, the vitamin A content of Romain lettuce is four times that of Iceberg lettuce.

Dietary Fibre

The stress on dietary fibre in diet is borne by the research done by Jensen (1983) and Burkitt (1980), who had conclusively shown that there was 8 times more risk of colon cancer in people using low fibre diet.

Fibre also affects the incidence of breast cancer. Women using adequate dietary fibre (say 28 g/day) excrete more estrogen, hence lesser estrogen is left to be re-absorbed. These changes in estrogen and other hormones level are associated with a reduced risk of breast cancer.

The insoluble cellulose in the fibre binds to water, increases the bulk in the intestine and so leaves very little room for harmful cancer-causing substances to act. Some cancer-causing compounds are formed from bile. Fibre binds to bile and thus discourages its conversion to harmful substances.

Similarly, pectin decreases the production of certain fatty acids that help accelerate the growth of cancer cells in the bowels. And lastly, a person can eat more food (with high fibre) and consume less calories. This helps maintain weight and also eliminates the feeling of hunger.

Best sources of dietary fibre are whole grain breads, cereals, dried beans and peas, nuts and seeds, apart from fresh vegetables and fruits. As such, three fourths of the menu should be from plant sources and these should preferably be unrefined, unprocessed food items. To ensure maximum supply of fibre, half of the grains in the diet should come from whole grains, rather than split or powdered cereals. The desirable amount of dietary fibre should amount to between 35 to 45 g/day, which can be computed from Table 22.12, which shows the amount of fibre present in different foodstuffs.

TABLE 22.12: HIGH FIBRE DIET FOR CANCER PATIENTS

	No. of servings	Quantity of fibre
1. Whole grain bread, cereals and pasta (1 serving—bread 1 slice, cooked cereals 1 cup)	six	13 g
2. Fresh fruits and vegetables (1 serving—1 cup raw or half cup cooked)	four	15-23 g
3. Dried beans or peas (1 serving—half cup cooked)	one	9 g
Total Dietary Fibre		**34-45 g**

Source: *Cancer and Nutrition* by David Heber *et al.*

Table 22.13 gives a full day menu for a high fibre diet for cancer patients.

TABLE 22.13: MENU FOR 45 g FIBRE DIET

	Foodstuffs	Amount	Fibre (g)
Breakfast	All bran	1/3 cup	7.9
	Banana	1 medium	1.3
	Milk low fat	1 cup	—
	Orange juice	6 oz	0.6
	Whole wheat bread	2 slices	5.4
	Jelly	I tsp	—
	Sub-total		**15.2 g**
Lunch	Salad—spinach	1 cup	2.2
	Carrots	¼ cup	0.8
	Tomato	¼ cup	1.8
	Cheese	2 oz	—
	Dressing	1-1½ tsp	—
	Whole wheat role	1	5.4
	Orange	1	3.8
	Sub-total		**14.5 g**
Afternoon Snack	Tangerine	1	1.8
	Rye crackers	2	1.5
	Sub-total		**3.3**
Dinner	Salmon fish	4 oz	—
	Baked potato with skin	1 medium	5.2
	Yogurt dressing	2 tbsp	—
	Broccoli	2/3 cup	3.2
	Dinner salad	1- 1½ cup	2.0
	Dressing	2 tsp	—
	Sub-total		**10.4 g**
Bedtime	Graham crackers	2	1.3 g
	Total dietary fibre		**44.7 g**

Heber *et al.*, *Diet and Nutrition*, CBS Pub.

Foods to Avoid

- Salt-cured, smoked and nitrites containing processed foods.
- Avoid cooking methods that promote the formation of cancer-causing substances, especially charred broiling.
- Excess fat meats, like organ meats and pork, as also over-cooked meats.
- Foods containing cancer-causing substances
- Foods high in pyridoxine as these stimulate malignant growths.
- Foods rich in phosphates.
- Moldy foods and old peanuts.
- Nuts that may contain aflatoxins
- Non-nutritive sweeteners, such as sachharines.
- Excessive use of alcohols.

Fats and Cholesterol

Many studies have reported that high-fat diets lead to a higher incidence of cancer of breast, ovaries, uterus, colon and prostate glands. Americans with an average of 42% of total calorie intake being provided by fats have reported high incidence of cancer, as compared to the Japanese on low-fat diet. Fried chicken contains one-third more calories than a broiled chicken. Non-fat milk contains half the calories than full cream milk.

A high-fat diet stimulates the production of more cholesterol and bile. In the presence of excess dietary fat, the altered bacteria produce certain compounds from excess bile. And these compounds promote colon cancer. A high-fat diet is also linked to breast cancer, since it changes the hormone levels of estrogen, and these changes are conducive to the development of breast cancer. As such, women should avoid red meat, pork and desserts.

The risk of ovarian cancer also increases two to three-fold on high-fat diet. When people consume diets like high fatty meats and low in fruits and vegetables, the risk of cancer increases eight-fold, as compared to the people on low-fat, high-fibre diet. Similarly, trans-fatty acids found in margarine and shortenings are reported to increase the risk of cancer development.

Cholesterol is also suspected to be involved in the link between dietary fat and cancers, especially cancer of colon.

As such, a person can positively control many factors that cause cancer. And many of these factors also reduce the risk of other degenerative diseases. Thus, anti-cancer diets could contribute a great deal to the overall fitness and sound health. As the eminent Medical educationist, Prof. Sue Rod Williams comments:

'Frequently, diet is the primary therapy itself.'

Special References for the Role of Vitamins and Minerals in Table 22.6.

1. Bjelke, E (1975). *Int. J. Cancer*, **15:** 561.
2. Graham *et al.* (1982). *Am.J. Epidem.*, **116:** 68.
3. Garrison and Somer (1985). *The Nutrition Desk Reference.* Keating Pub.
3a. *Medical News in JAMA* (1977). **238:** 15.
4. Basy, Tin (1979). *J. Human Nutr.*, **33;** 24.
5. Weber F (1983). *Proc. Nutr. Soc.*, **42:** 31.
6. Dungel and Sigurjonsson (1967). *Br.J.Cancer*, **21:** 270.
7. Hormozdier *et al.* (1975). *Cancer Res.*, **35:** 3493.
8. Tuyns, A. (1983). *Nutr. Cancer*, **5:** 195.
9. Yamanaka, W. (1985). *Postgrad. Med.*, **78:** 47.
10. Cameron *et al.* (1979). *Cancer Res.*, **39:** 663.
11. Willet and MacMahon (1984). *N. Eng. J. Med.*, **310:** 697.
12. Shamberger R. (1982). *The Cancer Bulletin*, **34:** 150.
13. Garland *et al.* (1985). *Lancet*, **1:** 307.
14. Cheney *et al.* (1985). *Food, Nutrition and Diet Therapy.* Pub. Saunders
15. Butterworth C. (1983). *Am. J. Clin. Nutr.*, **32:** 926.
16. Prior F. (1985). *Medical Hypothesis*, **16:** 421.
17. Shambergere R (1976). *Arch. Environ. Health*, **31:** 231.
18. NRC (1982). *Diet, Nutrition and Cancer.*
19. Spalhoz *et al.* (1981). *Selenium in Biology and Medicine.* AVI Pub.
20. Whelm *et al.* (1983). *Br. J. Urol.*, **55:** 552fc.

Dr. (Mrs.) USHA JAIN SUPPLEMENT

SPECIAL DIET CHART FOR CANCER

7.00 AM	Crushed Garlic with Honey	1 tsp
	Green Sun-charged Water	1 glass
8.00 AM	Wheat grass Juice	1 cup (40 leaves at a time)
	+ Carrot/Cucumber Juice	1 cup
9.00 AM	Overnight soaked Figs	2
	Almonds	5
	Munakkas (dried Currants)	5
	Raisins	15 plus
	Sprouts of Wheat with Grated Coconut	1 tbsp
	Seasonal Fruit Salad—Apples, Pears, Banana, Sapota	1 bowl
	Whole Milk with Dates 3	1 glass
11.00 AM	Seasonal Fruit/Vegetable Juice	1 glass
1.00 PM	Seasonal Green Vegetable salad	1 bowl
	Sprouts—Alfalfa, Bengal/Green grams	1 tbsp mixed with
	Curd	1 bowl
	Ashgourd Juice	1 cup or
	Butter Milk/Vegetable Soup	1 cup
3.00 PM	Seasonal Juicy Fruits/Vegetable Juice	1 bowl/glass
5.00 PM	Wheat grass Juice	1 cup with
	Carrot or Amla Juice	1 cup
7.00 PM	Seasonal Fruit salad	2 cups with
	Wheat Sprouts	½ cup
	Grated Green Coconut	½ cup with
	Soaked Figs 2, Raisin 5 and Dates 4	
9.00 PM	Soaked Apricots	3
	Milk	1 cup with
	Honey	1 tsp
	(*If very hungry, then give Papaya fruit*	*1 bowl*)

Dr. Gerson's Cancer Diet (Special Dietary Formulations)

For the first 6-12 weeks

- Fresh raw juice of fruits and vegetables with leaves
- Raw fruits and vegetables
- Vegetables and fruits stewed in their own juices
- Potatoes, Oatmeal, Saltless Rye Bread
- Fresh Calf Liver Juice (very high in oxidizing enzymes)

Subsequently, sodium-free, but high potassium diets like

- Saltless and Creamless Pot Cheese
- Unsalted Buttermilk
- Yogurt from skimmed unflavoured, unsweetened milk

Forbidden in the first month of treatment

- Milk, Meat, Fish, Butter, Cheese and Eggs.

To avoid

- Tea, Coffee, Cocoa. Tobacco, Refined Sugar, Candies and Chocolates, Soy products, Cakes, Cucumbers, Spices, Berries, Canned foods, Sulphured Peas, Lentils and Beans, Alcohol and Ice creams.

Medication to include

- Niacin (Nicotinic acid) 50 mg thrice a day
- Vitamin E (Natural) 400 IU once a day
- Vitamin A 50,000 IU each day (from fish oil)
- Vitamin C 500 mg twice a day.
- Pancreatin 2 tablets three times a day.
- Lugol's Solution one drop twice a day.
- Dessicated liver, defatted—each meal 2 tablets

Detoxification

- Coffee Enema every 4 hours for relieving pain, nusea and depression.

CHERIE CALBOM SUPPLEMENT

The following table gives Cherie Calbom's recommended Juice Regime for cancer.

Suggsted Juicing Recipes for cancer

Ginger Hopper

¼-inch slice ginger root
4-5 carrots, greens removed
½ apple, seeded

Push ginger through hopper with carrots and apple

Garden Salad Special

3 Broccoli flowerets
1 garlic clove
4-5 carrots or 2 tomatoes
2 stalks celery
½ green pepper

Push broccoli and garlic through hopper with carrots or tomatoes. Follow with celery and green pepper

Potassium Broth

Handful parsley
Handful spinach
4-5 carrots, greens removed
2 stalks celery

Bunch up parsley and spinach leaves, and push through hopper with carrots and celery

Cherie's Cleansing Cocktail

¼-inch slice ginger root
1 beet
½ apple, seeded
4 carrots green removed

Push ginger, beet, and apple through hopper with carrots

Garlic Express

Handful parsley
1 garlic clove
4-45 carrots, greens removed
2 stalks celery

Bunch up parsley and push through hopper with garlic carrots, and celery

Cantaloupe Shake

½ cantaloupe, with skin

Cut cantaloupe in strips, and push through hopper

Alkaline Special

¼ had cabbage (red or green)
3 stalks celery

Push cabbage and celery through hopper

Chlorophyll Cocktail

3 beet tops
Handful parsley
Handful spinach
4 carrots, greens removed
½ apple, seeded

Bunch up beet tops, parsley, and spinach, and push through hopper with carrots and apple

Calcium-Rich Cocktail

3 kale leaves
Small handful parsley
4-5 carrots, greens removed
½ apple, seeded

Bunch up kale and parsley, and push through hopper with carrots and apple

APPENDIX 4

(A) Nutrition During Radiation Therapy

Fortified Milk

1 quart whole milk
1 cup dry skim milk power
(210 caliries, 15 g protein per 1 cup)

Milkshake

1½ cups ice cream
4 tsp dry skim milk powder
1/4 cup whole milk
(500 calories, 15 g protein)

Peach Yogurt Shake

1 cup sliced peaches
1 cup plain yogurt
1 cup fortified milk
2 tsp honey
(525 calories, 15 g protein)

Orange Sherbet Shake

1 cup orange sherbet
¾ cup fortified milk
(380 calories, 8 g protien)

(B) Sample Supporting Diet

Breakfast

Orange Juice
Cream of Rice
Scrambled Egg
White toast with Butter or Margarine
Coffee with Milk and sugar

Snack

Creamy Peanut Butter on crackers

Lunch

Roast Beef sandwich on buttered
white bread
Banana
Decaffeinated Tea with Milk and sugar

Snack

Milkshake
Vanilla Wafers

Dinner

Broiled Chicken
Baked Potato (without skin)
Cooked Carrots with Butter
Chocolate Pudding
Grape juice

Snack

English Muffin with jelly and butter
Decaffeinated Tea with Milk and sugar

Source: Lisa Tartamella, MS, RD, Ambulatory Nutrition Specialist, Department of Food and Nutrition, Yale-New Haven Hospital, New Haven, Connecticut (USA).

(C) Clear Liquid Diet: Suggested Meal Plan

When the body cannot handle the softest foods or heavy or thick liquids. This type of diet is needed after surgery or before stomach or bond surgery.

Breakfast

> 1 cup Juice
> 2 cup clear Broth
> ½ cup Gelatin dessert
> Coffee or Tea* with sugar

Snacks

> 1 cup Fruit Juice or soft drink
> ½ cup Gelatin dessert

Lunch

> 1 cup Juice
> 1 cup clear Broth
> ½ cup gelatin Dessert
> Coffee or Tea* with sugar

Snacks

> 1 cup Fruit Juice or soft drink
> ½ cup Gelatin dessert

Dinner

> 1 cup Juice
> 1 cup clear Broth
> ½ cup Gelatin dessert
> Coffee or Tea* with sugar

Snacks

> 1 cup Fruit Juice
> ½ cup Gelatin dessert

Source: *Eating Hints for Cancer Patients*, National Cancer Institue, National Institutes of Health, USA.

(D) Fiber-Restricted Diet: Suggested Meal Plan

For patients whose gastrointestinal track cannot digest fiber in foods. It is recommended after G.I. surgery before patients can return to their regular diet.

Breakfast

½ cup strained Fruit Juice*
1 egg
1 slice White Toast
3 tsp Butter or Margarine
Jelly

Snack

1 cup Milk**
1 serving allowed Cereal
Sugar

Lunch

½ cup Soup***
2 oz Meat, Fish, or Poultry
½ cup allowed Vegetable
2 slices White Bread or roll
1 serving allowed dessert

Snack

2 slices White Toast
2 tsp Butter or Margarine
Jelly or Honey

Dinner

5 oz Meat, Fish, or Poultry
1 cup Milk**
3 tsp Butter or Margarine
1 Baked Potato, without skin
1 serving allowed dessert
½ cup Vegetable Juice

Snack

½ cup strained Fruit Juice
3 Plain Cookies

* 2 servings of fruit/juices allowed per day.
**2 servings or milk allowed per day.
***Count as ½ cup milk if made with milk.
Source: Eating Hints for Cancer Patients, National Cancer Institue, National Institutes of Health.

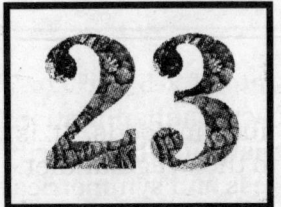

23

MISCELLANEOUS DISABLING DISEASES

This Chapter includes special debilitating diseases like

1. Arthritis
2. Tuberculosis
3. Anemia
4. Asthma
5. Sex disorders—Menorrhagia, Leucorrhea and Impotency

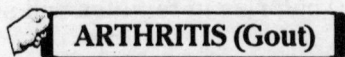 **ARTHRITIS (Gout)**

The term Arthritis is formed from two words: '*arth*' means joints and '*itis*' means inflammation. Hence, arthritis is a disease of one or more joints, which become swollen and painful. In USA, it is the principal crippling disease occurr ing mostly after the age of 45, with a higher incidence in the women. Middle aged men are more prone to arthritis. It is caused by deposition in the joints of urate crystals, associated with an increased concentration of urate in plasma, *i.e.* 'Hyperuricaemia'.

Arthritis may be acute or chronic, depending upon severity, location, deformation and cause. There are three types of arthritis, viz.

1. Rheumatoid Arthritis
2. Osteoarthritis
3. Gouty Arthritis.

Gout is a disease that affects older men and post-menopausal women. It is characterized by a disorder of purine metabolism, which results in abnormally high levels of uric acid in the blood and deposits of sodium urate in soft and bony tissues like joints, cartilage and tendonds. Sodium urates are formed and deposited as '*Trophi*' in joints. These deposits can destroy joint tissues, leading to chronic arthritis.

The plasma level of uric acid goes up from the normal rate of 2-5 mg% to 7 mg%, even upto 20 mg% in gout. There may be attacks of acute inflammation, accompanied by severe pains in joints like toe, knee and wrist joint. In majority of the cases, the onset of disease is insidious with pain, stiffness and symmetrical swelling of the small joints. Morning stiffness of joints is a common symptom. In about 10% of the patients, the attack of arthritis is sudden and acute with symptoms of fever, weight loss, profound fatigue and malaise. As the disease advances, pain, muscle-spasm and joint destruction result in the limitation of joint movement that could lead to deformities.

Rheumatoid arthritis is a systemic disease that could lead to eye problems (scleritis and keratitis), heart disease, pleurisy and nerve damage.

Diet Therapy

A purine-restricted diet will help reduce the excretion of uric acid by 200-400 mg per day and also lower the mean serum-uric acid level by 1mg/100ml. Dietary intervention must take into consideration three major factors, viz. energy, proteins and fluids.

1. Energy

It is necessary to control weight. Generally, obese patients suffer from acute symptoms of gout more severely. However, the weight loss exercise should be interrupted during the acute stage, since the catabolism of adipose tissue reduces uric acid excretion. In actual practice, a gradual weight loss on 1600 calories diet in males and about 1200 calories in females will suffice.

2. Proteins and Carbohydrates

Limit the proteins to 0.8-1.0 g/kg body weight. Meat should not exceed 3-4 oz per day. Ensure a high-carbohydrate and low-fat intake to enhance the excretion of urates. Fats should be limited to up to 60 g/day.

3. Fluids

To prevent urate precipitation in the kidneys, ensure a higher fluid intake (3 lit/day). Beverages like tea can be given in moderate doses. So also small amounts of alcohol up to 2 oz/day.

There should be liberal consumption of fruits and vegetables, which would help make the urine alkaline. Avoid large heavy meals late in the evening and maintain an alkaline urine to increase the solubility of uric acid in urine. In case of sodium retention, restrict the diet to 1000 mg sodium. Milk should be taken in large amounts.

Since the inflammatory process is initiated by the production of prostglandins (from arachidonic acid), an Omega-3 fatty acid diet decreases the severity of inflammation.

Table 23.1 gives a sample menu for gout.

TABLE 23.1: SAMPLE MENU FOR GOUT

8.00 AM	Cornflakes	1 cup
	Milk with sugar	1 cup
	Toast with honey	2 pcs
	Tea/coffee	1 cup
	Orange	1
12.00 Noon	Mixed vegetable salad	1 bowl
	Ridged gourd (turiya) or	
	Spinach cooked	1 cup
	Rice with dal	½ cup
	Buttermilk	½ cup
	Chapattis	3-4
	Banana/grapes	
	(*Chicken roast/ cold roast beef for non-veg.*)	
4.00 PM	Tea/coffee	1 cup
	Biscuits	2
7.00 PM	Tomato soup/potato and cabbage soup	1 cup
	Mashed potatoes with lady fingers	1 cup
	Mixed vegetables	1 bowl
	Chapattis	3-4
	Ice cream	
	(*Green pepper stuffed with minced meat for non-veg.*)	

Source: Dr. F. P. Antia.

DR. (Mrs.) USHA JAIN SUPPLEMENT

Avoid the following purine-rich foods:

Organ meats	Dried peas/beans	Fish/pork
Dried lentils	Meat extractives	Sweet breads
Mushrooms	Chocolates	Cauliflower
Alcohol	Spinach	Tea/coffee

Low-purine foods permitted:

Maize, tapioca	All Fruits	Wheat, rice
Milk	Cabbage, lettuce	Beet roots, brinjals
Butter, oil	Potatoes, pumkin	Cucumber
Cheese, cream	Sugar, sweets	Turnips
Tomatoes	Nuts	Carrots, lady fingers

In Naturopathy, Yoga and Magnet Therapy are found very useful if taken up in the early stages of arthritis.

Yogasanas are reported to increase the acetylcholine content of cerebral cortex, *i.e.* endogenous cortisones and this leads to a reduction in the severity of stimulation of the hypothalmus and sympathetic nerve endings, even though they are exposed to chronic stress.

Yoga

Yogasanas recommended for gout/rheumatoid arthritis are:

- Dhanurasana
- Chakrasana
- Trikonasana
- Shalabhasana
- Bhujangasana
- Supta Vajrasana

Magnet Therapy helps to prevent flare-ups of the disease, if undertaken regularly.

Acupressure on specific points goes a long way in effectively controlling Rheumatoid arthritis. Both the magnet Therapy and Acupressure are useful for Osteoarthritis patients.

To support and supplement the above, Dr. Jain recommends the following diet:

TABLE 23.2: DIET CHART FOR ARTHRITIS

7.00 AM	Crushed garlic with honey and green sun-charged water	1 clove
8.00 AM	Bitter gourd	1 large slice (to be chewed) or
	Bitter gourd juice	¾ cup with
	Amla Powder/juice	¼ cup
9.00 AM	Soaked figs	2 with
	Munakka with	
	Alfalfa and methi (fenugreek) and drink the soak water	1 tsp
	Seasonal fruit salad	1 bowl
	Mango shake	
12.00 Noon	Seasonal green vegetable salad	
	Amla chutney with honey	
	Fortified chapattis	4 (wheat bran 25%)
4.00 PM	Seasonal juicy fruits	
7.00 PM	Same as lunch	
9.00 PM	Soaked figs and amla powder	1 tsp

From Naturopathy, massage the joints with Red Oil, enema and steam bath, besides Acupressure are the additional support measures for treating Arthritis.

Avoid

- Salt
- Sugar
- Fried foods
- Flesh foods
- Tea
- Coffee
- Soft drinks
- Spices
- Maida
- Pickles

CHERIE CALBOM SUPPLEMENT

Dietary Modifications

1. **Try eliminating the Nightshade family**—tomatoes, peppers, potatoes, eggplant, and tobacco. If symptoms improve even slightly, continue to avoid these foods. Though not proven, there is a theory that a long-term low-level consumption of the solanum alkloids found in this family inhibits normal collagen repair in the joints or encourages inflammatory degeneration of the joints.

2. **Avoid the Citrus family**—lemons, limes, oranges, and grapefruits. This family, like the nightshade family, is thought to contribute to joints swelling.

3. **Avoid all Refined Foods** such as white flour, white sugar, and preserved and processed foods. Eat a nutritious diet that emphasizes whole grains, legumes (beans, split peas, and lentils), seeds, nuts, vegetables, and fruits, and includes only a small protion of low-fat animal products.

4. **Significantly decrease** your consumption of sweets and alcohol.

5. **Consider testing for Food Allergies.**

6. **Check** for hydrochloric acid deficiency. Seek medical advice in this regard.

7. **Try a Juce Fast,** which has been shown to be very helpful for arthritis.

Nutrients That Help

- **Niacinamide** may bring a noticeable improvement within two to six weeks. This nutrient is said to be especially beneficial for degenerative arthritis of the knee. (Warning! Niacinamide supplements may affect the liver or cause nausea.)
- **Pantothenic acid** may be helpful, as a deficiency of this nutrient has been associated with osteoarthritis.
- **Vitamin C** may be beneficial.
- **Vitamin E** may produce effects similar to those of nonsteroidal anti-inflammatory drugs.

- ☙ **Methionine** is important in cartilage structures.
- ☙ **Superoxide dismutase** may have therapeutic benefits.
- ☙ **Copper** may be helpful, as a deficiency of this nutrient has been associated with osteoarthirits.
- ☙ **Bioflavonoids** have been shown to be beneficial.
- ☙ **Bromelain** has anti-inflammatory properties.

Beneficial Juices

- ☙ Broccoli and kale—source of pantothenic acid.
- ☙ Kale, parsley, and spinach—source of vitamin C.
- ☙ Spinach and carrot—source of vitamin E.
- ☙ Carrot, ginger root, and apple—source of copper.
- ☙ Cherry and blueberry—source of bioflavonoids.
- ☙ Pineapple, the only source of bromelain.

Suggested Juicing Recipes for Arthritis

Garden Salad Special

3 broccoli flowerets
1 garlic clove
4-5 carrots or 2 tomatoes
2 stalks celery
½ green pepper

Push broccoli and garlic through hopper with carrots or tomatoes. Follow with celery and green pepper

Digestive Special

Handful spinach
4-5 carrots, greens removed

Bunch up spinach and push through hopper with carrots

Bromelain Special

¼ pineapple, with skin

Push pineapple through hopper.

Ginger Hopper

¼-inch slice ginger root
4-5 carrots, greens removed
apple, seeded

Push ginger through hopper with carrots and apple.

> ### *Gingerberry Fizz*
>
> 1 quart blueberries
> 1 medium bunch grapes
> ¼-inch slice ginger root
> Sparkling water
>
> Push blueberries through hopper, followed by grapes and ginger. Pour juice into ice-filled glass. Fill glass to top with sparkling water.

CHERIE CALBOM ON RHEUMATOID ARTHRITIS

Rheumatoid arthritis is a systemic disease characterized by inflammatory changes in joints and related structures. Its symptoms include fatigue, low-grade fever, weakness, and joint stiffiness and plain. There is often severe joint pain, with increased inflammation beginning in small joints and progressively affecting all joints in the body. Evidence exists that rheumatoid arthritis is an autoimmune reaction in which antibodies develop against components of joint tissues.

Dietary Modifications

1. **Consume a low-fat, low-calorie diet** excluding most animal sources (meat, dairy products, and so forth). Studies have shown that patients following this type of diet experienced remission of joint symptoms. A vegetarian diet, excluding all animal sources but fish, has been found to be very beneficial.

2. **Increase your consumption** of cold-water fish, e.g., mackerel, salmon, tuna, and sardines. Cod-liver oil may also be beneficial.

3. **Excluded refined sugar,** refined wheat flour, corn flour, salt, strong spices, alcohol, tea, and coffee from your diet.

4. **Identify Food Allergies.**

5. **Check** for low stomach acid (hydrochloric acid).

6. **One folk remedy** calls for drinking Basil as a tea. Basil has been used to ease rheumatoid pain.

7. **Try a Juice Fast,** which has been shown to help arthritis.

Nutrients that help

- **Vitamin C** has anti-inflammatory action.

- **Vitamin E** has anti-inflammatory action.

- **Vitamin K** may stabilize the membranes and cells of rheumatoid tissue.

- **Pantothenic acid** may be helpful, as deficiencies of this nutrient have been found to be directly related to the symptoms.

- ❧ **Copper** has anti-inflammatory action.
- ❧ **Iron** may be helpful, as an iron deficiency may be involved. (Supplementation is controversial. Food is the best source).
- ❧ **Manganese** may have therapeutic benefits.
- ❧ **Selenium** may be helpful, as a deficiency may be involved.
- ❧ **Sulfur** may be helpful, as a deficiency may be involved.
- ❧ **Zinc** may be helpful, as a deficiency may be involved.
- ❧ **Omega-3 fatty acids** have therapeutic benefits.
- ❧ **Superoxide dismutase** has anti-inflammatory properties.

Suggested Juicing Recipes for Rheumatoid Arthritis

Popeye's Favorite

Small handful spinach 4-5 carrots, greens removed ½ apple, seeded	Bunch up spinach and push through hopper with carrots and apple

Potassium Broth

Handful parsley Handful spinach 4-5 carrots, greens removed 2 stalks celery	Bunch up parsley and spinach leaves, and push through hopper with carrots and celery

Bromelain Special

¼ pineapple, with skin	Push pineapple through hopper

Garden Salad Special

3 broccoli flowerets 1 garlic clove 4-5 carrots or 2 tomatoes 2 stalks celery ½ green pepper	Push broccoli and garlic through hopper with carrots or tomatoes. Follow with celery and green pepper

Ginger Hopper

¼-inch slice ginger root 4-5 carrots, greens removed ½ apple, seeded	Push ginger through hopper with carrots and apple

Maureen's Spicy Tonic

¼ pineapple, with skin
½ apple, seeded
¼-inch slice ginger root

Push pineapple through hopper with apple and ginger.

Gingerberry Fizz

1 quart blueberries
1 medium bunch grapes
¼-inch slice ginger root
Sparkling water

Push blueberries through hopper, followed by grapes and ginger. Pour juice into ice-filled glass. Fill glass to top with sparkling water.

Cherie's Cleansing Cocktail

¼-inch slice ginger root
1 beet
½ apple, seeded
4 carrots, greens removed

Push ginger, beet, apple through hopper with carrots

Suggested Juicing Recipes for Gout

Cherry Cocktail

4 handfuls cherries, pitted
½ cup strawberries

Push cherries and strawberries through hopper

Green Surprise

1 large kale leaf
2-3 green apples, seeded
Lime twist for garnish

Bunch up kale leaf and push through hopper with apples. Garnish with lime twist. The surprise is that you won't taste the kale!

Wheatgrass Express

Handful wheatgrass
2 mint sprigs
3-inch slice pineapple, with skin

Bunch up wheatgrass and mint, and push through hopper with pineapple.

Waldorf Salad

1 green apple, seeded
1 stalk celery

Push apple and celery through hopper

Berry Cantaloupe Shake

½ cantaloupe, with skin
5-6 strawberries

Push cantaloupe and strawberries through hopper

Strawberry Apple Delight

1-2 apples, seeded
6 strawberries

Push apple and strawberries through hopper. Garnish with strawberry.

Chlorophyll Cocktail

3 beet tops
Handful parsley
Handful spinach
4 carrots, greens removed
½ apple, seeded

Bunch up beet tops. parsley, and spinach, and push through hopper with carrots and apple

---

TUBERCULOSIS

Tuberculosis is an infectious disease caused by the tubercle bacillus: *Mycobacteriun tuberculosis*, which invades the lungs. Many times, other organs like bones kidneys, larynx and lymph nodes are also affected. Over 10 million people in the USA are infected with TB.

Pulmonary or Lung TB is accompanied by cough, spitting of phlegm, fever, anorexia, exhaustion and wasting of tissues. It can lead to fatal pneumonia, else wasting of bones that produce deformities. Tubercular Meningitis, which affects brain, can be a fatal disease.

In the acute stages, the fever may be high, but in chronic TB, the temperature may be only slightly higher than the normal. If there is a persistent loss of weight, cough, rise in body temperature in the evening and spitting of blood, it poses grave danger.

Diet Therapy

Liberal intake of proteins (1.2-1.5 g/kg) is recommended to restore plasma proteins and promote wound healing. And it has to be a high calorie diet about 1.5 times the RDA, *i.e.* 3000-3500 kcal.

The diet must also supply adequate minerals, especially calcium, needed to help in the calcification of the lesions. Iron, plus other hematopoietic nutrients have to be liberally provided in case of bleeding. When Isoniazid is being administered, increase the supply of vitamin B_6 and folic acid.

One of the simple and effective drink is fresh Neera (from palm trees) to be taken before sunrise everyday. It is indeed very beneficial for TB patients and also enables them to gain weight.

Mrs. S A Joshi has recommended the following sample menu for TB:

TABLE 23.3: SAMPLE MENU FOR TB

7.00 AM	Tea	1 cup
9.00 AM	Egg-nog	1
	Banana	1 medium
11.00 AM	Cheese sandwich	1
	Sweet lime juice	or
	Orange juice	1 glass
1.00 PM	Chapatti	4
	Rice	1 cup
	Dal	1 cup
	Mung Usa l	½ cup
	Parwal-Cabbage curry	½ cup
	Curds	
4.00 PM	Tea	1 cup
	Egg sandwich	1
6.00 PM	Milk shake	1 glass
7.00 PM	Cream of tomato	
	Soup	1 bowl
	Green salad	
	Vegetable pulao	1 cup
	Chapattis	2
	Spinach-paneer	1 cup
	Potato-Bengal	
	Gram curry	½ cup
	Curds	1 cup

Source: Joshi S. A. *Nutrition and Dietetics.* Tata McGraw Hill, 1992.

DR. (Mrs.) USHA JAIN SUPPLEMENT

Dr. Usha Jain has recommended the following for TB both Lung and Bone

TB, Lung TB and Bone TB

1. Maximum exposure to the ultraviolet rays of sun.
2. Green sun-charged water to be taken.
3. Diet, more than the RDA for proteins, carbohydrates, vitamins and minerals.
4. Freshly drawn Goat's milk to be used.
5. Garlic is very good for its antibacterial action.
6. Raw Turmeric and sunflower petals chopped finely and mixed with Honey-These must be sun-charged for 40 days. This helps internal healing.
7. Green Amla grated with Honey to be sun-charged.

Avoid the following food:

- Spices
- Oils
- Fried foods
- Refined flour

Also avoid the Mucus-forming foods like:

- Sweet potato
- Rice
- Rajmash
- Urad
- Bhindi
- Banana
- Arbi

The diet menu given in Table 23.4 must be followed scrupulously.

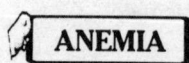 **ANEMIA**

The most widespread 'Deficiency disease', anemia is characterised by reduction in the size or number of red blood cells, the amount of hemoglobin or both, which eventually results in the decreased oxygen-carrying capacity of the blood. Even in USA, 10% of all the women in prenatal clinics suffer from anemia. Their hemoglobin concentration is less than 10 g/dL and a hematocrit count below 32%.

The technical definition of anemia has been set on hemoglobin level of less than 12 mg% in women (versus 14 mg% normal), and less than 14 mg% in men (vs 16 mg% normal).

TABLE 23.4: DIET CHART FOR TUBERCULOSIS

7.00 AM	Sun-charged Water	1 glass
	Garlic chutney with Amla juice and honey	
8.00 AM	Fresh vegetable juice	1 glass
	(*Beets, carrots, fresh amla and honey*)	
9.00 AM	Soaked Figs	2
	(*Very good for constipation*)	
	Raisins	10
	Almonds	5
	Drink the soak water	
	Goat's Milk—unheated or Cow's Milk (whole)	1 glass
	Seasonal fruits—Papaya, chikoo, apple, pear, black grapes, etc.	
11.00 AM	Fruit/Vegetable juice	1 glass
12.00 Noon	Seasonal vegetable soup	1 glass
	Green salad	
	Curd raita (if no cough)	
	Green Amla chutney	
	Fortified Chapattis	3-4
4.00 PM	Goat's Milk	1 glass
	Seasonal fruits	
	Soaked raisins	10 very rich in Fe and Ca
7.00 PM	Vegetable dalia	1 cup
	Seasonal vegetable soup	1 cup
	Green amla chutney with raw turmeric, ginger, coriander, mint and garlic	
9.00 PM	Milk with Dates	1 glass
	Amla + Turmeric juice	1 tsp each
	with honey + almond oil	½ tsp

N.B. Pomegranate and Amla juice with honey is recommended for healing of wounds and bleeding etc.

Such Diet should continue for at least 3 months;

Initial recovery in 3 months;

Full recovery in about 6 months.

Anemias may be classified as under:

1. Cell size

   - Macrocytic Anemia (Large Cells)
   - Microcytic Anemia (Small Cells)

2. Color Index of Blood

   - Hyperchromatic Anemia (High colored)
   - Hypochromatic Anemia (Low colored)

Anemias may be

- Non-nutritional Anemia, as in chronic diseases and sports
- Nutritional Anemia, due to deficiency in nutrients necessary in the formation of blood, e.g. iron, proteins, folic acid, vitamin B_{12} and vitamin C. Though needed in very small amount, copper and cobalt are also essential for blood formation.

There are three main causes of Anemia

1. Loss of blood from circulation, *i.e.* external or internal haemorrhage
2. Haemolysis, *i.e.* increased destruction of RBCs (erythrocytes)
3. Reduced production of erythrocytes and hemoglbin, *i.e.* Dyshaemopoiesis.

For the production of RBCs, a variety of nutrients are needed the most important being Fe, folic acid and Vitamin B_{12}. But others are also needed, e.g. proteins, pyridoxine, ascorbic acid, copper and possibly vitamin E.

Other causes of Anemia are infections, uremia, hepatic cirrhosis, malignant diseases and genetic defects.

TABLE 23.5: HEMOGLOBIN THRESHOLD LEVEL AND ANEMIAS

	Age	WHO 1972 (Hb g/dL)
Children	6 months-6 yrs	11
	6 yrs-14 yrs	12
Adults		
Men		13
Women		12
Pregnant women		11

Table 23.6 gives the normal range of finding in women deficient in Fe and folates.

In Tables 23.7 and 23.8 are given two diverse diet charts for Anemias from two different authorities.

TABLE 23.6: IRON AND FOLATE DEFICIENCY

	Normal range in women	Deficiency Iron	Folates
Basic measurement Hb g/dL	12-16	7	7
Packed cell volume—PCV %	36-47	28	22
Red Blood Cells—106 mm^3	3.9-4.6	3.7	2.0
Mean Corpuscular Volume (MCV)—µm	75-95	78	110

Source: Stanley Davidson *et al. Human Nutrition and Dietetics.*

TABLE 23.7: DIET CHART FOR ANEMIAS

8.00 AM	Stewed prunes	10
	Porridge with milk sugar/honey	1 cup
	Toast with butter	2
	Tea/coffee	1 cup
	Orange	1
	(*Scrambled egg for non-veg.*)	
12.00 Noon	Cooked cheese with lettuce salad	1 cup
	Cooked brinjals	1 cup
	Rice with dal	1 cup
	Chapattis	3-4
	Buttermilk	1 cup
	Banana/pear	
	(*Grilled live/lamb chop with tomatoes/potato chips*)	
4.00 PM	Tea/coffee	1 cup
	Raisin cake	
7.00 PM	Tomato soup/leak and potato soup	1 cup
	Curd	1 cup or
	Soya protein muggets cooked	
	Cooked carrots and potatoes	1 cup or
	French beans kebab	
	Dal and chapattis	3-4
	Pudding	
	(*Meat soup, fried fish or roast chicken or beef stick with boiled potato and green peas*)	

Source: Dr. F. P. Antia.

DR (Mrs.) USHA JAIN

TABLE 23.8: DIET CHART FOR ANEMIA

7.00 AM	Decoction of Curry leaves	1 glass with
	Lemon and honey	1 tsp
8.00 AM	Beet juice	½ cup with
	Carrot juice	½ cup with
	Green Amla juice	¼ cup with
	Honey	1 tsp
9.00 AM	Soaked Figs	2
	Munakkas (Dried Currants)	10
	Almonds	5
	Seasonal fruit salad	
	Sprouts of wheat	1 tbsp with
	Grated Coconut	2 tbsp
11.00 AM	Milk with Dates (3-4)	1 cup
	Spinach + tomatoes + carrot juice	1 cup
12.00 Noon	Seasonal green veg. salad	125 g
	Sprouts of moong + alfalfa	1 tbsp
	Vegetable Chapattis (fort.)	3-4
	Raita of green mint and coriander, etc	
	Amla chutney	
4.00 PM	Mango or seasonal fruit salad	
7.00 PM	Seasonal vegetable soup	1 cup
	Vegetable dalia	2 tbsp with
	Moong sprouts	2 tbsp
	Green cooked vegetable	250 g
	Raita and chutney	
	Eat the above with raita and chutney and salad	
9.00 AM	Soaked Almonds	5
	Milk	1 cup
	Dates	3-4

Table 23.9 gives Cherie Calbom's juice therapy for anemia.

TABLE 23.9: JUICING RECIPES FOR ANEMIA

Folic Acid Special

3 kale leaves
Small handful parsley
Small handful spinach
4-5 carrots, greens removed

Bunch up kale, parsley, and spinach, and push through hopper with carrots

Iron-Rich Drink

3 beet tops
4-5 carrots, greens removed
½ green pepper
½ apple, seeded

Bunch up beet tops, and push through hopper with carrots, followed by green pepper and apple

Spring Tonic

Handful parsley
4 carrots, greens removed
1 garlic clove
2 stalks celery

Bunch up parsley and push through hopper with carrots, garlic, and celery

Popeye's Favorite

Small handful spinach
4-5 carrots, greens removed
½ apple, seeded

Bunch up spinach and push through hopper with carrots and apple

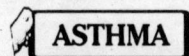 ASTHMA

Asthma, an allergic disorder, means difficulty in breathing or gasping for breath. Over one percent of the world population suffers from this disabling disease. The substances that produce allergy are:

Pollen of flowers
Household dust
Foods like eggs, fish or wheat.

Spores of fungi
Nickle and chromium

The substances that cause reaction in an allergy-prone individual is called 'Allergen' or antigen. The human body reacts to these antigens by producing antibodies. When the offending allergen and antibodies react, histamine and serotonin are released into the blood stream, which give rise to various manifestations of allergy, like spasm of muscles, exudation of fluid from the nasal mucosa in case of sneezing and swelling and redness of skin in urticaria.

Asthma may be Intrinsic asthma seen in patients who have no history of allergy. Or it may be Extrinsic asthma or Allergic asthma that occurs with exposure to an allergen. Occasionally, it may be Drug-induced asthma.

The commonly occuring asthma is the Bronchial asthma. The other type is the Cardiac asthma, due to heart failure.

The factors that pre-dispose a man to asthma are:

1. Heredity
2. Infection
3. Psychological factors
4. Climate
5. Occupational hazards
6. Drugs

Diet Therapy

Proper diet should be taken regularly at the scheduled hour in order to prevent the attack or minimise its severity. Food, especially dinner should be light, since heavy diet predisposes one to asthma attacks. Spicy foods, pickles, fried foods and milk products should be avoided at dinner time. Seasonal fruits and vegetables should be taken in plenty.

Asthmatics should drink lot of water between the meals, but not during the meals that would cause dilution of the gastric juices and cause heaviness of stomach. Alcohol and tobacco must be altogether avoided.

Table 23.10 gives the sample menu for asthma.

TABLE 23.10: DIET CHART FOR ASTHMA

7.00AM	Warm water	1 glass
	Light tea	1 cup
9.00 AM	Milk	1 cup
	Seasonal fruits	
	Toast/Khakhra	1
	(Half-boiled/scrambled egg for non-veg.)	
12.00 Noon	Green vegetable salad	1 bowl
	Cooked vegetables	1 cup
	Dal	1 cup
	Chapattis	3-4
	Curd/butter milk	1 cup
	(Meat/chicken for non-Veg.)	
4.00 PM	Tea	1 cup
	Biscuits/Khakhra	
6.00 PM	Seasonal fruits/fruit juice	1 glass
8.00 PM	Dinner as lunch	

Source: Dr. D. L. Gala: *Incurable Disease Don't Despair.* Gala Pub. Bombay.

DR. (Mrs) USHA JAIN SUPPLEMENT

In Naturopathy, Yogasanas and Pranayamas are quite helpful. Special mention be made of Neti Kriya (nasal cleaning), done with salt water, diluted milk or diluted honey. The result of this Neti Kriya have been very encouraging.

Both acupressure and magnet therapy help stave off fresh attack of Asthma. Dr. Usha Jain's recommendations on diet have been shown in Table 23.11

TABLE 23.11: SPECIAL DIET CHART FOR ASTHMA.

7.00 AM	Fresh Garlic chutney with Amla and honey	1 tsp	
	Sun-charged green Water	1 glass	
8.00AM	White Onion	½ cup	
	Lemon juice	¼ cup	Half of this special drink.
	Ginger juice	1 tsp	morning and evening
	Plus honey	1 tbsp	
9.00 AM	Soaked Figs	2	
	Munakkas (Dried Currants)	10	
	Almonds	5	
	Sprouts of moong	1 cup	
	Apple		
	Seasonal vegetable soup	1 cup	
1.00 PM	Seasonal vegetable salad	125 g	
	Vegetable chapattis	3-4	
	Green Amla chutney		
4.00 PM	Vegetable or sweet lime juice with honey	¾ cup with	
	Boiled water	¼ cup	
7.00 PM	Vegetable soup	1 cup	
	Vegetable dalia	2 tbsp	
	Moong Sprouts	2 tsp	
	Steamed seasonal vegetables	250 g	
	Amla chutney		
9.00 PM	Special drink (cf. 8 AM) with amla powder	1 tsp with	
	Turmeric	½ tsp with	
	Honey		

CHERIE CALBOM SUPPLEMENT

Cherie Calbom's recommendations for asthma are given below:

Suggested Juicing Recipes for Asthma

Digestive Special

Handful spinach
4-5 carrots, greens removed

Bunch up spinach and push through hopper with carrots

Energy Shake

Handful parsley
4-6 carrots, greens removed
Parsley sprig for garnish

Bunch up parsley and push through hopper with carrots Garnish with sprig of parsley

Magnesium Drink

1 garlic clove
Small handful parsley
4-5 carrots, greens removed
2 stalks celery
Parsley sprig for garnish

Wrap garlic in parsley, and push through hopper with carrots and celery. Pour juice into glass, and garnish with sprig of parsley

Vegetable Cocktail

1 garlic clove or small piece
  of onion
3 broccoli floweretes
2 kale leaves
5 carrots, greens removed
Dash cayenne pepper
Seasoning(s) of choice

Roll garlic (or onion) and broccoli in kale leaves, and push through hopper with carrots. Add pepper. Season to taste

SEX DISORDERS

One of the most disconcerting problem the modern man faces is the sex disorders. And this set of 'Disabling Diseases' do not readily respond to the conventional treatment. Indeed, in most of the Asian countries, sex problem quackery is a multi-billion business.

In the males, the major problem is sexual weakness or Impotency, while the females suffer from Leucorrhoea and Menorrhagia. Here is what Dr. Usha Jain has to say about the extraordinary efficacy of Diet therapy in curing sexual disabilities in the women.

1. Freshly crushed raw garlic with half a spoon of olive or soyabean oil be taken at bedtime.
2. Fresh coconut water and juice of radish and its tender leaves or fenugreek (Methi) leaves are very beneficial.
3. Yogurt and buttermilk of cow or goat's milk will reinstate a normal and favourable microbial balance in the body.
4. Yarrow herbal tea helps the entire reproductive system.

Other steps that Dr. Usha Jain recommends are:

1. Take enema 3-4 times a week to improve elimination.
2. Apply wet bandages on the abdomen 2-3 times a day. Wrap tightly a woollen bandage overlapping it and fasten it with a string. Go about your work for 30-45 minutes. Then open the bandage and rub that part of the body.

Yoga

Sex apparatus can be strengthened by practising Sarvangasan (whole body pose), Bhujangasana (serpent pose) and Dhanur-asana (bow pose). The following Yoga mudras help impart vigor to ovaries, uterus and the pelvic region:

1. Sitting with back straight and upright and exhaling completely.
2. Sitting straight-backed, place lefty heel on urethra and right one on pubis. Inhale gradually and simultaneously contract the sex nerve. After 5 seconds, relax with slow exhalation. Repeat 10 times, changing the position of heels.
3. Another version of Pranayama helps tone up the ovaries. Sit straight-backed and exhale completely. Now strain the navel backward and then inhale relaxing the tense region. Repeat it for 2-3 minutes.

Tables 23.12 and 23.13 give the diet charts for Menorrhagia (profuse bleeding) and Leucorrhoea in women.

DR. (Mrs.) USHA JAIN

TABLE 23.12: DIET CHART FOR MENORRHAGIA

7.00 AM	Soak 'Multani Mitti' (special mud) in a mud pot.	
	Decant the water and drink this soak water	
8.00 AM	Honey squash	½ cup
	Green Amla juice	1 tsp with
	Mishri (candy)	1 tbsp with
	Roasted 'Jeera' (spices) powder	1 tsp
9.00 AM	Pomegranate or Pineapple juice or beetroot and carrot juice	1 glass
	Boil 'Ashoka' tree bark in milk—1 cup and water—1 cup, till half the quantity is left. Take it with candy, dalia or carrot 'Kheer'	1 cup
11.00 AM	Pomegranate juice with lemon and honey	
12.00 Noon	Seasonal salad and sprouts	1 bowl
	Fortified Chapattis	3-4
	Amla chutney with grated green coconut and curry leaves	
	Apple	
4.00 PM	Milk with Ashoka bark water with seasonal fruits	
7.00 PM	Vegetable soup (tomatoes)	1 glass
	Green vegetable salad	1 bowl
	Dalia	1 cup
	Cuird raita	
	Amla chutney	
9.00 PM	Soak 1 tsp Amla powder in ½ cup of fresh Amla juice and candy	

TABLE 23.13: DR. (Mrs.) USHA JAIN'S DIET CHART FOR LEUCORRHOEA

7.00 AM	Sun-charged green water	1 glass
	Overnight soaked Bengal grams	1 tbsp
	Raisins	10 and
	Amla powder	½ cup
8.00 AM	Beetroot and carrot and Amaranth juice	1 glass with
	Fresh green Amla (if available) with honey	1 tbsp
9.00 AM	Soaked figs	2
	Raisin	10
	Prunes	10
	Almonds	5 alongwith soak water
	Ripe banana	
	Goat's milk unboiled	1 glass or
	Cow's milk with honey and Amla powder	
	Seasonal fruit	
12.00 Noon	Green salad	1 bowl
	Sprouts—Bengal gram, Alfalfa	½ cup
	Fortified chapattis	3-4
	Steam-cooked seasonal vegetables	1 cup
	Curd	
	Raita	
	Chutney	
4.00 PM	Seasonal fresh fruits	
	Milk with honey/dates	1 glass
7.00 PM	Seasonal green salad	1 bowl
	Vegetable juice	1 glass
	Dalia and sprouts	½ cup
	Steamed vegetables	250 g
	Eat with salad or chutney	
9.00 PM	Amaranth juice	1 glass with
	Amla powder and honey	1 tsp

N.B.

1. Amla powder 1 tsp with liquorice 1 tsp to be taken twice a day.
2. Acacia beans-air-dried in shade 1 tsp powder with honey at bed-time.
3. Wash the body parts with neem water or green water or alum powder.
4. Douche with neem water or *Acacia* leaves water.

TABLE 23.14: DR. (Mrs.) USHA JAIN'S DIET CHART FOR MALE IMPOTENCY

7.00 AM	Drumstick leaves	1 cup
	Drumstick soup with honey and amla powder	
8.00 AM	Aerial roots of Banyan tree—air-dried in shade—1 tsp of this powder with milk and honey	1 tbsp
	with Ashwagandha powder	1 tsp
9.00 AM	Milk with dates	1 glass
	Soaked figs	2
	Prunes	10
	Almonds	5
	Seasonal fruit salad	
11.00 AM	Seasonal vegetable juice	1 glass
12.00 Noon	Green vegetable soup	1 cup
	Fresh vegetable salad	1 bowl
	Fortified chappatis	3-4
	Curd	
	Amla chutney	
4.00 PM	Fresh fruit juice/coconut water	1 glass
7.00 PM	Green vegetable salad	1 bowl
	Vegetable soup	1 cup
	Fortified chapattis	3-4
	Dalia	1 cup
	Curd	1 cup
	Amla chutney	
9.00 PM	Chavanparash	1 tsp with
	Ashwagandha powder	1 tsp
	Milk	1 glass

CHERIE CALBOM SUPPLEMENT FOR SEX DISORDERS

Suggested Juicing Recipes for Menopausal Symptoms

Sweet Calcium Shake

1 pint strawberries
6 oz. silken tofu

Juice strawberries, place juice and fofu in blender or food processor, and blend until smooth. Garnish with strawberry

Super-Eight Stress Reliever

1 kale leaf
1 collard leaf
Small handful parsley
1 stalk celery
1 carrot, greens removed
½ red pepper
1 tomato
1 broccoli floweret
Celery stalk for garnish

Bunch up leaves and parsley, and push through hopper with celery and carrot. Follow with red pepper, tomato, and broccoli. Garnish with celery stalk.

Sweet Magnesium Smoothie

1 pint blackberries
1 ripe banana
2 oz. silken tofu
1 Tbsp Brewer's yeast

Juice berries. Place juice, banana, tofu, and yeast in blender or food processor, and blend until smooth. Garnish with blackberries. Drink 1 hour before bedtime

Popye's Garden Tonic

Handful spinach
3 stalks celery
2 stalks asparagus
1 large tomato
1 cherry tomato for garnish

Bunch up spinach and push through hopper with celery. Juice asparagus and tomato. Mix juices in a tall glass and garnish with cherry tomato

Calcium-Rich Cocktail

3 kale leaves
Small handful parsley
4-5 carrots, greens removed
½ apple, seeded

Bunch up kale and parsley, and push through hopper with carrots and apple

Spiced Orange Foam

¼-inch slice ginger root
2 large oranges, peeled (leave white pithy part)
½ apple. seeded
Orange twist for garnish

Push ginger through hopper with orange and apple. Serve with twist of orange.

Garden Tonic

¼ head cabbage
2 stalks celery
1 stalk broccoli
Parsley sprig for garnish

Juice vegetables and garnish with sprig of parsley

Orange Spice Tea

½-inch ginger root
1 orange, peeled (leave white pithy part)
Water
Cinnamon stick for garnish

Push ginger and ornage through hopper. Pour 2 oz. of juice into teacup and fill with boiling water. Garnish with cinnamon stick.

CHERIE CALBOM SUPPLEMENT FOR MENSTRUAL PROBLEMS

Long, heavy peroids are a problem for many women, causing a loss of many important minerals. Fortunately, this disorder responds well to nutritional intervention. The dietary suggestions that follow can help to lessen menstrual bleeding and to alleviate menstrual pain.

Suggested Juicing Recipes for Menstrual Problems

Mineral Tonic

Handful parsley
2 turnip leaves
1 kale leaf
4-5 carrots, greens removed

Roll up parsley in turnip and kale leaves, and push through hopper with carrots

Sweet Magnesium Smoothie

1 pint blackberries
1 ripe banana
2 oz. silken tofu
1 Tbsp. Brewer's yeast

Juice berries. Place juice, banana, tofu, and yeast in blender of food processor, and blend until smooth. Garnish with blackberries. Drink 1 hour before bedtime.

Maureen's Spicy Tonic

¼ pineapple, with skin
½ apple, seeded
¼-inch slice ginger root

Push pineapple through hopper with apple and ginger

Sweet and Sour Red Pop

½ lemon
1 pint cherries, pitted
Sparkling water

Juice lemon. Pour juice into ice cube tray, add water, and freeze, Juice cherries. Pour juice into tall glass, add lemon-juice cubes, and fill to top with sparkling water

Garden Tonic

¼ head cabbage
2 stalks celery
1 stalk broccoli
Parsley sprig for garnish

Juice vegetables and garnish with sprig of parsley

K-Cooler

1 turnip green
1 stalk broccoli
1 red apple. seeded
Parsley sprig for garnish

Juice vegetables and apple. Pour juice into ice-filled glass, and garnish with parsley

Magnesium Drink

1 garlic clove
Small handful parsley
4-5 carrots, greens removed
2 stalks celery
Parsley sprigh for garnish

Wrap garlic in parsley, and push through hopper with carrots and celery. Pour juice into glass, and garnish with sprig of parsley

PART 4

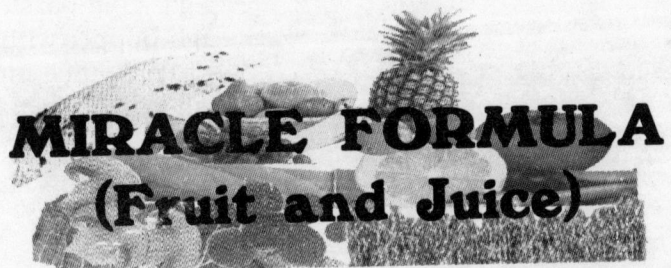

MIRACLE FORMULA
(Fruit and Juice)

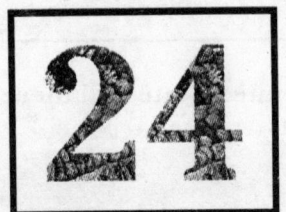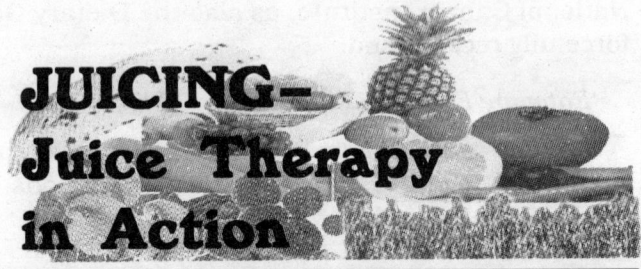

JUICING –
Juice Therapy
in Action

The juice of fresh fruits and vegetables is the richest available source of vitamins, minerals and enzymes, besides some half-known 'Anutrients'. And it is a natural concoction that is digested and assimilated within a span of 20-30 minutes, thus proving to be an instant 'Energy Booster'.

Fruits differ from other foods in that their nutritive elements exist in the soluble forms of organic sugars, dextrin and fruit acids, which are found almost exclusively in their juices. An eminent authority, Dr. Joy Kurdich (nicknamed the 'Juiceman') has rightly pontificated:

'All Life on Earth emanates from the Green of the Plant.'

Technically speaking, this 'Green' (Chlororphyll) is the most concentrated 'Sun-power'. From the medical angle, chlororphyll boosts the function of heart, effects circulatory system, intestines, uterus and lungs. In practice, chlorophyll, which forms the rock-foundation of Bio-Nutrition, is the greatest ever tonic that keeps the body and soul going in the top gear all the time.

As such, raw fruits and vegetables are the Nature's way of giving us life. A still more powerful endorsement comes from Dr. Bircher-Benner, the founder of the world-famous Bircher-Benner Clinic at Zurich in Switzerland, who had said:

'Nothing more therapeutic exists on the earth than Green Juice.'

That way, juice is a concentrated form of nutrients packaged in the best natural proportion to offer synergistic effect of all the nutrients working in concert to enhance man's health and spirits. In essence, this vitamin and mineral mixture may rightly be called the 'Green or Golden Cocktail' (cf. Poem: Green Gold in Chapter 1).

Already, the leading Health authorities in the USA, viz. Surgeon General (Report 1989), the Secretary of Health and Human Services (Health America 2000), the

National Cancer Institute, as also the Dietary Goals for United States-all these forcefully recommend:

> '*Eat more Fruits and Fresh Vegetables.*'

Somehow, this truism has been relegated by the market forces of globalisation and the bane of the 'Pizzas and Pleasure Foods.' And all this costs a fortune in medical bills.

PHYTOCHEMICALS (Anutrients)

By now, it has been well recognised that the orange-red vegetables offer a high level of carotenes, which have anti-cancer properties. Citrus fruit provides vitamin C and bioflavonoids—the immune-strengthening nutrients. And dark green leafy vegetables are rich in folic acid—a vitamin B Complex known for the proper maintenance of red blood cells and the nervous system. In fact, *Naturopathy and Bio-Nutrition offer an infinite range of sure-shot and efficacious juice remedies even for chronic maladies like Cancers*. This emphasis on fresh produce and 'Diet that is unrefined' is indeed become the dominant trend in contemporary nutrition and Clinical Dietetics. In reality, this raw juice healing goes back to the nineteenth century, when the juice making process involved the cumbersome squeezing of crushed vegetables through muslin cloth. So much for its inherent wisdom!

CURING CANCER

Apart from the pioneering work of Dr. Benner, credit must also be given to the eminent cancer specialist, Dr. Max Gerson, who has done very extensive research and successfully cured many terminally-ill cancer parties, all of which have been recorded in his book, A Cancer Therapy: Results of Fifty Cases (1958). He was fully convinced that cancer did not require any specific treatment. The main point is that the whole body must be detoxified with raw fruit and vegetables juices. The much acclaimed β-carotenes apart, new α-carotenes have been discovered which show protective effect against vulvar cancers. And then we have the phytochemicals like phenols, indoles, aromatic isothiocyanates, terpenes and organo-sulfur compounds-collect-ively called 'Anutrients', which have specific anti-cancer properties.

A very interesting custom is reported from Europe, *i.e. Grape Cure*. People go all the way and stay to recuperate in grape-growing areas. Once they are there, they eat nothing but grapes for days and days. Thus begins the process of elimination of the accumulated catarrh and other toxic materials from the body. And once this 'Cleansing' has been effected, new healthy tissue is regenerated in place of the old worn out body parts. Dr. Bernard Jensen, another great authority on cancers, has been specially cultivating grapes at his sanatorium to provide this million-dollar 'Technically congenial' ambience. He specifically reports the case of a nurse who came from the Salt Lake City with advanced breast cancer. Within 30 days of starting with this Grape Juice therapy, all the signs of cancer had disappeared. He specially recommends grapes with seeds. On the outer coat of the seeds, there is the special layer, *Cream of Tartar*, which is the greatest thing to cut the mucus and catarrh so that these can be rapidly eliminated from the body.

The alphabetically-arranged repertoire of Juicing (cf. Chapter 1) sums up the beauty and bounty of the Green Gold, Chlorophyll, the greatest benefactor of the Mankind.

As the famed Dietician: Dr. Cherrie Calbom says,

'Sickness or Health, the choice is yours'.

The physical condition you have tomorrow starts with what you do for your body today. And today is the time when you begin with the Miracle Formula called Juicing. Let us go back 2400 years to the prophetic words of Hippocrates, the Father of Medicine:

'Let living (natural) food be thy medicine.'

Into this repertoire of Green Gold, Dr. (Mrs) Usha Jain, the eminent 75-years old 'Practising Dietician of Delhi' has forcefully added the Miracle Juice, Ashgourd (Hindi-Petha, the vegetable normally used for making sweets). This has proved very efficacious in Cancer, TB, Liver disorders and Gout. To further enrich and fortify this Chlorophyll power, she advises sprouts, especially Alfalfa sprouts. For speeding up the regeneration process, she recommends soaked figs and munakka (dried currants), to be taken early morning. Even the 'Soak Water' (in which these were kept overnight) must be religiously consumed for added benefits. Another panacea in Dr. Jain's Naturopathy kit is Amla (Gooseberry) powder/juice to be taken regularly with honey, as also a clove of garlic.

Wheatgrass juice is another 'Wonder Remedy'. And there are umpteen such beneficial experiences reported both by the nutritionists and the 'Raw Foodists'. Juice Fasting is another effective formula, wherein very serious cases are put on an exclusive Juice diet for 5-7 days. The juice is to be taken every 2-3 hours, with no solids allowed. A report in the New York Times (2002) had shown as to how a 'Raw Foodist' is living happily on such a raw diet for 5 years. Though his calorie intake was only 800 kcal. otherwise deemed to be a starvation diet, this 40+ adult was doing wonderfully well.

It would be worthwhile recounting a few more outstanding success stories of the Bio-Nutrition, nay Fruit and Vegetable Juice Therapy.

1. **Dr. Bernard Jensen** (California, USA) was asked to treat a lady, who was dying of cancer of the breast. She could not speak or move her body and her toes were getting blue (cyanosed due to lack of blood). He gave her some Whex (Dried Goat Whey) dissolved in warm broth, one tablespoonful every hour. Whex is a natural formulation that is very high in sodium, potassium, phosphorus and calcium. For the previous 5 days, she had

even stopped eating—she just could not swallow anything. The whole night, the dedicated doctor sat with the patient, giving a tablespoonful every 60 minutes. Next morning, the lady had new energy and she was much better than before. She gradually improved on this liquid diet and in three months, she had recouped 20 pounds of her weight. When she went back to her own doctor, the latter could not believe this transformation and the total absence of any signs of cancer in his old patient. And after six months, she had fully recovered, having become active like any other normal person.

2. **Dr. Harry Hoxsey**, a herbalist of USA, first tried to cure cancer patients with Herbal Medicines and Fruit juices. He had this prescription from his father, who had successfully cured animals using only Herbal medicines. Dr Hoxsey was arrested and convicted on the charges of quackery. But his conviction was later on quashed when he proved before the judges that cancer of the skin, tongue, face and legs could be cured with herbs and fruit juice therapy. The judges were satisfied with his regime of treatment and released him with honour. His main treatment consisted of applying one piece of crushed garlic with a sticking plaster on the affected part and renewing the same every four hours. The cancerous growth of skin disappeared altogether within a short time. The doctor kept his patients solely on fruit and vegetable juice, without allowing any cereals during this period of treatment. His revolutionary theory ushered in a new hope for the suffering mankind.

He has recorded these miraculous healing powers in his widely-acclaimed book: *'You don't have to die!'*

3. **Dr. Eva Hill**, a Cancer specialist, would often rhapsodize:

'Eat your food the way God has made it,

i.e. in their raw state. Cancer is caused due to consumption of irrational, cooked foods or dead foods. Cancer is nothing but a vitamin deficiency disease.'

Dr Hill was herself suffering from cancer of the face. She completely cured herself by taking only the raw fruit and vegetables for some time.

4. **Dr. S. Firenczi**, a Hungarian Cancer specialist, found remarkable results in treating tumour patients with raw beet juice, administering one kg daily. Of the 16 patients he recorded in 1950s, 15 patients had recovered and gained weight ranging from 6 to 21 pounds and furthermore, their blood count had improved considerably.

5. **Dr. John B. Lust** of USA successfully cured colitis with lime, lemon, garlic, orange and carrot juice. He said, 'Fresh fruit juices are the cleanser of the human system and are regenerative and builders of the body.'

6. **Dr. Paul Bragg** had this to say of his field experiences: 'The continuous and persistent practice of getting the liquid life of fruits and vegetables into the system is one of the secrets of keeping young. They revitalize the bloodstream, giving a sparkle to the eyes, color to the lips and a spring to the steps.

As such, one realises the worth of Dr. Bernard Jensen's wisdom:

> *'Nature cures,*
> *When given the opportunity*!'

Yet another renowned authority, Prof. Bauer of the University of Heidelburg vindicates the inordinate emphasis on fruit and vegetables with the words: 'We are justified in concluding that the nutritive foods, whatsoever their nature, can protect us from cancers.'

DOCTORS NOT NEEDED

As such, diet more than the doctor is eventually the best friend of the man, the builder, the protector and the 'Real Restorer'. This brings us to the more assuring words of another pioneer in medicine, Dr Victor G. Rocine who had expounded the simple, but prophetic quote:

> *'If we eat wrongly,*
> *No doctor can cure us.*
> *If we eat rightly,*
> *No doctor is needed.'*

Dr Henry Lindlar sums up the essence of Bio-Nutrition in his memorable words:

> 'The greatest achievement of Nature Cure philosophy lies in the
> fact that it has reduced the treatment of acute and sub-acute
> diseases to the greatest simplicity...(Cure sans medicine).'

As such, the Fruit and Vegetable Juice Therapy is the *'Final Savior'* that is now catching up all over.

Bio-Nutrition redeems!

JUICE THERAPY IN ACTION

The Greek philosopher, Plato, who was a contemporary of Hippocrates, believed that the test of truly knowing what is right is 'To Act on What you Know!' We all can certainly put this gem of a philosophy to work right now with the inbuilt faith: 'Foods that Heal.'

Today, the value of Organic and Natural Foods is being positively affirmed by the most respected health authorities all over in USA. People are now waking up to the truism:

'We are what we eat'.

This is, in essence, the ultimate victory of this new Medical philosophy: Bionutrition.

In the second part of this concluding chapter, we are more than tempted to quote from the world-renowned Practising Nutritionist, Cherie Calbom's book: *'Juicing for Life'*. We are putting this practical wisdom and life-long experience of an octogenarian in an alphabetic order, those not covered earlier in this book, for the benefit of the interested readers. In the book, she has covered about 70 disorders and diseases and there are about 5-8 juice diet charts for each entry. We advise the readers to look up the book. In India, this book (351 pages, priced Rs.70 only) has been published by:

Health and Harmony
1921, St. No.10,Chuna Mandi,
Pahar Ganj, New Delhi-110055
Phone: 27770430, 27536418 Fax 011-7510471
E mail: bjain @ vsnl.com

Two more addresses which would be helpful are:

Dr.(Mrs) Usha Jain,
M-15, Lajpat Nagar-III,
New Delhi- 110024
Phone: 29845529.

Dr. Dhanlal Gala,
Gala Publishers,
70,Princess Street, Bombay or
Gomtipur, Ahmedabad (Guj).

CHERIE CALBOM SUPPLEMENT

CHERIE CALBOM'S JUICE DIETS

Malady	Ingredients	Preparation
1. Allergies		
Molybdenum Drink	A handful of spinach, garlic clove 1 carrots 4, small cauliflower buds 4	Bunch up spinach with garlic. Push thru' hopper with carrots and cauliflower
Cherie's Cleansing Cocktail	¼-inch slice ginger root, beet 1, ½ apple seeded, carrots 4	Push ginger, beet and apple thru' hopper with carrots
2. Backache		
Vegetable Express	Lettuce leaves 2, cabbage small piece, carrots 4, broccoli flowerets 3, ½ apple seeded	Bunch up lettuce leaves. Push thru' hopper with cabbage, carrots, broccoli and apple
Ginger Hopper	¼-inch slice ginger root, carrots 4, ½ apple, seeded	Push ginger thru' hopper with carrots and apple
3. Bronchitis		
Bromelain Special	¼ Pineapple, with skin	Push pineapple thru' hopper.
Ginger Tea	½ inch slice ginger root, ¼ lemon, water 1 pint, cinnamon 1 stick, cloves 4, dash of nutmeg/cardamom	Juice ginger and lemon. Put juice in saucepan, add water, cinnamon and cloves. Gently simmer. Add nutmeg/cardamom
4. Cataract		
Eye Therapy Express	Endive leaves 2, handful parsley, carrots 4, celery stalks 2	Bunch up endive and parsley. Push thru' hopper with carrots and celery.
Harvest Soup	Garlic cloves 2, kale leaf 1, tomato 1, celery stalks 2, collard leaf 1 chopped, 1 tbsp croutons	Roll garlic in kale leaf. Into hopper with tomato and celery. Put juice in saucepan, collards, heat and garnish
5. Cholesterolemia		
Anticholesterol Cocktail	Handful parsley and spinach, garlic clove 1, carrots 4, dash of Tabasco sauce	Bunch up parsley and spinach, push thru' hopper with garlic and carrots. Add sauce
Sprout Salad Express	Handful each of spinach and alfalfa sprouts, carrots 4, 1 apple, seeded	Push spinach and sprouts thru' hopper with carrots and apple
Monkey Shake	Orange peeled ½, papaya peeled ½, banana 1, orange twist for garnish	Push orange thru' hopper with papaya. Put juice and banana in blender until smooth. Garnish
6. Common Colds		
Gazpacho Express	Tomatoes 4, ½ cucumber, ¼ green pepper, garlic clove 1, celery stalks 2, Dash of Tab. Sauce	Push tomatoes, cucumber, green pepper and garlic thru' hopper with celery. Add Tab. Sauce

	Harvest Soup	Garlic cloves 2, kale leaf 1, tomato 1, celery stalks 2, collard leaf 1 chopped, 1 tbsp croutons	
	Ginger Tea	½ inch slice ginger root, ¼ lemon, water 1 pint, cinnamon 1 stick, cloves 4, dash of nutmeg/cardamom	
7.	**Constipation**		
	Evening Regulator	Apples 2, seeded, pear 1	Alternately pushing apple and pear slices thru' hopper.
	Tropical Squeeze	Papaya firm 1 peeled, pear 1 ½ inch slice ginger root	Juice papaya. Push ginger thru' hopper with carrots.
8.	**Depression**		
	Garden Salad Special	Kale leaves 2, handful each parsley and spinach, carrots 4, greens removed	Bunch up kale, parsley and spinach. Push thru' hopper with carrots
	Green Surprise	Kale leaf large 1, green apples 2 seeded, lime twist for garnish twist	Bunch up kale leaf. Push thru' hopper with apples. Garnish with lime
	Potassium Broth	Handful each of parsley and spinach, carrots 4, celery stalks 2	Bunch up parsley and spinach. Push thru' Hopper with carrots and celery
9.	**Diarhoea**		
	Cabage Cocktail	½ cabbage head, tomatoes 2	Push cabbage and tomatoes thru' hopper
	Spring Tonic	A handul parsley, carrots 4, garlic clove 1, celery stalks 2	Push parsley thru' hopper with carrots, garlic and celery
	Vegie Cocktail	A handful parsley, bet tops 3, celery stalks 2, carrots 4	Push parsley and beet tops thru' hopper with celery and carrots.
10.	**Eczema**		
	Cucumber Cooler	Tomato 1, cucumber 1, celery stalks 2, parsley sprig for garnish	Pour tomato juice into ice cube tray and freeze. Pour cucumber and celery juice into tall glass, add tomato cubes and garnish with parsley sprig
	Potassium Broth	Handful each of parsley and spinach, carrots 4, celery stalks 2	Bunch up parsley and spinach. Push thru' hopper with carrots and celery
	Garden Salad Special	Kale leaves 2, handful each parsley and spinach, carrots 4, greens removed	Bunch up kale, parsley and spinach. Push thru' hopper with carrots
11.	**Hair Loss**		
	Hair Growth Cocktail	Green lettuce leaves 2, handful alfalfa sprouts, carrots 4	Push lettuce and alfalfa thru' hopper with carrots
	Green Surprise	Kale leaf large 1, green apples 2 seeded, lime twist for garnish	Bunch up kale leaf. Push thru' hopper with apples. Garnish with lime twist
	Potassium Broth	Handful each of parsley and spinach, carrots 4, celery stalks 2	Bunch up parsley and spinach. Push thru' Hopper with carrots and celery

12. Hypoglycemia

Warm Apple Pie	Tarp aple 1, ater, apple pie sauce, cinnamon stick for garnish	Boib 2 oz. Apple juice and 4 oz. water in a pan. Season with spice. Garnish with cinnamon stick
Low-sugar Pop	Apple 1 seeded, ¼ lime, sparkling	Pour apple and lime juice into tall, ice-filled glass. Fill glass to top with sparkling water
Cucumber Cooler	Tomato 1, cucumber 1, celery Stalks 2, parsley sprig for garnish	Pour tomato juice into ice cube tray and freeze. Pour cucumber and celery juice into tall glass, add tomato cubes and garnish with parsley sprig.

13. Indigestion

Heartburn Quencher	¼ head cabbage, celery stalk 1, carrots 2	Juice vegetables. Drink 3 times a day
Tropical Squeez	irm papaya 1, ¼ inch slice ginger root, pear 1	Juice papaye. Push ginger thru' hopper with pear. Mix and drink
Gnger Fizz	¼ inch slice ginger root, apple 1 seeded, sparkling water	Push ginger thru' hopper with apple. Pour into ice-filled glass an fill the glass to top with sparkling water. Juice vegetables and garnish with a sprig of parsley
Garden Tonic	¼ heads cabbage, celery stalks 2, broccoli stalk 1, parsley sprig for garnish	

14. Insomnia

Traditional Sleep Potion	Lettuce leaves 4, celery stalk 1	Puh letuce thru' hopper with celery. Drink 30 minutes bhefore bed time
Popeye's Garden Tonic	A handful spinach, celery stalks 3, asparagus stalks 2, tomato large 1, cherry tomato for garnish	Push spinach thru' hopper with celery. Juice asparagus and tomato. Mix juice and garnish with cherry tomato.
Garden Salad Special	Kale leaves 2, handful each parsley and spinach, carrots 4, greens removed	Bunch up kale, parsley and spinach. Push thru' hopper with carrots.
Bromelain Special	¼ Pineapple, with skin	Push pineapple thru' hopper.
Sweet Magne-sium Smmothie	Blackberries 1 pint ripe banana 1, Silken tofu 2 oz, brewer's yeast 1 tbsp	Blend berries juice with banana, tofu Until smooth. Garnish with blackberry. Drink one hour before bed-time.

15. Memory Loss

Peach Nectar	Firm peaches 2. ½ lime, ripe , banana 1 Brewer's yeast 1 tbsp	Put lime and peach juice with yeast in a blender and blend until smooth
Brain Booster	Large tart apple 1 seeded, cashew nuts 1 cup	Blend apple juice with cashew nuts until smooth, chill until it thickens. Serve on whole with wheat crackers

16. Muscle Cramps

Summertime Punch	Large bunch green grapes, ½ lime, clery stalks 2, water	Juice grapes and celery. Mix juice with equal amount of water.
Magnesium Drink	Garlic clove 1, handful parsley, carrots 4, celery stalk 2, parsley sprig for	Push parsley thru' hopper with carrots and celery. Pour jice in glass and garnish with parsley sprig
Cucumber Cooler	Tomato 1, cucumber 1, celery stalks 2, parsley sprig for garnish	Pour tomato juice into ice cube tray and freeze. Pour cucumber and celery juice into tall glass, add tomato cubes and garnish with parsley sprig.

17. Osteoporosis

Red Crush	Red grapes—meduim bunch, cheries pitted ½ cup, blueberries ½ cup	Juice grapes, cheries and berries. Pour into a bowl over finely curshed ice
Cabbage Cocktail	½ Cabbage head, tomatoes 2	Push cabbage and tomatoes thru' hopper
Magnesium Drink	Garlic clove 1, handful parsley, carrots 4, celery stalk 2, parsley sprig for	Push parsley thru' hopper with carrots and celery. Pour jice in glass and garnish with parsley sprig.

18. Obesity

Warm Apple Pie	Tarp aple 1, ater, apple pie sauce, Cinnamon stick for garnish	Boib 2 oz. Apple juice and 4 oz. water in a pan. Season with spice. Garnish with cinnamon stick
Cumber Cooler	Tomato 1, cucumber 1, celery Stalks 2, parsley sprig for garnish	Pour tomato juice into ice cube tray and freeze. Pour cucumber and celery juice into tall glass, add tomato cubes and garnish with parsley sprig
Harvest Soup	Garlic cloves 2, kale leaf 1, tomato 1, celery stalks 2, collard leaf 1 chopped, 1 tbsp croutons	Roll garlic in kale leaf. Into hopper with tomato and celery. Put juice in saucepan, collards, heat and garnish
Low Sugar Pop	Apple 1 seeded, ¼ lime, sparkling	Pour apple and lime juice into tall, ice-filled glass. Fill glass to top with sparkling water

19. Prostate Enlargement

Strawberry Shake	Strawberry 1 pint, firm pear ½, ripe banana 1, Brewer's yeast 1 tbsp	Push strawberry and pear thru' hopper. Blend juice with banana and yeast until smooth
Ginger Ale	Lemon wedge 1, ¼ inch slice ginger root, green grapes mdium bunch 1, sparkling water	Juice lemon. Push ginger thru' hopper with grapes. Pour into tall ice-filled glass. Fill glass with sparling water

20. Soar Throat

Hot scotcher	½ lemon, Honey 1 tsp, hot water	Add honey to lemon juice. Mix with hot water. Sip slowly (not for kids)
Soothing Pops	Pineapple ringhs with skin 3, ¼ inch slice ginge root, firm pear 1	Push ginger thru' hoper with pear. Pour juice into cups and freeze

Instant Soup	Garlic cloves 3, spinach, ½ cucumber, celery stalk 1, finely chopped spinach and celery, parsley sprig for garnish	Push garlic and spinach thru' hopper with cucumber and celery. Put juice in pan, add chopped vegetables and heat gently. Garnish with parsley sprig. Serve while hot
Ginger Roger	Pineapple rings with skin 3, ¼ inch slice ginger root	Push pineapple slices and ginger thru' hopper

21. Stress

Super-8 Stress Reliever	Kale leaf 1, collard leaf 1, parsley, carrot 1, red pepper ½, tomato 1, broccoli floeret 1, celery stalk 1	Push leaves and parsley thru' hopper with celery and carrot. Follow with red pepper, tomato and broccoli. Garnish with celery stalk
Magnesium Drink	Garlic clove 1, handful parsley, carrots 4, celery stalk 2, parsley sprig for garnish	Push parsley thru' hopper with carrots and celery. Pour jice in glass and garnish with parsley Sprig
Garlic Express Express	A handful parsley, garlic clove 1, carrots 4, Celery stalks 2	Bunch up parsley. Push thru' hopper with garlic, carrots and celery
Potassium broth	Handful each of parsley and spinach, carrots 4, celery stalks 2	Bunch up parsley and spinach. Push thru' Hopper with carrots and celery

22. Thrombosis

Garden Salad Special	Kale leaves 2, handful each parsley and spinach, carrots 4, greens removed	Bunch up kale, parsley and spinach. Push thru' hopper with carrots.
Calcium-rich Cocktail	kale leaves 3, handful parsley, carrots 4, ½, apple seeded	Push kale and parsley thru' hopper with carrots and apple.
Ginger Hopper	Pineapple rings with skin 3, ¼ inch slice ginger root	Push pineapple slices and ginger thru' hopper.

23. Ulcers

Healing Smoothie	Kiwi firm 1 peeled, cantaloupe with skin ¼, ripe banana 1	Push kiwi and parsley thru' hopper. Blend juice with banana until smooth. (this drink protects and heals the stomach lining)
Sweet and Sour Cherry Cream	Cheries 1 cup, non-fat yogurt 4 oz.	Juice cherries. Blend juice and yogurt until smooth

24. Varicose Veins

Garlic Express	A handful parsley, garlic clove 1, carrots 4, celery stalks 2	Bunch up parsley. Push thru' hopper with garlic, carrots and celery
Maureen's Spicy Tonic	Pineapple with skin ¼, apple seeded ½, ¼ inch slice ginger root	Push pineapple thru' hoppe with apple and ginger
Healing Smoothie	Kiwi firm 1 peeled, cantaloupe with skin ¼, ripe banana 1	Push kiwi and parsley thru' hopper. Blend juice with banana until smooth. (this drink protects and heals the stomach lining)

JUICE FASTING

Juice fasting is one of the safest and the easiest mode to detoxify or cleanse the body. In this 'Most Efficacious Tool of Naturopathy', an individual, and a healthy one at that, subsists solely on fruit and vegetable juices. No other solid diet, raw or cooked, is allowed and one has to take juice every two hours.

Fasting, as a technique for optimum health, has been recommended by every religion in the world. However, in both Christianity and Hinduism, it has been elevated to a sacred ritual, nay it is considered a way of life. Juice fasting goes still farther in the recuperation and restoration of the human system. Juice offers large quantities of the essential nutrients to support our immune system, hence Juice fasting is a powerful tool, as authentically supported by the wide-ranging choice it offers in different diseases, as shown in the Cherie Calbom's Supplement in this book.

In the normal course, one's work situation permitting, it should be taken up for 3 days every month. But if it is more than 5 days, and some people do it for one or more weeks, then it should be undertaken under the strict supervision of a qualified dietician.

Beet root is considered to be the most effective cleansing agent. One can start with three oz on the first day, gradually go on increasing this amount up to 6 oz. One may select cabbage, wheatgrass, lemon carrot, celery or apple juice, depending upon the market availability. Equally important is the manner in which you break fast. No animal products should be taken for one day after breaking the fast. Fish and whole grains may be added on the 2nd day after that.

Two special cleansing diets has been described in Special Supplement by Cherie Calbom.

JUICING TIPS

Here are a few more relevant tips to make the Juice Therapy a still more potent tool of Health and Disease Prevention.

1. Preferably use fruits and vegetables which are organically grown.
2. Peel and wash the fruits and vegetables thoroughly to remove any molds or damaged portions.
3. The skins of oranges and grapefruits contain a toxic substance, hence these should not be consumed in large quantity.
4. Since the skins of many fruits and vegetables are somewhat bitter, it is best to peel these before juicing. However, leave the white pithy part of the peel intact as it contains valuable bioflavonoids and vitamin C. The skins of other fruits like lemons and lime should be left untouched.
5. All pits, viz., peach pits, plum pits etc.—should be removed before juicing. Seeds, viz., lemon, lime, melon and grape seeds, may be placed in the juicer with the fruits. But apple seed, since it contains some cyanide, must not be juiced.

6. One must not hesitate in using the stem and leaves of fruits and vegetables. But carrot green and rhubarb green should be removed, as they contain toxic matter.

7. Fruits like banana and avocados cannot be placed in the juicer, since their water content is very low. For mixing these with other juices, transfer these fruits into a blender with the already extracted juice and blend them all together.

8. It is always better to make fresh juice every time that one has to take it. Never store the fresh juice in a fridge.

DR. (Mrs.) USHA JAIN SUPPLEMENT

Herewith, we give the very philosophy and techniques of the art and science of Naturopathy, as eminently enunciated by the top Practising Dietician of Delhi:

1. Naturopathy believes that the human body has an inbuilt ability to heal itself with the help of its own vital force, which has got very subtle vibrations.
2. Naturopathy offers complete cure for the person as a whole, and not just for the disease only.
3. Nature has created the human body virtually self-sufficient in itself. It is indeed a very perfect machine. Rather, it is an evolving system that is ever active and ever-vigilant against outside forces. We ought to allow Mother Nature to do its job in its own inimitable manner, although the scientific mind, for the time being, may not be able to rationalize it fully well.
4. The gross body is made of five elements, viz., Aakash (ether), air, fire, water and earth. It is the gross imbalance of these elements that results in disease. Man must let this balance remain restored fully.
5. Besides the Yogasanas, brisk long morning walk always helps.
6. One must avoid all sort of stress and strain. Learn to relaxe and enjoy good sleep at night.
7. Juice fasting is the 'Gateway to Health!' Try practising it once a month, if not once a week. All the great religious leaders had this most telling compulsion to do it regularly.
8. Restrict the intake of salt, sugar and fats to the barest minimum.
9. Avoid smoking and alcohol.
10. Always make it a habit of taking raw onions and garlic, raw vegetables along with lemon and honey.
11. Always insist on taking fresh juice, it should never be stored.
12. Take unrefined cereals and whole grains, as also pulses. Always take them with the bran. Apart from being rich in many minerals, especially iron, bran also helps fight diseases
13. Take maximum amount of water that you can. Start the day with a glass of water, preferably green, sun-charged water. Better don't take water along with the meals, or two hours before and half an hour after the meals.
14. Never eat fast. Try eating in a relaxed manner, masticating the food well. There should be a gap of minimum four hours between two meals.
15. Adopt the 'Diaphragmatic System' of breathing, just like an infant. With every inhale, the abdomen should go up and on exhale, it should go down. Always practise deep breathing, preferably in a green, open atmosphere.
16. Keep your skin healthy and clean. It does help in the proper functioning of your heart and lungs. Regular body massage and occasional steam bath also help a great deal in warding off many a disease.

CHERIE CALBOM SUPPLEMENT

The Seven-Day Liver-Cleansing Diet

For this diet, follow the Basic Diet adding the following foods to your daily diet plan.

Seven-Day Liver-Cleansing Diet Guidelines

- **Eat Carrot Salad every day.** Take one cup of very finely shredded carrots or carrot pulp. The carrots should be shredded to a mushy consistency with a food processor or fine grater, or you can use the carrot pulp left over from making carrot juice. If the pulp seems to dry, moisten it with a little carrot juice. Combine 1 tablespoon of olive oil with 1 tablespoon of fresh lemon juice (You may add more lemon or olive oil, but not less). Pour over the carrot pulp or grated carrots as a dressing and mix well. If you like, add pineapple or raisins to taste. Eat this salad every day for seven days. If you miss a day, you must begin all over again. This salad is very helpful in cleansing the liver.

- **Eat one to two cups of vetetable Broth each day.**

2-3 cups chopped green beans	Steam green beans, zucchini, and celery in water until soft, but still green. Put the vegetables in a blender and puree until smooth. The broth should be fairly thick. Add butter and chopped parsley. Season to taste.
2-3 cups chopped zucchini	
2-3 stalks celery, chopped	
1 tbsp. unsalted butter	
1-3 tbsp chopped parsley	
Season with ginger, cayenne, herbs, garlic, or vegetable broth as desired.	

- **Drink two glasses of Green Drink each day.** Make one cup of green juice from any green vegetables. Suggested vegetables include beet tops, spinach, parsley, zucchini, kale, cucumbers, green leafy lettude, dandelion leaves, collard greens, and wheatgrass. Add to your green drink mixture and equal part of a mild-tasting juice like carrot, apple, tomato, or pineapple, (We dont't recommend drinking green juices straight because they are too strong and can be irritating to the throat.) This drink has been used traditionally as an aid for digestion. It is high in chlorophyll, which is said to help detoxify the body and cleanse the blood.

- **Drnik three ounces of beet juice each day.** If you have more than three ounces per day when you begin the cleansing program, you may cleanse your body a little faster than you want. After the first couple of days, you can increase the amount of beet juice one ounce at a time.

- **Take the herb milk thistle each day.** Milk thistle contains some of the most potent liver-cleansing and protecting substances known. The active nutrient in milk thistle, Silymarin, enhances liver function and inhibits factors that cause hepatic damage. Silymarin prevents free radical damage through its antioxidant properties. A traditional remedy recommends one tablet with each meal for seven days.

- **Avoid all alcohol.**

- **Avoid all junk foods and sweets.**

The Six-Week Cleansing Diet

This diet is designed to detoxify the body slowly over time. It can be used in cojunction witha one to five-day juice fast. The goal is to avoid all animal products during this period, as well as refined and processed foods. Please note that you may wish to eat more on this temporary cleansing diet because it is low in calories.

CHERIE CALBOM'S MENU FOR SIX WEEK CLEANSING DIET

8.0 AM	Fruit juice
	Cereal with soymilk/juice
	Whole wheat/rye toast
	Herbal tea
11.00 AM	Fruit juice/fresh fruits
1.00 PM	Salad
	Vegetable soup
	Baked potato
	Steamed vegetables
	Herbal tea
4.00 PM	Vegetable juice or vegetable slicks
7.00 pm	Vegetarian bean bake
	Salad
	Vegetable soup
	Brown rice/millets
	Cooked vegetables
	Fruit
	Herbal tea
9.00 pm	Juice
	Herbal Tea

A Bio-Nutritionist's Farewell:

MAY THIS 'BODY BEAUTIFUL'

THE FINEST CREATION OF MOTHER NATURE -

SUSTAIN and MAINTAIN ITSELF

WITH THE BEST NATURAL PRODUCT -

viz.

THE GREEN GOLD

IN THE FORM OF

FRUIT and VEGETABLE JUICE!

Dr. S. Paul

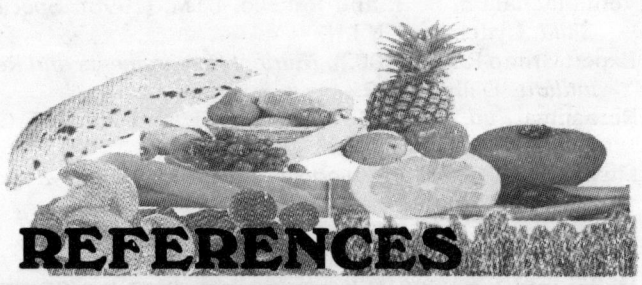

REFERENCES

Wardlaw, Gordon M and Insel Paul, M. (1996). *Perspectives in Nutrition*. New York Mosby.

Watson, Ronald R. (1994). *Handbook of Nutrition in Aged*. London, CRC Press.

Whitney, Elanor N. *et al.* (2001). *Nutrition for Health and Health Care*. Belmont, Wadsworth.

Shils, Maurice E. *et al.* (1994). *Modern Nutrition in Health and Disease*, Vol. 1-3. London, Lea and Febiger.

Cho, Susan Sungsoo and Dreher, Mark L. (2001). *Handbook of Dietary Fibre*. New York, Marcel Drekker.

Wolinsky, Ira and Driskell, Judy A. (1997). *Sports Nutrition—Vitamins and Trace Elements*. London, CRC Press.

Driskell, Judy, A. (1999). *Sports Nutrition*. London, CRC Press.

Karleskind, A. (1992). *Oils and Fats Manual*. Paris, Lavoisier Pub.

Cho, Susan Sungsoo, Dreher, Mark, L. and Prosky, Leon (1999). *Complex Carbohydrates in Foods*. New York, Marcel Drekker.

Mitchell, Rynberger, Anderson and Dibble (1976). *Nutrition in Health and Disease*. New York, J. B. Lipinsky and Co.

Howe, Phyllis Sulliva (1981). *Basic Nutrition in Health and Disease*. London, W. B. Saunders and Co.

Johnston, Ivan, D. A. (1983). *Advances in Clinical Nutrition*. Boston, MTP Press.

Garrow, J. S., James, W. P. T. and Ralph, A. (2000). *Human Nutrition and Dietetics*. London, Curchill Livingstone.

Krause, Marie, V. and Mahaan, L. Kathleen (1984). *Food, Nutrition and Diet Therapy—A Text Book of Nutritional Care*. London, W. B. Saunders and Co.

Fleck, Henrietta (1971). *Introduction to Nutrition*. New York, Macmillan.

Coulston, Ann, M. Rock, Cherryl, L. and Monsen, Elanor, R. (2001). *Nutrition in Prevention and Treatment of Disease*. London, Academic Press.

Cottrell, Richard (ed.) (1987). *Food and Health—Now and the Future*. New Jersey, Parthenon Pub.

Chenault, Alice, A. (1984). *Nutrition and Health*, New York, Holt, Rinehart and Winston.

Wildman, Robert, E.C. and Medeiros, Denis. M. (2000). *Advanced Human Nutrition*. London, CRC Press.

Thomas, H. and Corbett, M. D. (1978). *Cancer and Chemicals*. Chicago, Nelson-Hall.

Venkatachalam, P. S. and Rebello, L. M. (1996). *Special Report: Nutrition for Mother And Child*, Hyderabad, N.I.N.

Expert Group Report (2002). *Nutrient Requirements and Recommended Dietary Allowances For Indians*. Delhi, ICMR.

Narasinga Rao, B. S., Deosthale, Y. G. and Pant, K. C. (1996). *Nutritive Value of Indian Foods*. Hyderabad, N.I.N.

Mishra, S. K. (1986) *Ayurveda—the Science of Life—A Profile on Research and Development*. Delhi, CCRAS.

Lakshmipathi, A. (1973). *One Hundred Useful Drugs*, Madras, Arogya Ashram Samithi. Gala, Dhanlal: Incurable Diseases? Don't Despair, Ahmedabad, 1992, Gala Pub.

Mahindru, S. N. (2001). *Know Your Foods*, Delhi, CBS Pub.

Sharma, Rekha (1999). *Diet Management*. Delhi, B. I. Churchill Livingstone.

Subba Rao, Kalluri (1994). *Aging*. Delhi, NBT.

Jensen, Bernard (2002). *Foods That Heal*. Delhi, Health and Harmony.

Calbom, Cherie and Keane (1999). *Maureen Juicing for Life*. Delhi, Health and Harmony.

Hayens, R. Brian and Leenen, Frans, H. H. (2001). *Conquering Hypertension*. Delhi, Health and Harmony.

Tietze, Harald, W. (1998). *Living Food for Longer Life*. Delhi, Health and Harmony.

Hobert, Ingfried and Tietze, Harald, W. (2001). *Guava—Medicine for Modern Diseases*. Delhi, Health and Harmony.

Saha, N.N. (2001). *Fruit and Vegetable Juice Therapy*. Delhi, Health and Harmony.

Saha, N.N. (2000) *Raw Juice Therapy*. Delhi, Health and Harmony.

Panda, K. N. (1998). *Juice Therapy and The Miracles of Wheat Grass Juice*. Delhi, Author.

Panda, K. N. (1998). *Sprouts for Health*. Delhi, Author.

Joshi, S. A. (2000). *Nutrition and Dietetics*, Delhi, Tata McGraw-Hill.

Khader, Vijaya (2001). *Food, Nutrition and Health*. Delhi, Kalyani Pub.

Health Media of Nutrition Series (1994). *Cancer and Nutrition*. Delhi, CBS Pub.

Health Media of Nutrition Series (1994). *Calcium and Nutrition*, Delhi, CBS Pub.

Health Media of Nutrition Series (1994). *Skin, Hair, Nails and Nutrition*. Delhi, CBS Pub.

Health Media of Nutrition Series (1994). *Weight Loss and Nutrition*, Delhi, CBS Pub.

Health Media of Nutrition Series (1994). *Seniors and Nutrition*, Delhi, CBS Pub.

Health Media of Nutrition Series (1994). *Women and Nutrition*, Delhi, CBS Pub.

Health Media of Nutrition Series (1994). *Children, Adolscent and Nutrition*. Delhi, CBS Pub.

Health Media of Nutrition Series (1994). *Stress and Nutrition*, Delhi, CBS Pub.

Health Media of Nutrition Series (1994). *Heart Disease, Hypertension and Nutrition*. Delhi, CBS Pub.

Health Media of Nutrition Series (1994). *Vitamins, Minerals and Nutrition*, Delhi, CBS Pub.

Williams, Sue Rodwell (1990). *Essentials of Nutrition and Diet Therapy*. Boston, Mosby College Pub.

Lagua, Rosalinda, T. and Claudio, Virginia, S. (1998). *Nutrition And Diet Therapy Reference Dictionary*, Delhi, CBS Pub.

Potter, Norman, N. and Hotchkins, Joseph, H. (1996). *Food Science*. Delhi, CBS Pub.

Simopoulous, A. P. and Gopalan, C. (2003). *Plants in Human Health and Nutrition Policy*. Basel, Karger.

Narasinga Rao, B. S. (1996). *Nutritional Requirements of Sportsmen and Athletes in Proceedings of Nutrition Society of India*, Vol.43.

Weijian, W. and Junshi, C. (1996). *Traditional Chinese Medicine in Nutrition Review* Vol. 54 II.

Kutumbiah, P. (1974). *Ancient Indian Medicine*. Madras, Orient Longman.

Sharma, Ramkaran (1984). *Rejuvenative Health Care in Ayurveda*, Author.

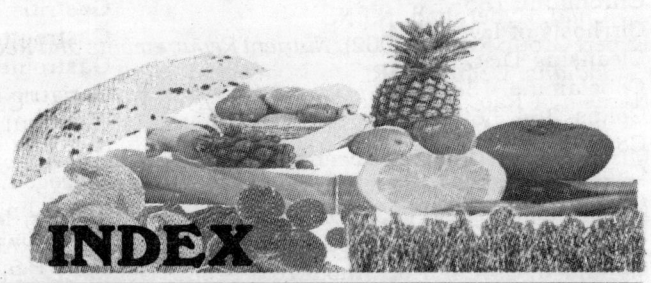

INDEX